IADVL
Bedside Companion for
Dermatology Residents

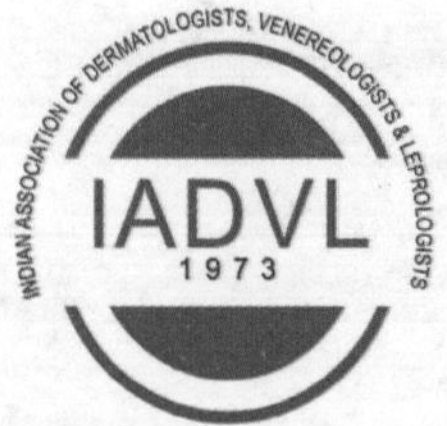

Indian Association of Dermatologists, Venereologists and Leprologists

IADVL
Bedside Companion for
Dermatology Residents

Editor

Biju Vasudevan
MD(Dermatology, Venereology, and Leprology) Fellowship(Dermatosurgery)
Professor and Head
Department of Dermatology
Armed Forces Medical College
Pune, Maharashtra, India

Associate Editor

Bhabani Singh MBBS MD(Skin and VD)
Associate Professor
Department of Dermatology, Venereology and Leprology
Institute of Medical Sciences and SUM Hospital
Bhubaneswar, Odisha, India

Assistant Editor

Shrikant Kumavat DDVL
Consultant
Department of Dermatology
Dr Kumavat Skin Clinic
Nashik, Maharashtra, India

Foreword

S Radhakrishnan

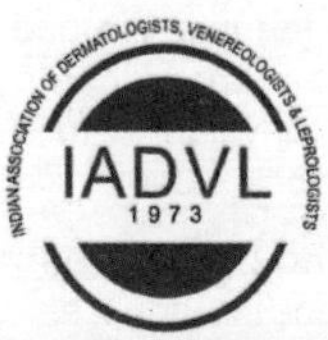

Under the Aegis of IADVL Academy

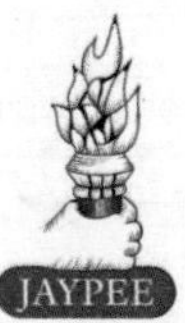

JAYPEE BROTHERS MEDICAL PUBLISHERS
The Health Sciences Publisher
New Delhi | London

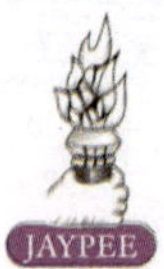 **Jaypee Brothers Medical Publishers (P) Ltd**

Headquarters

EMCA House
23/23-B, Ansari Road, Daryaganj
New Delhi 110 002, India
Landline: +91-11-23272143, +91-11-23272703
+91-11-23282021, +91-11-23245672
E-mail: jaypee@jaypeebrothers.com

Corporate Office

Jaypee Brothers Medical Publishers (P) Ltd.
4838/24, Ansari Road, Daryaganj
New Delhi 110 002, India
Phone: +91-11-43574357
Fax: +91-11-43574314
E-mail: jaypee@jaypeebrothers.com

Overseas Office

JP Medical Ltd.
83, Victoria Street, London
SW1H 0HW (UK)
Phone: +44-20 3170 8910
Fax: +44(0)20 3008 6180
E-mail: info@jpmedpub.com

Website: www.jaypeebrothers.com
Website: www.jaypeedigital.com

Inquiries for bulk sales may be solicited at: jaypee@jaypeebrothers.com

IADVL Bedside Companion for Dermatology Residents / **Biju Vasudevan**

First Edition: **2024**

ISBN: 978-93-5696-682-6

Printed in India at Sterling Graphics Pvt. Ltd.

Dedication

Dedicated to my wife Deepa Biju and daughter Parnika Biju for the time which they have given me so that I could complete the book in time. Also dedicated to my parents, teachers, colleagues, and students.

Contributors

Abhinav Kumar Verma MBBS MD
Junior Resident
Department of Dermatology
Armed Forces Medical College
Pune, Maharashtra, India

Abirami C MD
Senior Resident
Department of Dermatology,
Venereology and Leprology
SRM Medical College Hospital
and Research Centre
SRM Institute of Science and
Technology
Potheri, Tamil Nadu, India

Anand Mannu MBBS MD
Senior Resident
Department of Dermatology
Armed Forces Medical College
Pune, Maharashtra, India

Aneez Ali MBBS
Junior Resident
Department of Pathology
Armed Forces Medical College
Pune, Maharashtra, India

Ankan Gupta MBBS MD
Associate Professor
Department of Dermatology
Christian Medical College
Vellore, Tamil Nadu, India

AW Kashif MBBS MD(Pathology)
DNB(Pathology) PDCC(Renal
Transplant Pathology) ACME
Professor
Department of Pathology
Armed Forces Medical College
Pune, Maharashtra, India

Bhabani Singh MBBS MD(Skin
and VD)
Associate Professor
Department of Dermatology,
Venereology and Leprology
Institute of Medical Sciences
and SUM Hospital
Bhubaneswar, Odisha, India

Biju Vasudevan
MD(Dermatology,
Venereology, and Leprology
Fellowship(Dermatosurgery)
Professor and Head
Department of Dermatology
Armed Forces Medical College
Pune, Maharashtra, India

Binu Kunwar MBBS
Junior Resident
Department of Dermatology
Armed Forces Medical College
Pune, Maharashtra, India

Chakravarti R Srinivas MD
Professor
Department of Dermatology,
Venereology, and Leprology
Kalinga Institute of Medical
Sciences (KIMS)
Bhubaneswar, Odisha, India

Dilip Paudel MBBS(General
Medicine)
Resident
Department of Dermatology
Armed Forces Medical College
Pune, Maharashtra, India

Durga Madhab Tripathy MD
DNB MRCP SCE
Assistant Professor
Department of Dermatology
Military Hospital
Agra, Uttar Pradesh, India

Jamyang Choden MBBS
Junior Resident
Department of Dermatology
Armed Forces Medical College
Pune, Maharashtra, India

Karthi Kishore MBBS MD DVL
Graded Specialist
Department of Dermatology
Military Hospital
Shillong, Meghalaya, India

Kavita Bala Anand MBBS MD
Professor
Department of Microbiology
Armed Forces Medical College
Pune, Maharashtra, India

K Lekshmipriya MBBS MD DVL
Associate Professor
Department of Dermatology
Armed Forces Medical College
Pune, Maharashtra, India

Lalita Kumari MBBS
Junior Resident
Department of Dermatology
Armed Forces Medical College
Pune, Maharashtra, India

Nidhi Sharma MBBS MD
Senior Resident
Department of Dermatology
Government Medical College
Jammu and Kashmir, India

Nishu Bala MBBS MD DVL
Specialist, Department of
Dermatology, Command
Hospital (Southern Command)
Pune, Maharashtra, India

Nitin Kumar Sharma MBBS
MD DVL
Resident
Department of Dermatology
Armed Forces Medical College
Pune, Maharashtra, India

Pankaj Das MD(Dermatology,
Venereology and Leprology)
Associate Professor
Department of Dermatology
Armed Forces Medical College
Pune, Maharashtra, India

Prachi Verma MD(Dermatology)
Specialist
Department of Dermatology
Military Hospital
Dehradun, Uttarakhand, India

Prince Malla MBBS
Junior Resident
Department of Dermatology
Armed Forces Medical College
Pune, Maharashtra, India

Rahul Thombre
MD(Dermatology)
Associate Professor
Department of Dermatology
Command Hospital (Southern
Command)
Pune, Maharashtra, India

S Radhakrishnan MBBS MD
Professor
Department of Dermatology
Army College of Medical
Sciences and Base Hospital
Delhi Cantt, New Delhi, India

Sampoorna Choudhary MBBS
Junior Resident
Department of Dermatology
Command Hospital (Central
Command)
Lucknow, Uttar Pradesh, India

Santhosh Battula MBBS MD
Specialist
Department of Dermatology
Dr BAMH Central Railways
Mumbai, Maharashtra, India

Senkadhir Vendhan
MD(Dermatology)
Specialist
Department of Dermatology
Dr BAMH Central Railways
Mumbai, Maharashtra, India

Shekhar Neema MBBS
MD(Dermatology)
Associate Professor
Department of Dermatology
Military Base Hospital
Lucknow, Uttar Pradesh, India

Shrikant Kumavat DDVL
Consultant
Department of Dermatology
Dr Kumavat Skin Clinic
Nashik, Maharashtra, India

Siddhartha Dash MD
Assistant Professor
Department of Dermatology
SCB Medical College and
Hospital
Cuttack, Odisha, India

Siddharth Mani MBBS MD DVL
Assistant Professor
Department of Dermatology
INHS Sanjivani
Kochi, Kerala, India

Sidharth Bhat MBBS MD
Assistant Professor
Department of Dermatology
INHS Asvini
Mumbai, Maharashtra, India

Silky Priya MBBS
Junior Resident
Department of Dermatology
Armed Forces Medical College
Pune, Maharashtra, India

Siva Chaitanya Senapathi
MD(Pediatrics) MBBS MD
Graded Specialist
Department of Pediatrics
Military Hospital
Shillong, Meghalaya, India

Smriti Sharma MBBS
Junior Resident
Department of Dermatology
Armed Forces Medical College
Pune, Maharashtra, India

Sonal Jain DVL MBBS MD DNB
Assistant Professor
Department of Dermatology
IIMSAR and Dr Roy Hospital
Haldia, West Bengal, India

Sreechithra Menon MBBS
Junior Resident
Department of Dermatology
Armed Forces Medical College
Pune, Maharashtra, India

Sunmeet Sandhu MD DVL DNB
MNAMS
Senior Medical Officer
Department of Dermatology
Air Force Station
Amritsar Cantt, Punjab, India

Sushmita Mishra MBBS
Resident
Department of Dermatology
Armed Forces Medical College
Pune, Maharashtra, India

Vijayshankar Palaniappan
MD
Assistant Professor
Department of Dermatology,
Venereology, and Leprology
Sri Manakula Vinayagar
Medical College and Hospital
Puducherry, India

Vinay Gera MBBS MD
Head
Department of Dermatology
Command Hospital (Southern
Command)
Pune, Maharashtra, India

Bedside investigations in dermatology are an integral part of clinical dermatology and have a huge impact on patient care, making early institution of definitive treatment possible even before more elaborate and expensive investigation reports are received. It is one of the essential basics of training which needs to be imparted to dermatology postgraduate residents early in their training period.

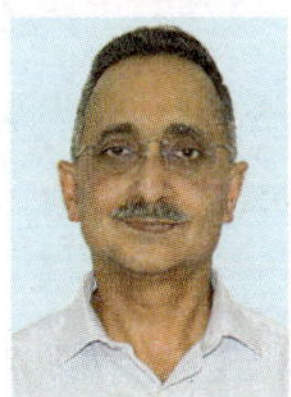

These investigations are extremely cost effective, are relatively easy to perform, and require very little equipment and resources in most cases. However, the learning curve is steep and residents need to be persistent in their learning of these procedures, with constant motivation and validation by the faculty.

I personally have been extremely passionate learning these bedside investigations over the years from great teachers and peers alike and found them indispensable in day-to-day clinical dermatology practice. While I was fortunate to be holding the prestigious appointment of the Professor and Head, Department of Dermatology, AFMC, Pune, a few years back, we utilized the opportunity of an excellent academic facility, availability of brilliant faculty, and, most importantly, extremely motivated and equally passionate postgraduate residents who not only developed expertise in these bedside procedures, but also took them to a whole new level as will be evident from their contributions illustrated in this book.

I consider myself extremely fortunate to have contributed to this book and would like to place on record my gratitude to all faculty members and the passionate residents, without whose efforts compiling this book would not have been possible.

S Radhakrishnan MBBS MD
Professor
Department of Dermatology
Army College of Medical Sciences
and Base Hospital
Delhi Cantt, New Delhi, India

Preface

Bedside tests are the most important tools that a dermatologist can utilize to diagnose various dermatological disorders at the bedside. This realization was not fully there when we did our residency. However, Dr S Radhakrishnan who has been a mentor always guided me and many other juniors and students to do bedside tests for all patients and the results we obtained gave us a great amount of satisfaction. This experience induced the idea of bringing out a book on bedside tests as we found that literature on the above was scant.

This book contains bedside tests and investigations that would be handy for residents, practicing dermatologists, and faculty in institutions. The relevance, procedural steps, and findings of the tests in various situations are highlighted in the text using appropriate images, key messages, tables, and text. Bedside tests like KOH (Potassium hydroxide) mount, Slit-skin smear, Tzanck smear, and Tissue smear are invaluable tools described in detail along with the stains used, namely Ziehl–Neelsen, Gram stain, Giemsa stain, and many others.

Bedside tests would help to make an early probable diagnosis while bedside investigations would help us reach an early confirmatory diagnosis many times. These processes are simple, easy to replicate, and do not require expensive equipment or techniques. The results are available at bedside when the patient has just presented to the OPD. This reduces precious time wasted in diagnosis, thus leading to early management and maximum satisfaction to a patient with minimal wastage of time, expenses, and hardly any discomfort. This would bring satisfaction to the dermatology resident/dermatologist for having made a bedside diagnosis by following the simple procedures highlighted in the book. It would also help postgraduate residents and examiners in their pursuit of exams.

I hope that the book would make a substantial contribution in aiding early diagnosis by its readers.

Biju Vasudevan

Acknowledgments

I am grateful to Dr Vijay Zawar, President IADVL for taking on this project as a President project and the IADVL Academy for giving me this opportunity to edit this book.

I acknowledge the contribution of teachers Drs Rajan Grewal, Rajesh Verma, MPS Sawhney, YK Sharma, S Radhakrishnan, and Manas Chatterjee.

I also acknowledge the contribution of colleagues Drs Shekhar Neema, AW Kashif, Kavita Bala Anand, Deepak Vashist, Pankaj Das, K Lekshmipriya, Vinay Gera, Rahul Thomre, and Nishubala.

I extend my thanks for the contribution of residents Drs Senkadhir, Anand, Santhosh, Surendra, Sushmita, Silky, Abhinav, Prince, Smriti, Lalita, Binu, Jamyang, Sreechitra, Nitin, Dilip, and Thinley.

Last but not the least, I would also like to extend my special gratitude to Shri Jitendar P Vij (Group Chairman), Mr Ankit Vij (Managing Director), and MS Mani (Group President), Ms Chetna Malhotra (Senior Director—Professional Publishing, Marketing & Business Development), Ms Pooja Bhandari (Director—Production) and Ms Himani Pandey (Development Editor), for their help and assistance in completing the project within the time frame.

Biju Vasudevan

Contents

Bedside Tests in Dermatology: Introduction

Biju Vasudevan, Pankaj Das, Sreechithra Menon

INTRODUCTION

Bedside testing is the medical diagnostic testing at or near the point of care that is, at the time and place of patient care. It includes clinical bedside tests and investigational bedside tests. Clinical bedside tests help in arriving at a provisional diagnosis at the bedside thus helping early management and prevention of complications. Bedside laboratory tests help us to confirm the provisional diagnosis thus aiding evidence-based management at the earliest point of contact with the patient. This is in contrast with the historical pattern in which testing was mostly or wholly confined to the medical laboratory, which entailed sending off specimens away from the point of care and then waiting hours or days to obtain the results, during which the care must continue without the desired information.

Correctly performing bedside diagnostic tests is an important fundamental skill for practicing dermatologists. Even with the advent of new technologies, bedside diagnostic tests have a very important and emergent place in contemporary practice. When properly implemented, these tests can efficiently and cheaply aid in diagnosis and treatment. This book reviews the commonly utilized bedside diagnostic procedures in dermatology while considering them in their historical context, outline the procedure for performing the test, discuss the relevance of the tests in today's clinical practice and include relevant images for better comprehension.

WHAT CONSTITUTES BEDSIDE TESTS IN DERMATOLOGY?

Bedside tests that are discussed in the chapter are summarized in **Tables 1 to 3**.

TABLE 1: Clinical tests.

Tests	Diseases
Grattage test and Auspitz sign	Psoriasis
Koebner phenomenon **(Fig. 1)**	Psoriasis, vitiligo, lichen planus, and Darier disease
Pseudo-koebner phenomenon	Molluscum contagiosum and verruca vulgaris
Bulla spread/Asboe-Hansen sign	Pemphigus vulgaris and bullous pemphigoid
Nikolsky's sign	Pemphigus disorders
False Nikolsky's/Sheklakov sign	Bullous pemphigoid, epidermolysis bullosa acquisita, dermatitis herpetiformis, and bullous SLE

Continued

Continued

Tests	Diseases
Pseudo-Nikolsky's sign	SJS/TEN, burns, and bullous ichthyosiform erythroderma
Dermographism	Urticaria and related disorders
Temperature test	Heat urticaria
Skin prick test	Spontaneous urticaria
Darier's sign	Mast cell disorders
Diascopy	Petechiae, sarcoidosis, and lupus vulgaris
Hair pull test	Telogen effluvium and androgenic alopecia
Wash test/Rebora test	Telogen effluvium and female pattern hair loss
Hair feathering	Trichorrhexis nodosa, monilethrix, pili torti, trichorrhexis invaginata, trichothiodystrophy, and bubble hair
Trichometry	Postpartum effluvium and androgenic alopecia
Trichotillometry	Loose anagen syndrome and malnutrition
Alcohol swab test	Terra firma-forme dermatosis
Buerger's postural test	PAOD
Love's pinhead test and Hildreth's test	Glomus tumor
Brodie–Trendelenburg test and Cough impulse test	Chronic venous insufficiency
Homan's sign and Moses sign	Deep vein thrombosis lower limbs
Two glass test and three glass test	Urethritis
Buschke–Ollendorff sign	Secondary syphilis
Blotting paper test	Frey's syndrome
Minor's starch iodine test	Hyperhidrosis
Calculation of MED	Phototherapy
Transillumination test	Parameatal cyst
Patch test	Allergic contact dermatitis

(MED: minimal erythema dose; PAOD: peripheral arterial occlusive disease; SJS/TEN: Stevens–Johnson syndrome/toxic epidermal necrolysis; SLE: systemic lupus erythematosus)

TABLE 2: Intradermal tests.

Tests	Diseases
Frei's test	Lymphogranuloma venereum
Lepromin test	Leprosy
Tuberculin test **(Fig. 2)**	Tuberculosis and atypical mycobacterial infections
Kveim test	Sarcoidosis
Schick test	Diphtheria
Histoplasmin test	Histoplasmosis
Leishmanin/Montenegro test	Leishmaniasis
Autologous serum skin test	Urticaria and related disorders
Intradermal sensitivity test	Immediate and delayed drug hypersensitivity
Autoerythrocyte sensitization test	Gardner–Diamond syndrome
Pathergy test	Behçet's disease

TABLE 3: Laboratory tests.

Tests	Diseases
Tzanck smear	Bullous disorders
KOH (Potassium hydroxide) mount **(Fig. 3)**	Fungal infections
Tissue smear	Donovanosis, leishmaniasis, and molluscum contagiosum
Gram-stain	Bacterial infections like pyoderma, and gonorrhea
Wet mount examination	Trichomoniasis, genital candidiasis, and gonorrhea
Slit-skin smear and Ziehl–Neelsen stain **(Fig. 4)**	Hansen's disease
Dark-field microscopy	Syphilis and Demodex mites
Light microscopy	Scabies and pediculosis
Polarizing microscopy	Trichothiodystrophy, trichorrhexis nodosa, thallium poisoning, and Fabry's disease

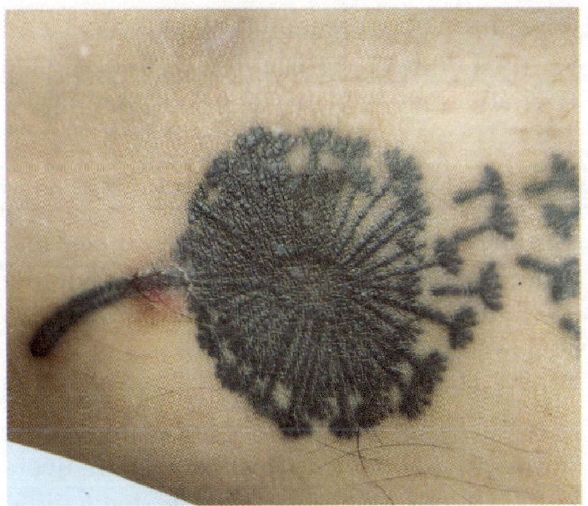

FIG. 1: Koebner phenomenon in a case of psoriasis following intradermal tattoo.

FIG. 3: KOH (Potassium hydroxide) mount showing candidal hyphae and spores.

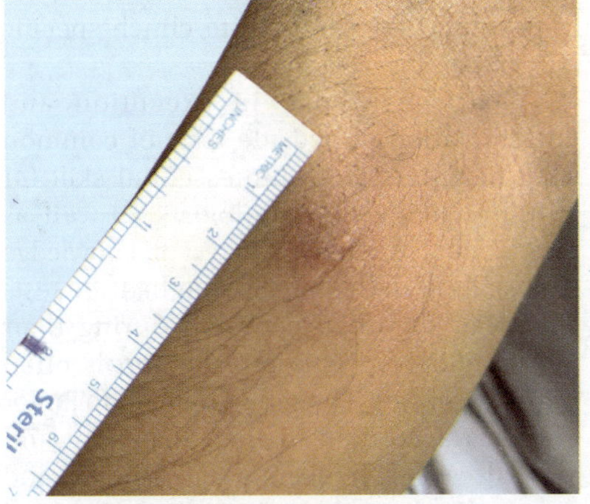

FIG. 2: Tuberculin test showing induration and erythema.

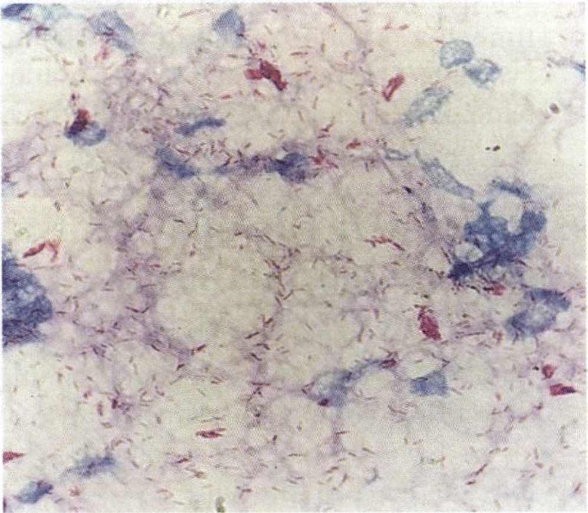

FIG. 4: Ziehl–Neelsen stain of slit-skin smear showing acid-fast bacilli in clumps.

ADVANTAGES OF DOING BEDSIDE TESTS

- Bedside clinical tests are part of clinical examination, easy to do, involve no cost, and give an early clue to diagnosis.
- Bedside diagnostic tests provide rapidly interpretable test results so that appropriate treatment can be implemented, leading to improved clinical or economic outcomes when compared to laboratory testing.
- Provides quick answers to important clinical questions, leading to diagnosis of wide variety of benign and malignant dermatologic conditions and common and uncommon infectious diseases.
- These techniques are reliable, specific, easy to perform, and interpret.
- These tests often complement more expensive and time-consuming tests. The bedside tests are repeatable and well-tolerated. They may be particularly valuable in resource-limited settings, inpatient ward, and in the clinic.
- Each technique is easily performed but requires expertise in interpretation.
- As these tests are "patient-centric" and are conducted in and around patients, they typically enhance patient satisfaction and experience by eliminating the need for sample transport, reducing turnaround time for laboratory-based tests, and avoiding procedural delays. It enables patient counseling, prevents unnecessary treatment escalation.

ISSUES FACED BY DERMATOLOGISTS WHILE PERFORMING THE TESTS

- Bedside tests require a certain amount of training and expertise. Adequate training is a critical component as preanalytical errors have an inverse association with the experience of clinician.
- It is the same person who often performs the collection and test execution. This can lead to task overload and errors in collection, preparation, transport, and analysis.
- Due to the portable nature of the tests, the reagents and samples are often exposed to conditions that may differ from those in a traditional laboratory setting.
- Errors in the preanalytical phase can occur during patient identification and in the specimen's identification, collection, handling, processing, transport, and storage.
- It may be less accurate than traditional laboratory testing. This can be attributed to variable personnel training and control over preanalytical, analytical, and postanalytical variables, which can be better managed in a laboratory setting.

CONCLUSION

Despite their limitations, bedside clinical and laboratory tests are not only a useful adjunct to the routine clinical examination but also essential clinical skills for a dermatologist. When used appropriately, these techniques provide unique efficiency and operational autonomy. Numerous tests and maneuvers can be employed to help narrow down differential diagnoses in dermatology, and their use may even obviate the need for biopsy. The clinical signs are not 100% sensitive, but if present, they can help to clinch specific diagnoses.

Basic knowledge in execution and interpretation of bedside tests of common skin disorders is a quintessential skill for any practicing dermatologists as well as postgraduate students. At present, knowledge and skills of dermatologists on bedside tests are what they had acquired during their postgraduation. This information is often verbally conveyed by senior trainees to junior trainees according to their exposure and expertise which frequently gets modified and manipulated over the years. Lack of substantial literature on the method and interpretation of these tests often prevent the clinicians from performing these tests and resort to more expensive and elaborate laboratory-based tests. Decision to address this shortcoming has led to the birth of this comprehensive book on Bedside Tests in Dermatology, which will negate the hassle of using multiple textbooks for reference, as none of them encompass sufficient data on the procedure as well as clinical images to guide the clinicians.[1-3]

Key Messages

- Bedside clinical and laboratory tests are immensely useful in diagnosis of common dermatological conditions.
- They provide rapid, easy, and replicable results for early management of these conditions.
- It is a very important tool in the hands of a dermatologist while handing challenging and common cases alike.
- It is a skill every dermatology resident and dermatologist should possess or learn to possess as part of daily clinical practice.

REFERENCES

1. Wanat KA, Dominguez AR, Carter Z, Legua P, Bustamante B, Micheletti RG. Bedside diagnostics in dermatology: Viral, bacterial, and fungal infections. J Am Acad Dermatol. 2017;77(2):197-218.
2. Schoenberg E, Keller M. Classic bedside diagnostic techniques. Clin Dermatol. 2021;39(4):563-72.
3. Goldenberg M, Liao YT, Libson K, Adame S, Spaccarelli N, Korman A, et al. Bedside Diagnostic Techniques in Dermatology. Curr Dermatol Rep. 2021;10:89-96.

Light Microscopy in Dermatology

Kavita Bala Anand, Silky Priya

INTRODUCTION

Light microscopy (LM) has remained a bedrock of dermatologic diagnosis for centuries, offering invaluable insights into the morphology and architecture of skin lesions at a cellular level. While advancements in sophisticated technologies such as immunofluorescence and confocal microscopy are transforming our understanding of cutaneous pathology, LM retains its unique advantages—noninvasiveness, affordability, accessibility, rapid turnaround time, and the ability to examine a wide spectrum of skin conditions. The technique has been used to diagnose a wide range of skin conditions; including infections, inflammatory disorders, and neoplastic diseases.[1] This chapter delves into the fundamentals of LM in dermatology, its diverse applications, and its limitations in the context of bedside diagnostics.

MECHANISM OF LIGHT MICROSCOPY

Light microscopy utilizes visible light to illuminate a tissue specimen, magnified through a series of lenses to visualize fine details invisible to the naked eye. **Figure 1** shows a labeled diagram of a light microscope. Basic LM mechanism includes.[2]

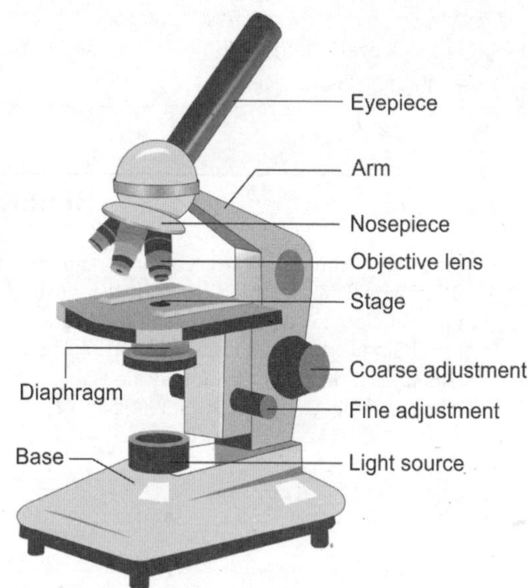

FIG. 1: Labeled diagram of a light microscope.

Illumination and Focusing

Light Source

The journey begins with a bright light source, typically a light-emitting diode (LED) or halogen bulb, illuminating the specimen.

Condenser

This lens system focuses the light onto the specimen, ensuring even illumination and optimal resolution.

Objective Lens

This crucial lens, positioned closest to the specimen, magnifies the image by bending light rays. Different objective lenses offer varying magnifications, allowing you to zoom in on specific features **(Fig. 2)**.

Interaction with the Specimen

Light Transmission

Visible light passes through the translucent specimen, interacting with its different structures.

Selective Absorption

Certain components of the specimen, such as melanin or collagen, absorb specific wavelengths of light, influencing the image contrast.

Refraction

As the light encounters, the structures with different refractive indices (e.g., air-tissue interface), its direction changes, further contributing to the image formation.

Image Formation and Observation

Ocular Lenses

These eyepieces further magnify the image formed by the objective lens, projecting it onto your retina.

Diaphragm

This adjustable opening controls the amount of light entering the eyepieces, optimizing brightness, and contrast.

Enhancing Contrast and Resolution

Staining

Staining techniques utilize dyes to selectively highlight specific structures within the specimen, enhancing contrast, and revealing hidden details.

Phase Contrast

This technique exploits the differences in refractive index within the specimen to create contrast without staining, ideal for visualizing live cells.

SPECIMEN PREPARATION

Accurate diagnosis hinges on optimal specimen preparation. The common techniques in dermatology include as described underneath.

Potassium Hydroxide Mount

Used for rapid identification of fungal elements, especially hyphae, and spores. A drop of potassium hydroxide (KOH) is placed on a glass slide with the specimen, clearing

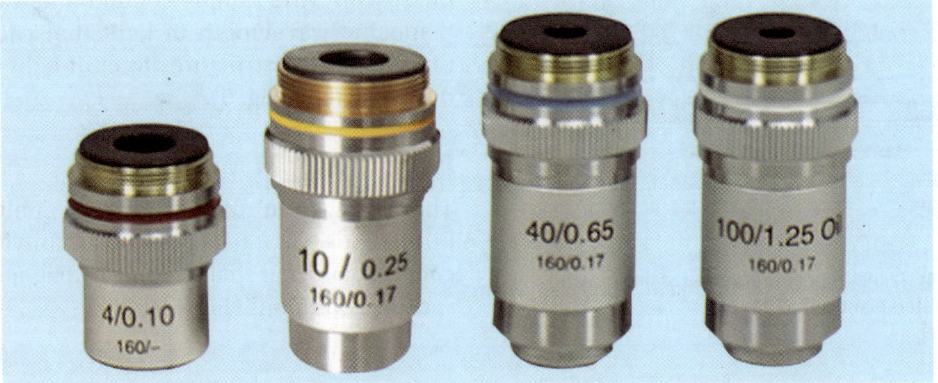

FIG. 2: Light microscope objective lens.

the surrounding tissue and highlighting fungal structures **(Fig. 3)**.[3]

Tzanck Smear

Diagnoses viral infections like herpes simplex by visualizing multinucleated giant cells. Skin scraping is smeared onto a glass slide and stained, showcasing characteristic giant cells with multiple nuclei **(Fig. 4)**.[4]

FIG. 3: Potassium hydroxide (KOH) mount with fungal hyphae (40×).

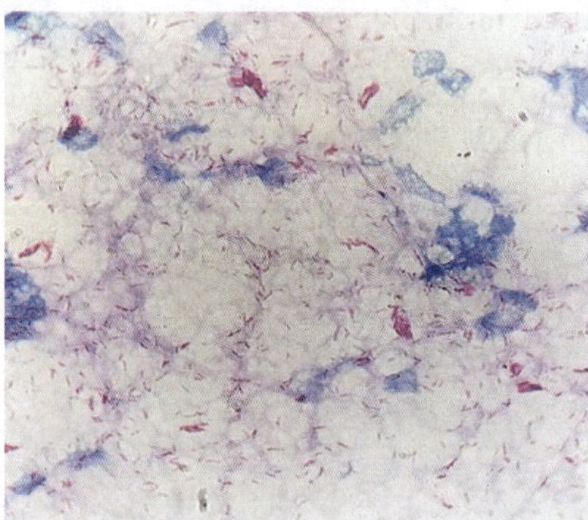

FIG. 4: Tzanck smear on Giemsa stain showing multinucleated giant cells (100×).

Types of Light Microscopy

There are several types of LM used in dermatology, including bright-field microscopy, dark-field microscopy, and fluorescence microscopy.

Bright-field Microscopy

This is the most commonly used type of LM in dermatology. It is a simple technique that uses a bright light source to illuminate the sample. The light passes through the sample and is then magnified by a series of lenses. This allows for the visualization of the cellular components of the sample.

Dark-field Microscopy

This is a type of LM that is used to visualize structures that are difficult to see with bright-field microscopy. It is particularly useful for the visualization of spirochetes, such as those that cause syphilis and Lyme disease. In dark-field microscopy, the sample is illuminated with a cone of light that is directed at an angle to the sample. This causes the light to scatter, making the structures visible.

Fluorescence Microscopy

This is a type of LM that is used to visualize structures that are fluorescent. It is particularly useful for the visualization of fungi, such as those that cause ringworm. In fluorescence microscopy, the sample is illuminated with a specific wavelength of light that causes the fluorescent structures to emit light of a different color **(Fig. 5)**.[5]

Polarized Light Microscopy

This is a type of microscopy that analyses birefringent materials, such as amyloid, collagen, and hair shafts, aiding in diagnosing specific conditions **(Fig. 6)**.[6]

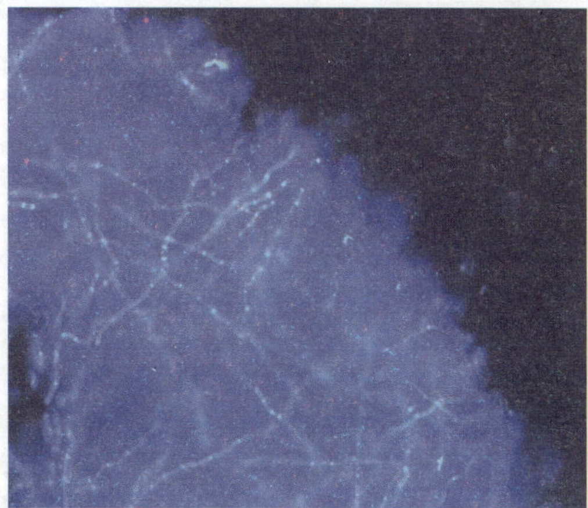

FIG. 5: Scraping from Tinea cruris stained with calcofluor white showing septate hyphae under fluorescence microscope.

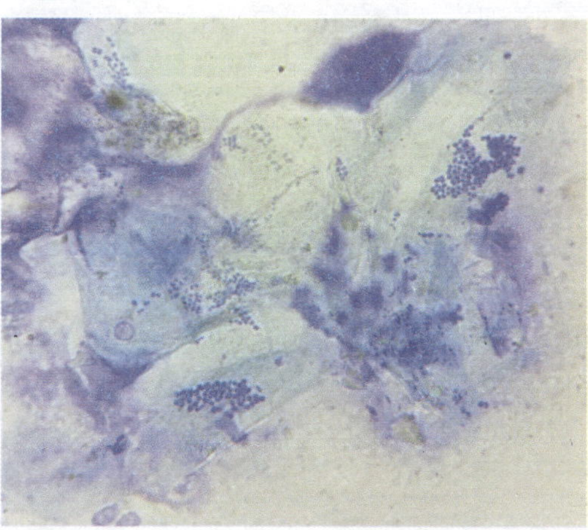

FIG. 7: Gram's staining of tissue smear showing bacterial cocci (100×).

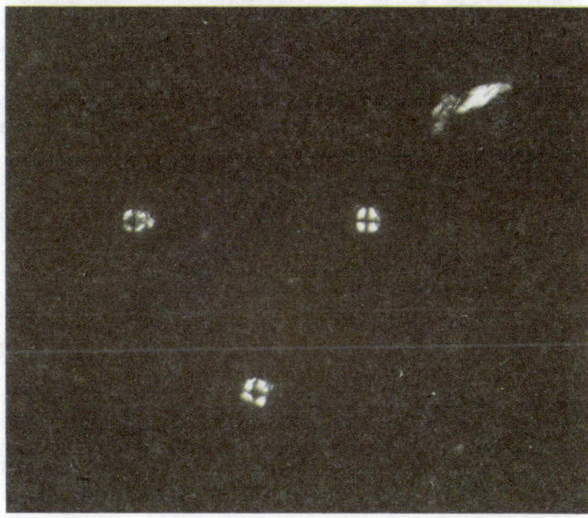

FIG. 6: Polarized microscopy of urine sample of a patient of Fabry's disease showing Maltese cross.

APPLICATIONS OF LIGHT MICROSCOPY IN DERMATOLOGY

Light microscopy plays a crucial role in the diagnosis of numerous skin conditions, serving as an indispensable tool for dermatologists at the bedside. Some key examples are discussed further.

Infectious Diseases

Bacterial Infections

Light microscopy can identify bacteria directly in smears from pustules or abscesses, aiding in the diagnosis of impetigo, folliculitis, and furunculosis **(Fig. 7)**.[7]

Fungal Infections

Potassium hydroxide mounts readily reveal fungal elements such as hyphae and spores in tinea infections, candidiasis, and dermatophytosis **(Fig. 3)**.[8]

Parasitic Infections

Direct examination of skin scrapings can identify scabies mites, lice, and larvae of filarial worms **(Fig. 8)**.

Viral Infections

Tzanck smears are diagnostic for herpes simplex **(Fig. 9)**, while *Cytomegalovirus* inclusions can be seen in skin biopsies of immunosuppressed patients.[9]

Hair and Nail Disorders

Netherton Syndrome

Light microscopy reveals the presence of trichorrhexis invaginata and/or bamboo hair and additional features, such as trichoschisis (longitudinal splitting of the hair shaft), irregular pigmentation, and abnormal medulla (central core of the hair) **(Fig. 10)**.[10]

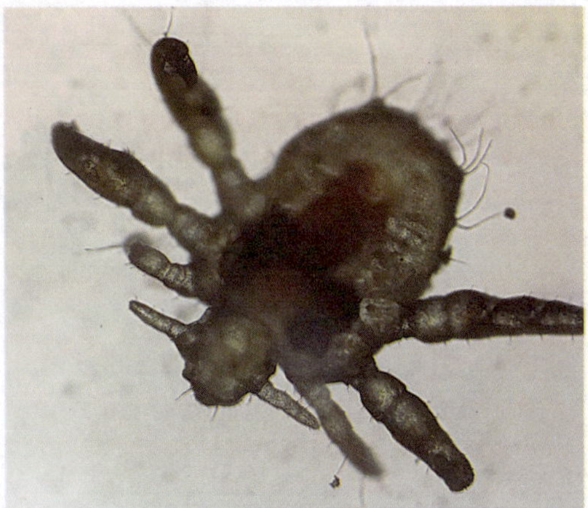

FIG. 8: Scabies mite under light microscope (40×).

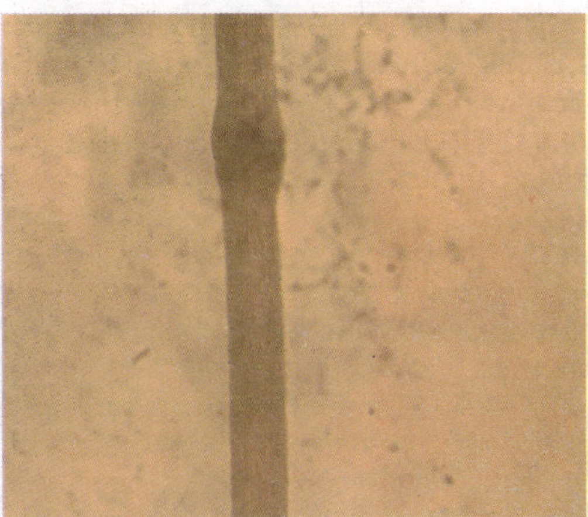

FIG. 10: Bamboo hair in a child of Netherton syndrome under LM.

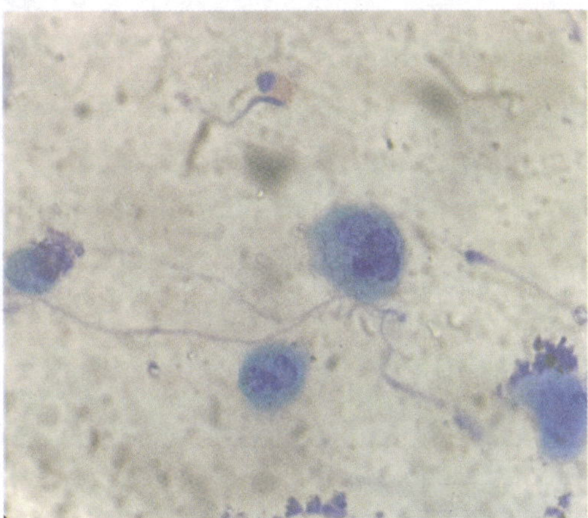

FIG. 9: Tzanck smear with multinucleated giant cells (100×).

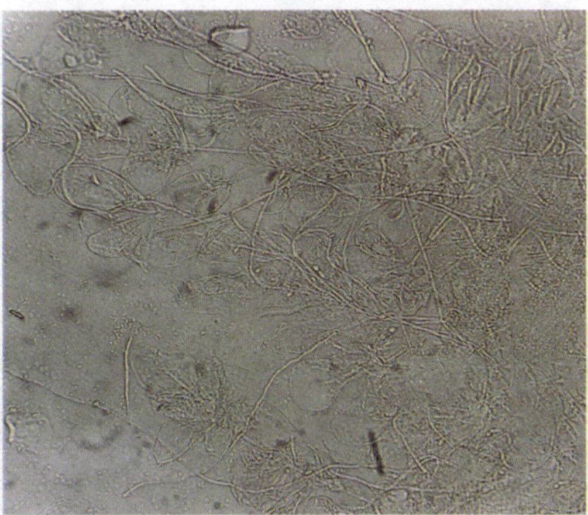

FIG. 11: Potassium hydroxide (KOH) mount from onychomycosis showing fungal hyphae (40×).

Onychomycosis

Potassium hydroxide mounts of nail clippings can reveal fungal hyphae and spores, confirming fungal infection as the cause of nail dystrophy **(Fig. 11)**.

BEYOND DIAGNOSIS: SPECIALIZED TECHNIQUES

Light microscopy can be combined with additional techniques for enhanced diagnostic accuracy and deeper understanding of skin diseases:

- *Polarized LM*: Distinguishes amyloid deposits from other dermal constituents in conditions like lichen amyloidosis.[6]
- *Mohs micrographic surgery*: Utilizes LM for real-time margin control during tumor excision, ensuring complete removal of malignant cells.
- *Dermatophathometry*: Quantifies features such as cell size and density with digital

image analysis tools, aiding in research and diagnosis.

LIMITATIONS OF LIGHT MICROSCOPY

Despite its invaluable role, LM has limitations:
- *Limited depth of penetration*: Cannot visualize deep structures, such as subcutaneous fat and muscle.
- *Static images*: Do not capture dynamic cellular processes.
- *Subjectivity*: Interpretation can be influenced by observer experience and training.
- *Limited specificity*: Certain morphologies may overlap in different diseases, requiring additional investigations for definitive diagnosis.[1]

THE FUTURE OF LIGHT MICROSCOPY IN DERMATOLOGY

Technological advancements are continuously enhancing the capabilities of LM in dermatology:
- *Digital pathology*: Offers advantages, such as teleconsultation, image sharing, and archiving of slides.
- *Computer-aided diagnosis (CAD) systems*: Utilize algorithms to analyze digitized images, assisting in identifying suspicious features and improving diagnostic accuracy.
- *Confocal microscopy*: Provides high-resolution 3D images of skin, offering deeper insights into cellular morphology and tissue architecture.
- *Super-resolution microscopy*: Enables visualization of structures beyond the diffraction limit of light, revealing finer details of cellular components and interactions, potentially leading to earlier and more accurate diagnosis of skin diseases.

CONCLUSION

Light microscopy remains a cornerstone of dermatologic diagnosis, providing readily accessible, cost-effective, and informative insights into skin pathology. Its versatility allows for the examination of a wide spectrum of skin conditions, guiding accurate diagnoses and timely treatment decisions. As technology continues to evolve, LM will integrate with advanced modalities, further solidifying its place as an essential tool in the dermatologist's armamentarium.

Key Messages

- LM is crucial for dermatologic diagnosis, revealing cellular-level morphology. Its advantages include noninvasiveness, affordability, accessibility, and rapid results.
- LM mechanism involves illumination, focusing, image formation, and contrast enhancement through staining.
- Types of LM (bright-field, dark-field, fluorescence, and polarized) serve specific purposes.
- LM is vital for diagnosing infections, and hair/nail disorders, and using specialized techniques.
- Techniques such as KOH mounts and Tzanck smear are vital for accurate diagnosis.
- Limitations include limited depth, static images, subjectivity, and limited specificity.
- Prospects include digital pathology, CAD systems, confocal, and super-resolution microscopy.
- LM remains essential in dermatologic diagnosis, providing cost-effective insights and evolving with technology.

REFERENCES

1. Sanderson J. Fundamentals of Microscopy. Curr Protoc Mouse Biol. 2020;10(2):e76.
2. Goodwin PC. A primer on the fundamental principles of light microscopy: Optimizing magnification, resolution, and contrast. Mol Reprod Dev. 2015;82(7-8):502-7.
3. Agrawal I, Panda M, Sahoo D, Panda AK, Puhan MR. Potassium hydroxide mount as an easy bedside test for early detection of cutaneous mucormycosis. J Cosmet Dermatol. 2022;21(8):3619-21.
4. SG, Srinivasan S, Kumar A, K M, Rajeev K. Tzanck Smear-Revisiting the basics. QJM. 2023;hcad265.
5. Mescon H, Grots IA. Fluorescence microscopy in dermatology. J Invest Dermatol. 1963;41:181-96.
6. Dongre A, Bhisey P, Khopkar U. Polarized light microscopy. Indian J Dermatol Venereol Leprol. 2007;73(3):206-8.
7. Bakos RM, Reinehr C, Escobar GF, Leite LL. Dermoscopy of skin infestations and infections (entomodermoscopy) - Part I: dermatozoonoses and bacterial infections. An Bras Dermatol. 2021;96(6):735-45.
8. Howell SA. Dermatopathology and the Diagnosis of Fungal Infections. Br J Biomed Sci. 2023;80:11314.
9. Rivero-Segura NA, Morales-Rosales SL, Rincón-Heredia R. Microscopy Principles in the Diagnosis of Epidemic Diseases. In: Gomez-Verjan JC, Rivero-Segura NA (Eds). Principles of Genetics and Molecular Epidemiology. Cham: Springer International Publishing; 2022. pp. 87-105.
10. Utsumi D, Yasuda M, Amano H, Suga Y, Seishima M, Takahashi K. Hair abnormality in Netherton syndrome observed under polarized light microscopy. J Am Acad Dermatol. 2020;83(3):847-53.

Potassium Hydroxide Mount

Biju Vasudevan, Nitin Kumar Sharma

INTRODUCTION

Potassium hydroxide (KOH) examination for fungal infections is a simple and cost-effective procedure and has a high sensitivity when performed by an experienced individual. It can be performed at a clinic on an outpatient basis, and the results are available within 1 hour. In experienced hands, a KOH mount is one of the most useful procedures in medical mycology, as it provides a rapid and accurate diagnosis in clinical settings where the diagnosis is in doubt. It has been adjudged more reliable than culture for the demonstration of dermatophytes. It is also helpful in the selection of appropriate culture media for the isolation of etiological fungal agents. In dermatology, a KOH mount of a skin scraping is a common procedure performed to demonstrate the evidence of fungal infection in skin, hairs, nails, and mucosa.

PRINCIPLE

Potassium hydroxide, a potent alkali, has the ability to soften, digest, and clarify tissues such as skin, hair, nails, or sputum when combined with specimens. This action targets the surrounding tissues, including keratin present in the skin, facilitating visibility of fungal hyphae and conidia (spores) under a microscope. Aqueous KOH effectively softens and digests protein debris, dissolving the cement substance-binding keratinized cells. As a result, fungal elements within clinical specimens become distinctly visible and easily observable.[1]

Procedure to make 100 mL of KOH 10% w/v solution:
- Weigh 10 g of KOH pellets
- Transfer the chemical to a screw-cap bottle
- Add 50 mL of distilled water and mix until the chemical is completely dissolved. Then, add the remaining distilled water to achieve a final volume of 100 mL.
- Label the bottle and mark it as corrosive. Store it at room temperature. The reagent remains stable for up to 2 years.

Caution: Potassium hydroxide is a highly corrosive deliquescent chemical. Handle it with great care and ensure the stock bottle of the chemical is tightly stoppered after use.

In a solution of KOH (10%), glycerol (10%) is added to prevent drying, as it is hygroscopic in nature and permits observations of the slide for up to 48 hours. The concentration of KOH may be increased depending upon the nature of the clinical material, as solid specimens require more than a 10% concentration, possibly up to 40%. Dimethyl sulfoxide (DMSO), a colorless organosulfur compound, can also be added to a KOH (20%) solution, which acts as a useful cleansing agent for fungi (KOH—20 g, DMSO—40 mL, and distilled water—60 mL). The wet mount with DMSO can be examined immediately without waiting for dissolution.

PREREQUISITE/MATERIAL REQUIRED

- *Equipment*: Microscope
- *Reagents and laboratory wares*:
  - Glass petri dishes
  - Clean and grease-free glass slides
  - Cover slips
  - Straight or bent wire
  - Needle
  - Bunsen burner
  - 10–20% KOH combined with a contrast dye of choice (KOH with DMSO optional)
- *Specimens*: It may vary according to the site of infection.

PROCEDURE OF POTASSIUM HYDROXIDE MOUNT

The standard method involves the following steps:[2,3]

1. The procedure should be explained to the patient in a language he or she understands, and written informed consent should be obtained beforehand.
2. The area is cleansed with water or spirit to eliminate dirt or any topical applications.
3. Utilize the blunt edge of a scalpel (No. 15 blade) to gather the specimen onto a clean glass slide and collect the scraping from the active margin in adequate quantity.
4. Alternatively, the specimen can be gathered on presterilized black chart paper, black card, or cellophane tape for transportation purposes.
5. The quantity and quality of the material examined significantly impact the availability of optimal results.
6. Once the scrapings are on the glass slide, add 1–2 drops of 10–20% KOH for hair and skin samples and 20–40% KOH for nail samples. Gently cover with a glass slip, lightly pressing and using a side-to-side technique to flatten the scale layer and mobilize excess solution to the edge. Any surplus solution can be gently blotted away using a paper towel, lens paper, or tissue.
7. Before microscopic visualization, the slide should be heated with a methanol burner to hasten keratinocyte digestion. However, caution is essential to avoid overheating the specimen, which can induce KOH crystallization and lead to artifacts. Sampling from hair and nails might necessitate prolonged heating to digest the denser keratinous material. In cases of thicker skin or hair lesions, leaving them for an hour enables adequate digestion of debris and intercellular substances. For nail specimens, a longer digestion time of up to 24 hours may be necessary.
8. To identify fungal elements, examine the slide under 10× magnification and study fungal morphology under 40× magnification. Partially close the condenser to lower the light intensity, providing better contrast. An excessively intense light source might diminish contrast, leading to potential oversight of unstained fungal elements.

PRECAUTIONS

- Ensure the KOH drop is not so large that it causes the cover slip to float.
- If kept outside a moist chamber, KOH dries, forming crystals that restrict the visibility of the fungus.
- After clearing, apply gentle pressure on the cover slip's top using a fold of filter paper or the handle of a teasing needle. This ensures even spreading of the material onto the slide.
- Fungal spores or hyphae may contaminate the laboratory's KOH solution, potentially yielding false-positive results. Therefore, a daily negative control should be established.

- Wash off any applied medication or cloth fibers with distilled water before collecting the sample.
- Excessive scales collected may heap up dissolved keratin, potentially interfering with the results. To prevent this, avoid mounting scales excessively when placing them on the glass slide.
- Avoid excessive heating of the slide to prevent KOH crystal formation.
- Inadequate sample collection or previous treatment with antifungals might result in false-negative outcomes. If clinical suspicion remains high, consider repeating the test.[3,4]

APPLICATIONS (TABLE 1)[5]

In dermatology, the KOH mount is primarily used to diagnose superficial fungal infections. Many other cutaneous disorders that resemble fungal infections in clinical morphology, such as psoriasis, various forms of eczema, and pityriasis rosea, can be quickly ruled out by a positive KOH test. This negates the need for a biopsy in many cases. The KOH mount is also valuable in ruling out fungal infections in conditions, such as erythema annulare centrifugum, lichen planus, cutaneous T-cell lymphoma, and parapsoriasis, which might otherwise be mistaken for superficial fungal infections.

TABLE 1: Potassium hydroxide (KOH) mount application with finding under light microscopy.

Suspected conditions	Specimen	Diagnostic characteristics
Dermatophytes	Skin scrapings, nails	Long branching septate hyphae, arthroconida or spherical yeast cells, depending on the etiologic agents involved
Tinea capitis infection	Hair	May show either endothrix pattern in which spores are seen in the hair shaft or ectothrix pattern where spores arealso seen on the external surface of the hair shaft
Tinea versicolor	Skin scrapping	Clusters of short hyphae and spores; referred to as "spaghetti and meatballs" or "banana and grapes"
Tinea nigra	Skin scrapping	Brown branching septate hyphae and budding cells of *Hortaea werneckii*
Bacterial vaginosis	Vaginal fluid	Few KOH drops to vaginal discharge give fishy odor. On light microscopy, "clue cells" will be seen
Blue neck syndrome	Skin scrapings	Nematode larvae can be seen
Mycotic keratitis	Debrided epithelium from corneal ulcers appearing as whitish flakes	Examined for molds (*Aspergillus*, *Fusarium*, or *Nocardia* species)
Mucormycosis	Exudates from infected lesions or tissue	Aseptate hyphae
Chromoblastomycosis	Scrapings from crusted lesions	Muriform cells (aggregation of dark brown cells that resemble stones in a wall) or round and brown sclerotic bodies of 4–10 µm diameter with fission planes. They resemble copper pennies
Candidiasis	Curdy white discharge from infection site	Pseudohyphae (nonseptate hyphae) and round to oval yeast bodies
Aspergillus infection	Sputum	Septate hyphae with V-shaped branching
Blastomyces dermatitidis infection	Pus, sputum, or skin specimens	Yeast cells (large budding yeast cells with distinct broad base) of *B. dermatitidis*. *B. dermatitidis* is a dimorphic fungus with yeast cells in tissue

Various indications and methods of collecting specimens are briefly explained herewith:[6]

- *Dermatophyte infection*: Dermatophytes are ascomycetes with septate hyphae that cause mostly superficial diseases in humans and other mammals. There are three genera of dermatophytes, (1) *Trichophyton*, (2) *Microsporum*, and (3) *Epidermophyton*. Although the species were historically divided into these genera by morphology and physical attributes, recent analysis by ribosomal ribonucleic acid (rRNA) sequencing indicates that the dermatophytes as a whole are a cohesive group with no clear distinction between the three genera. The diseases that result from a dermatophyte infection are known as tineas. The location of the disease on the body further defines the disease, so that tinea pedis is a dermatophyte infection of the feet, tinea cruris of the genitals, tinea corporis of the torso, and tinea capitis of the head. There are at least 40 species of dermatophytes that infect humans, and many of these fungi can cause disease in more than one body location. The most prevalent cause of tinea pedis is *Trichophyton rubrum*, and the most prevalent causes of tinea capitis are *Trichophyton tonsurans* and *Microsporum canis*. *Tinea nigra* is an uncommon dermatomycosis typically presenting on palmoplantar surfaces of the body and rarely occurs on interdigital surfaces. *Hortaea werneckii*, the underlying fungus, develops a melanin-like substance in the stratum corneum, resulting in the development of asymptomatic brown macules and patches with irregular borders. These pigmented lesions are concerning for melanocytic nevi or melanoma.[7]

  - *Dermatophyte skin infection:* Lesions suspected to harbor underlying fungal pathology are identified. The advancing border, known for its heightened fungal activity, serves as the optimal site, yielding superior results. In the majority of tinea plaques, an advancing rim characterized by erythematous papules and vesicles presents the ideal locations for scrapings. For enhanced accuracy, it is advisable to collect samples from multiple sites. Skin scrapings can be collected using the edge of a clean glass slide or the blunt end of a surgical blade (**Fig. 1**). Collecting an adequate sample is crucial to obtain a higher yield of fungal elements. Insufficient sampling may lead to false-negative results. KOH examination reveals refractile and branching fungal hyphae of dermatophytes (**Figs. 2 and 3**). In cases of tinea nigra, KOH examination of scrapings shows colonies of brown, septating, and branching hyphae with spores.

  - *Dermatophytic infection of hairs*: Various samples, including plucked hair, epilated hair, hair stubs, and matted hair crusts, hold significant value for examination. Ensure to incorporate skin scrapings from the surrounding infected scalp when preparing your hair mount. When dealing with lusterless hair close to the surface, use sterile epilation forceps

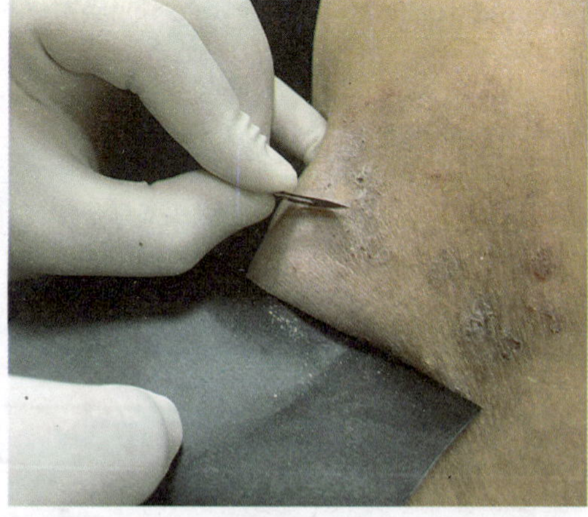

FIG. 1: Fungal sample collection technique.

to pluck it along with its root. Woods lamp can be used to identify infected hair strands, manifesting yellow-green fluorescence for *Microsporum* species and bluish-green for *Trichophyton schoenleinii*. To aid in clearing, keep the hair shaft length under 5 mm. In the case of tinea capitis, gather scale scrapings from the base of broken hair and the affected scalp. Dermatophyte infection of hair reveals spores on a KOH mount, either within the hair shaft (endothrix) or outside it (ectothrix). Ectothrix spores appear grouped and attached outside the hair cortex. Conversely, in endothrix, these spores are not only densely packed inside the hair cortex but might also extend outside the cortex, potentially associated with hair shaft dystrophy **(Figs. 4 to 6)**. *T. tonsurans* commonly causes tinea capitis in children, recognized as "black dot ringworm" due to short and dark broken hairs resembling black dots. Ensure to sample and examine these hairs for endothrix spores.

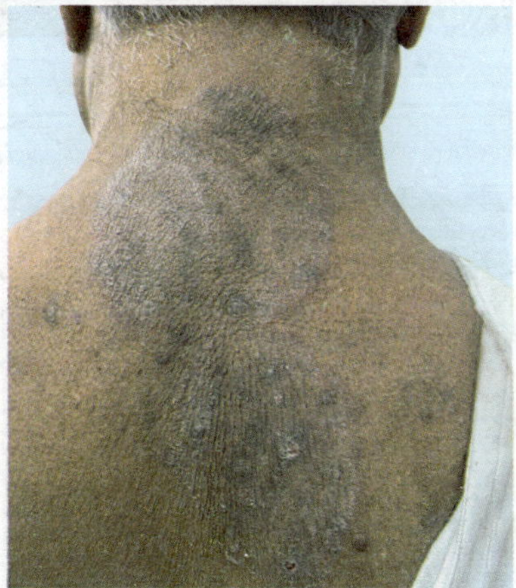

FIG. 2: Clinical image of tinea corporis.

○ *Dermatophytic infection of nails*: Fungal infection of the nail unit can impact any part of the nail structure be it the nail plate, nail matrix, or nail bed. Its presentation involves various discolorations, such as white or yellow-brown, violaceous, green, or black patches on the nail. Clinical signs also encompass subungual hyperkeratosis, separation of the nail from the nail bed (onycholysis), and thickening of the nail plate (onychauxis). The condition of onychomycosis can be categorized into five distinct clinical subtypes based on the pattern of invasion: (1) distal lateral subungual onychomycosis, (2) white superficial onychomycosis, (3) proximal subungual onychomycosis, (4) endonyx onychomycosis, and (5) total dystrophic onychomycosis. Nail clippings, avulsed nails, subungual debris, and the under surface of nail plates are suitable samples for diagnosing onychomycosis. For better visualization, nail clippings should not exceed 2–3 mm in thickness. Preferably, collect clippings from proximal areas targeting white or yellow, crumbly regions, as these areas commonly

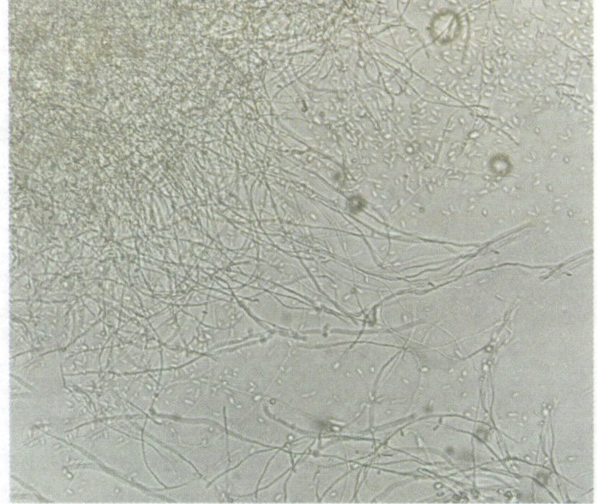

FIG. 3: Potassium hydroxide (KOH) mount showing refractile and branching fungal hyphae of dermatophytes (40×).

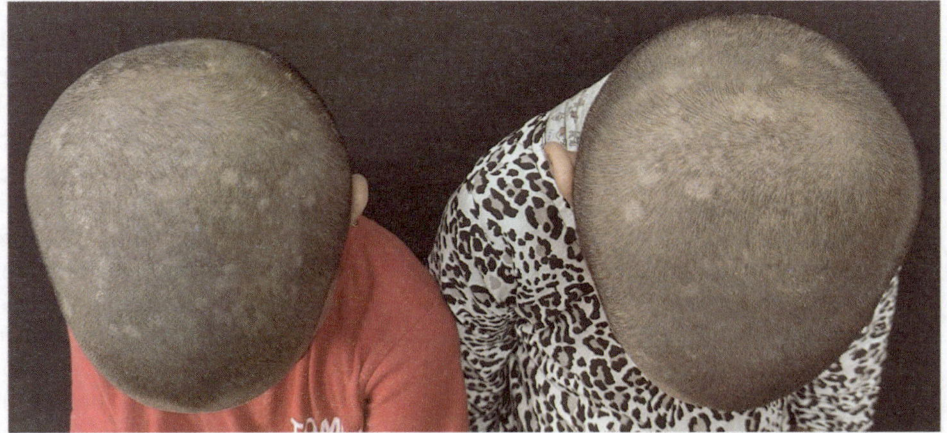

FIG. 4: Clinical image of tinea capitis in siblings.

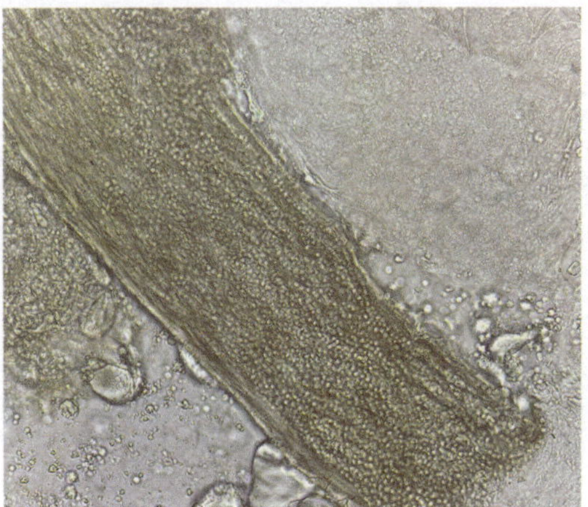

FIG. 5: Potassium hydroxide (KOH) mount of hair with ectothrix (40×).

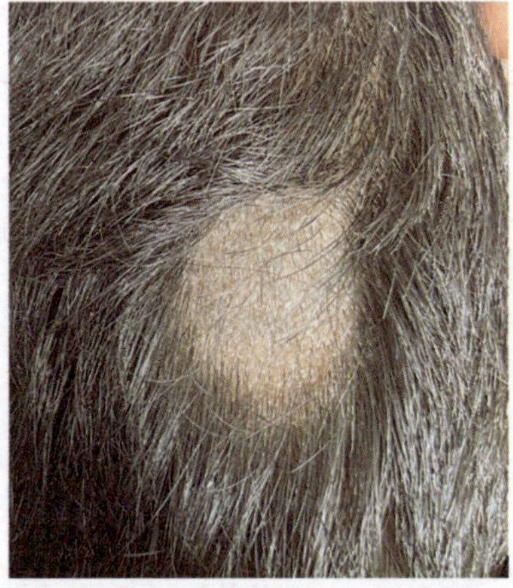

FIG. 6: Clinical image of tinea capitis.

indicate active infection. If no distinct affected area is visible, sampling from the distal subungual debris is suitable, aiming to obtain material from the most proximal involved area. If suspecting paronychia, a *Candida* skin infection impacting the periungual skin, collect pus from beneath the nail fold for microscopic examination. This can be achieved by compression or incision using a number 11 scalpel blade on the inflamed tissue. The collected sample should be immersed in 40% KOH on a clean grease-free glass slide for 2 hours or more (up to 48 hours) until softening or digestion of the specimen occur (gentle heat should be applied to facilitate keratin clearance). Examination under low- and high-power objectives reveals the presence of hyphae or pseudohyphae **(Figs. 7 and 8)**.

- *Pityriasis versicolor*: Tinea versicolor, also known as pityriasis versicolor, is

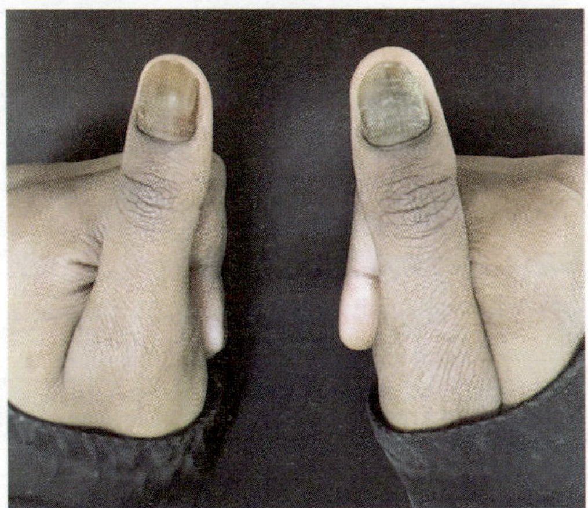

FIG. 7: Clinical image of onychomycosis both thumbs.

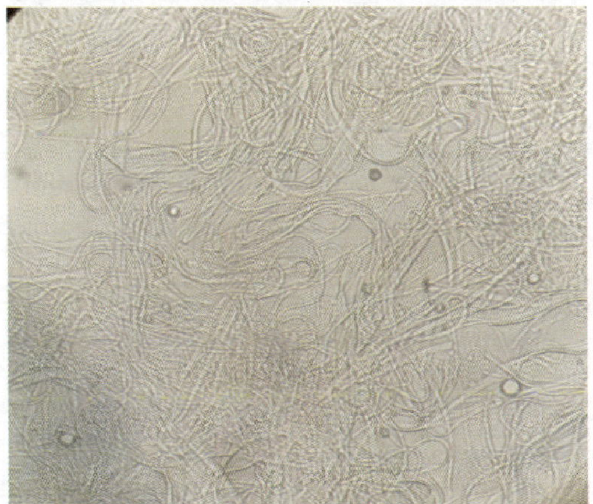

FIG. 8: Potassium hydroxide (KOH) mount of nail showing branching fungal hyphae (40×).

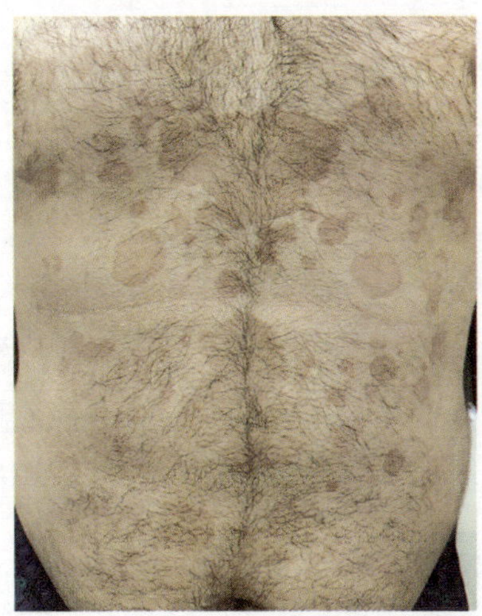

FIG. 9: Clinical image of pityriasis versicolor (anterior of trunk).

cause by dimorphic lipophilic and lipid-dependent yeasts of the genus *Malassezia* (formerly known as *Pityrosporum*) species, notably *Malassezia globosa* (*M. globosa*) and *Malassezia furfur*. Patients with tinea versicolor typically present with asymptomatic hypopigmented (thought to result from damage to melanocytes and inhibition of tyrosinase by azelaic acid) or hyperpigmented (may result from a hyperemic inflammatory response elicited by *Malassezia* species), finely scaled, oval or round macules/

patches on the trunk and upper arms. Patients can have pruritus, particularly when the condition is more extensive. The term "versicolor" refers to the variable colors of the skin lesions that may occur in this disorder. Clinical manifestations of tinea versicolor are myriad, and the differential diagnoses are broad. Scaly hypopigmented or hyperpigmented lesions are identified and scratching the lesion can accentuate the scales (known as Besnier's sign). Collecting scrapings from the scaly edges often yields good results. When subjected to a KOH examination, scrapings from these lesions exhibit a distinctive appearance, described as "banana and grapes" or "spaghetti and meatballs" appearance which corresponds to the hyphae and spores, respectively **(Figs. 9 to 12)**.[8]

- *Candidiasis*: Candidiasis, an opportunistic infection caused by *Candida*, a eukaryotic fungus found in various forms, such as yeasts, molds, or dimorphic fungi. Diverse species of *Candida* exist, such as *Candida albicans*, *Candida glabrata*, *Candida krusei*, *Candida parapsilosis*, *Candida pseudotropicalis*, *Candida stellatoidea*,

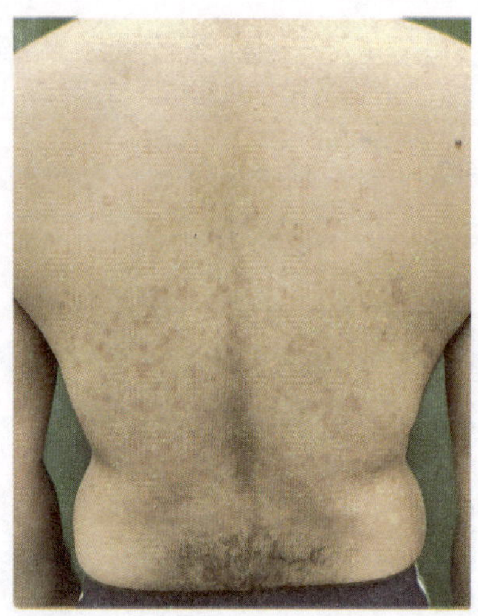

FIG. 10: Clinical image of pityriasis versicolor (posterior of trunk).

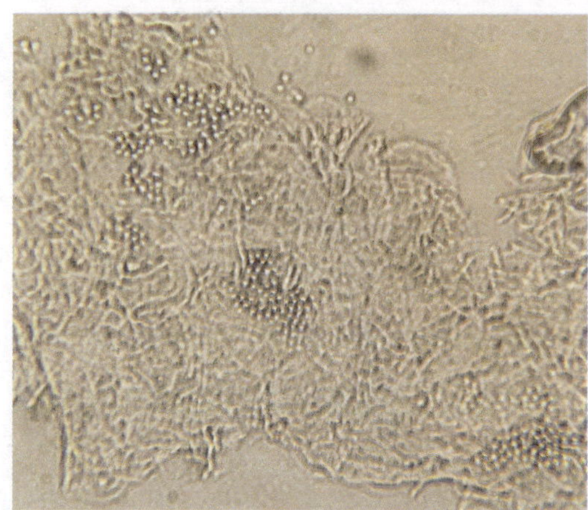

FIG. 12: Potassium hydroxide (KOH) mount of skin scrapping showing "spaghetti and meatballs" appearance which corresponds to the hyphae and spores (40×).

FIG. 11: Potassium hydroxide (KOH) mount of skin scrapping showing "spaghetti and meatballs" appearance which corresponds to the hyphae and spores (40×) (in another patient).

and *Candida tropicalis*. This infection commonly manifests as a secondary ailment in immunocompromised individuals, affecting oral cavity, vagina, penis, or other body parts. Oral candidiasis, often referred to as thrush, typically exhibits as white patches on the tongue and throat, accompanied by soreness and difficulty swallowing. It may manifest in various forms, such as pseudomembranous, erythematous, or chronic hyperplastic candidiasis. Vaginal candidiasis presents with symptoms, such as genital itching, burning sensations, and curdy white "cottage cheese" like discharge from the vagina. Yeast infections affecting the penis are less common and may show up as an itchy rash. Samples are collected based on the site of infection. For instance, curdy white discharge may be gathered from the oral cavity, vagina or glans penis, satellite pustules of cutaneous lesions, diaper area, web spaces, and nail clippings can be obtained. KOH mount will demonstrate budding yeasts, hyphae, pseudohyphae (nonseptate hyphae), and round to oval yeast bodies **(Figs. 13 and 14)**.[9]

- *Demonstration of fungi from cutaneous lesions of deep fungal infections*: Deep fungal skin infections are chronic diseases, caused by various groups of fungi. The clinical spectrum of these infections can be classified into (1) subcutaneous mycoses and (2) systemic mycoses. *Subcutaneous mycoses* occur when fungi like sporotrichosis, mycetoma,

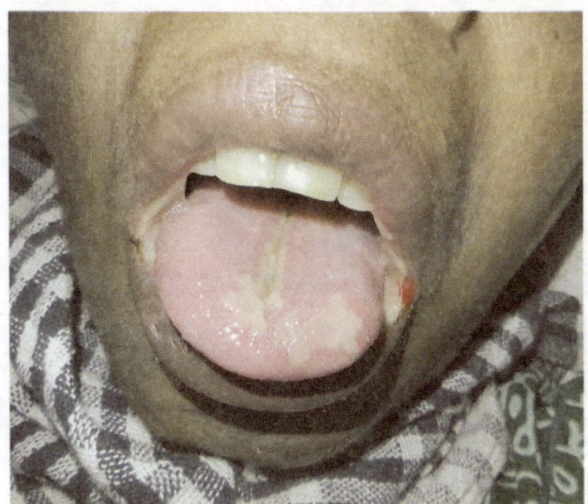

FIG. 13: Clinical image of oral candidiasis.

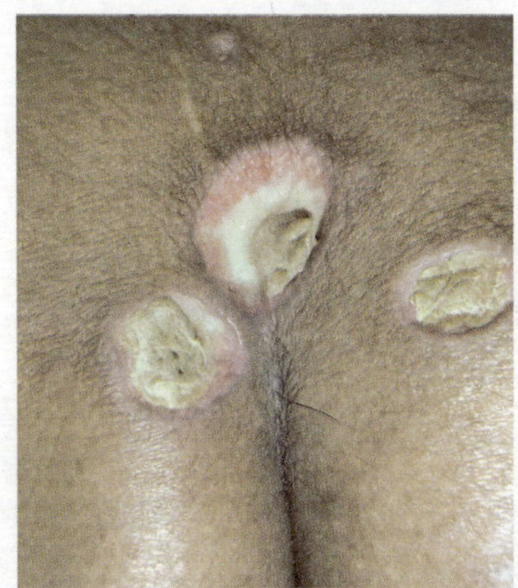

FIG. 15: Clinical image of pheohyphomycosis.

FIG. 14: Potassium hydroxide (KOH) mount of scrapping showing budding yeasts, hyphae, pseudohyphae (nonseptate hyphae), and round to oval yeast bodies (40×).

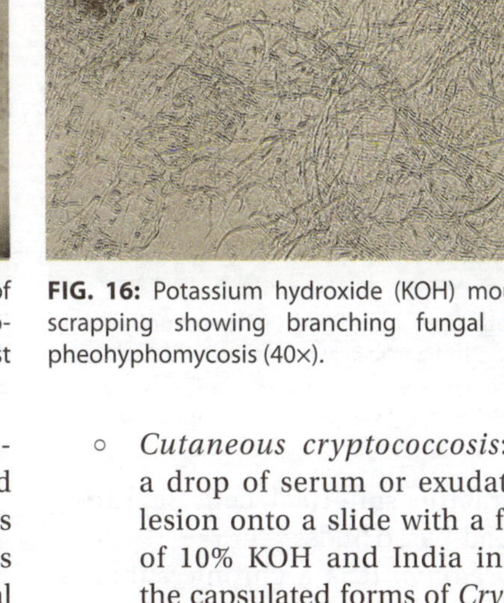

FIG. 16: Potassium hydroxide (KOH) mount of skin scrapping showing branching fungal hyphae of pheohyphomycosis (40×).

chromomycosis, and lobomycosis traumatically introduced into the skin and subcutaneous tissue. Systemic mycoses are caused by "true" fungal pathogens and opportunistic fungi. The "true" fungal pathogens are agents of histoplasmosis, blastomycosis, coccidioidomycosis, and paracoccidioidomycosis. The opportunistic deep mycoses comprise a spectrum of diseases including zygomycosis, cryptococcosis, aspergillosis, pheohyphomycosis **(Figs. 15 and 16)**, and hyalohyphomycosis.

○ *Cutaneous cryptococcosis*: Placing a drop of serum or exudate from a lesion onto a slide with a few drops of 10% KOH and India ink reveals the capsulated forms of *Cryptococcus* **(Figs. 17 and 18)**.

○ *Chromoblastomycosis*: Examining a KOH mount of skin scrapings from lesion surfaces displays sclerotic or muriform fungal cells **(Figs. 19 and 20)**.

○ *Blastomycosis*: Observing a KOH mount of pus, skin scrapings, or sputum showcases round and

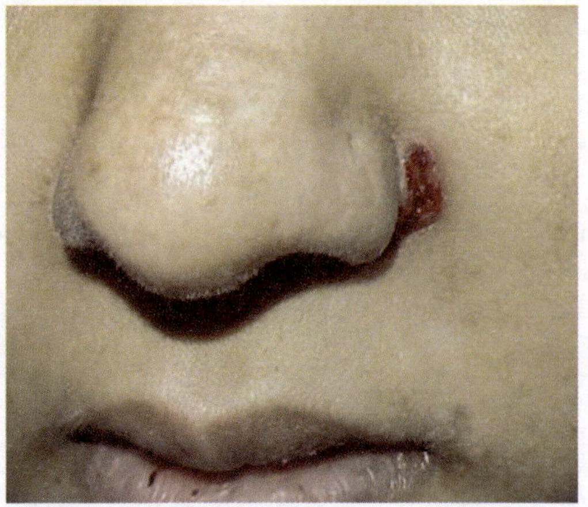

FIG. 17: Clinical image of cutaneous *Cryptococcus* infection.

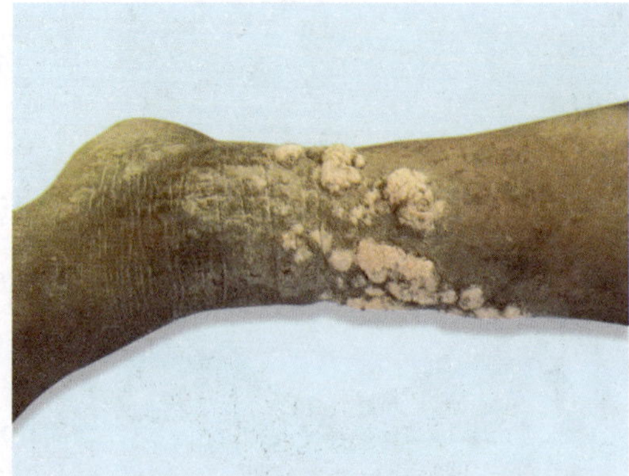

FIG. 19: Clinical image of chromoblastomycosis.

FIG. 18: Potassium hydroxide (KOH) mount of skin scrapping and India ink showing the capsulated forms of *Cryptococcus*.

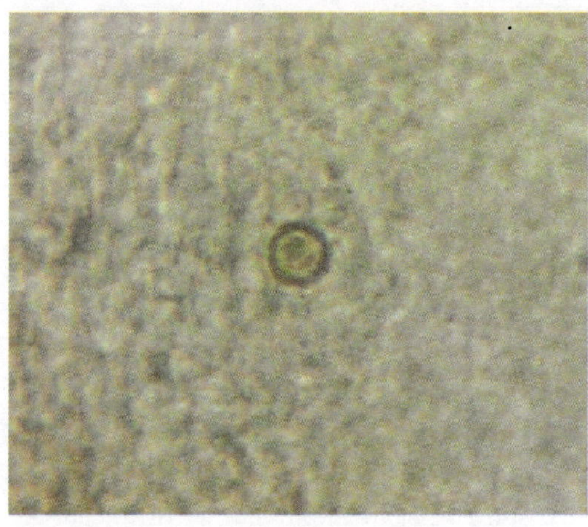

FIG. 20: Potassium hydroxide (KOH) mount of skin scraping showing the copper penny body of chromoblastomycosis.

refractile spherical cells featuring broad-based buds.

○ *Mycetoma*: It is a chronic subcutaneous granulomatous inflammatory disease caused by several true fungi and bacteria, and hence, it is classified as eumycetoma and actinomycetoma, respectively. The disease is characterized by numerous deformations and disabilities, high morbidity, and in its late stage it is potentially fatal. The triad of a painless subcutaneous mass, multiple sinuses, and discharge that contains grains of different colors, sizes, and consistency is characteristic of mycetoma. The grains can be directly examined under light microscope using 10% KOH, which can help in ruling out actinomycotes as causative agents by additional characteristic features identification **(Fig. 21)**.

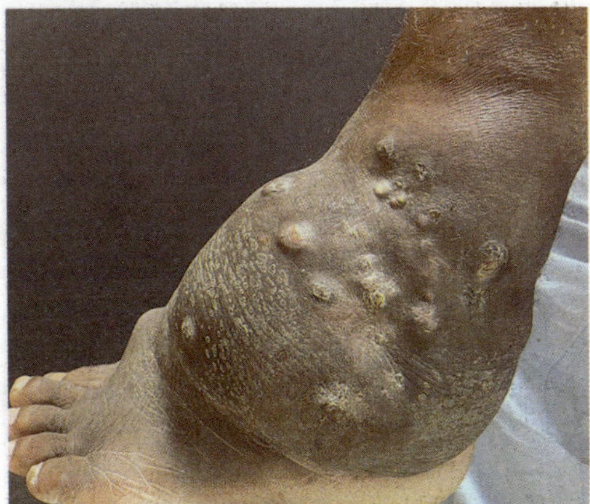

FIG. 21: Clinical image of mycetoma.

- *Bacterial vaginosis*: Bacterial vaginosis frequently occurs in sexually active women of childbearing age and is a common cause of vaginitis. To diagnose it, the vaginal fluid collected after removing the speculum should undergo pH testing. Few drops of 10% KOH should to be added to the discharge on a glass slide, and then sniffed to detect a fishy odor and wet mounts examined under light microscopy will demonstrate clue cells' of *Gardnerella*.
- *Mycotic keratitis*: A strong clinical suspicion, meticulous corneal scraping (deep scrapping) using a No. 15 blade on a Bard–Parker handle, and a comprehensive microscopic analysis of direct smears result in a high sensitivity of the 10% KOH smear. Samples of debrided epithelium from corneal ulcers, manifesting as whitish flakes, are directly mounted in 10% KOH for examination to detect molds (such as *Aspergillus* and *Fusarium*), yeasts, or *Nocardia* species.
- *Blue neck syndrome*: This condition is prevalent in Northern Kerala. The affected skin displays a dry, dull, and matte surface with a characteristic bluish-black hue, showcasing distinctive pigmentation of skin surface and clearly visible nonpigmented grooves in the skin folds. When skin scrapings from the neck are examined under a microscope using KOH mounts, nematode larvae are visible.

ADVANTAGES

- Economical, swift, and easy-to-perform test
- Minimally invasive procedure
- Requires minimal infrastructure
- KOH is a reliable outpatient procedure that yields quick results. Although fungal culture is a good confirmatory test for identifying fungus, it is more expensive and takes a minimum of 3 weeks to obtain results.
- KOH can serve as a primary screening tool for detecting fungal elements in hair, skin, nails, and sputum samples.[4]

LIMITATIONS

- Sensitivity of test depends on the operator's expertise
- Pus and sputum may contain artifacts that superficially resemble hyphal and budding forms of fungi. These artifacts may be produced by cotton or wool fibers, starch grains (in pleuritis), or cholesterol crystals.
- It only provides an idea about the presence of hyphal elements but cannot distinguish different fungi.
- Preparations cannot be kept for too long, although drying can be prevented by keeping the slides in a moist chamber.
- Wrong interpretations may lead to false-positive or false-negative results.[3]

CHICAGO SKY BLUE AND CALCOFLUOR-WHITE STAINS

Potassium hydroxide mount is the standard bedside laboratory technique for confirming dermatophytosis while culture is used to identify the species. However, KOH mount results in a lot of false negative results while culture takes a long period of about 4–6 weeks to yield results but identifies the species. Calcofluor-white staining observed under a fluorescent microscope has been found to detect dermatophytes with good efficacy in a few studies previously. Chicago sky blue stain is a new contrast stain for detecting dermatophytes rapidly and at a low cost. Chicago sky blue stain is a contrast stain that can help to distinguish between hyphae and epithelial cells and is used together with KOH as a clearing agent. When stained, fungal filaments appear distinct blue against a pale or purple background.

Calcofluor-white stain is a nonspecific fluorochrome that binds with cellulose and chitin contained in the cell walls of cellulose-containing organisms and facilitates the visualization of pathogenic elements.

This diagnostic test has showed significantly higher sensitivity, specificity, positive predictive value, negative predictive value, and accuracy, with very low rates of false-positive and false-negative results **(Figs. 22 and 23)**.[10]

CONCLUSION

In conclusion, the KOH mount procedure stands as a fundamental and cost-effective tool in dermatology for diagnosing fungal infections in skin, hair, nails, and mucosa. Its simplicity, rapid results, and minimal invasiveness make it invaluable in clinical settings where timely and accurate diagnoses are crucial. While the KOH mount offers high sensitivity, it does come with certain limitations, such as dependency on operator expertise and the potential for false-positive or false-negative results. However, advancements in complementary staining techniques like Chicago sky blue

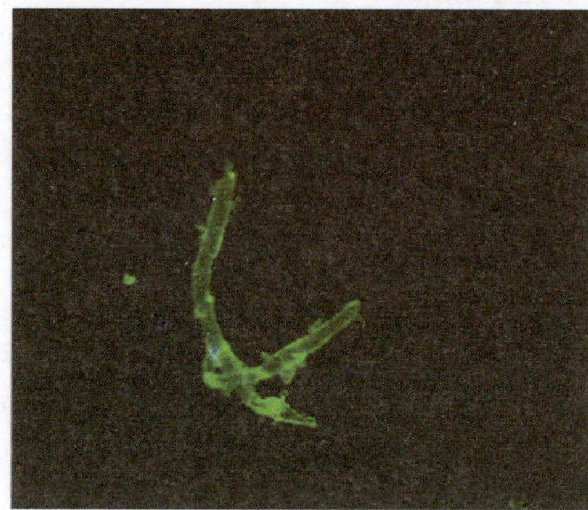

FIG. 22: Calcofluor-white staining observed under a fluorescent microscope demonstrating fungal elements.

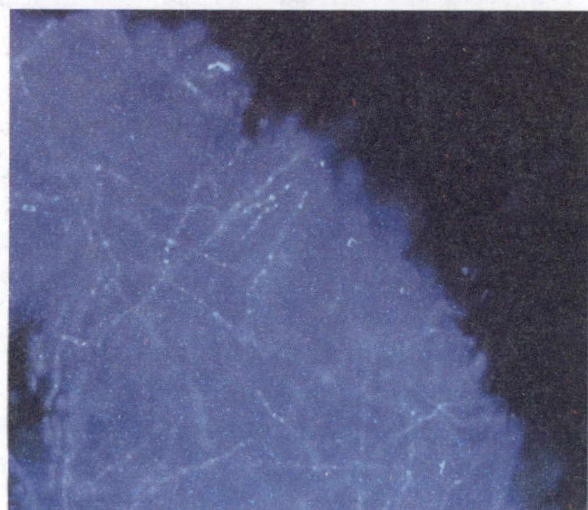

FIG. 23: Calcofluor-white staining observed under a fluorescent microscope demonstrating fungal elements.

and Calcofluor-white stains are promising additions, enhancing accuracy and reducing diagnostic errors. The versatility of the KOH mount extends beyond fungal infections, aiding in distinguishing various cutaneous disorders and guiding appropriate treatment paths. Despite its limitations, when performed meticulously and in conjunction with other diagnostic tools, the KOH mount remains an indispensable initial screening method, providing critical insights for dermatological diagnosis.

Key Messages

- KOH mount is an easy-to-perform, simple, and cost-effective procedure and has a high sensitivity for clinical diagnosis in dermatology.
- It majorly helps in diagnosis of fungal infection in skin, hairs, and nails.
- However, it has certain limitations like false-positive results in various cases.

REFERENCES

1. Zaias N, Taplin D. Improved preparation for the diagnosis of mycologic diseases. Arch Dermatol. 1966;93:608-9.
2. Manjyot G, Saloni B. Mount the Menace!—Potassium Hydroxide in Superficial Fungal Infections. Indian J Paediatr Dermatol. 2020;21(4):343-6.
3. Brodell RT, Helms SE, Cosulich MT, Jackson JD, Abramovits W, Bhatia AC, et al. Tips and Tricks in Procedural Dermatology: Efficient and Effective Approaches to Achieving Optimal Diagnostic and Therapeutic Results. New Delhi: Jaypee Brothers Medical Publishers; 2019.
4. Chander J. A Textbook of Medical Mycology. New Delhi: Mehta Publishers; 2002.
5. Kurade SM, Amladi SA, Miskeen AK. Skin scraping and a potassium hydroxide mount. Indian J Dermatol Venereol Leprol. 2006;72:238-41.
6. Tille PM. Bailey & Scott's Diagnostic Microbiology. St. Louis, Missouri: Elsevier; 2022.
7. White TC, Findley K, Dawson TL Jr, Scheynius A, Boekhout T, Cuomo CA, et al. Fungi on the skin: dermatophytes and Malassezia. Cold Spring Harb Perspect Med. 2014;4(8):a019802.
8. Leung AK, Barankin B, Lam JM, Leong KF, Hon KL. Tinea versicolor: an updated review. Drugs Context. 2022;11:2022-9-2.
9. R AN, Rafiq NB. Candidiasis. 2023. In: StatPearls [Internet]. Treasure Island (FL): StatPearls Publishing; 2024.
10. Afshar P, Larijani LV, Rouhanizadeh H. A comparison of conventional rapid methods in diagnosis of superficial and cutaneous mycoses based on KOH, Chicago sky blue 6B and calcofluor white stains. Iran J Microbiol. 2018;10:433-40.

Slit-skin Smear and Ziehl–Neelsen Stain

S Radhakrishnan, Binu Kunwar, Anand Mannu

INTRODUCTION

Slit-skin smear (SSS) is one of the most simple and valuable cytodiagnostic techniques used in the diagnosis of various cutaneous dermatoses. This safe and simple side laboratory procedure entails carefully taking a sample from a tiny cut in the afflicted area of skin, staining it and examining under a microscope.

HISTORICAL ASPECTS OF SLIT-SKIN SMEAR

Patrick Manson diagnosed leprosy in 1884 using the squeeze and pierce method. Subsequently, Alvarez created smears by surgically extracting and grinding the nodules.[1] Muir prepared smears by using the skin clip process. It was not until 1963 that Wade introduced the SSS method for the diagnosis of leprosy.[2]

Demonstration of *Mycobacterium leprae* in SSS was an essential component in the early phases of the multidrug therapy (MDT) program. Based on SSS positivity, the World Health Organization (WHO) (1981) classified leprosy as either paucibacillary (PB) or multibacillary (MB), with patients receiving treatment for MB if their bacteriological index (BI) was >2 and MB for all other patients. However due to the lack of enthusiasm and requisite experience in smear taking,

fixing, staining, or scoring, Georgiev and McDougall (1988) suggested to abandon SSS in leprosy control programs.[3] In 1988, the WHO simplified the classification of leprosy, categorizing all cases with positive smears into MB group and those with negative smears into PB group. SSS is no longer mandatory for the diagnosis of leprosy in leprosy control programs.

INDICATIONS OF SLIT-SKIN SMEAR

It can be used as a diagnostic modality in following indications.

Leprosy

Slit-skin smear is used to:
- Confirm the diagnosis of leprosy
- Classify the disease
- Determine the disease activity in a patient
- Assess progress of the disease
- Diagnose relapse of leprosy
- Follow up patients on treatment

Cutaneous Mastocytosis

Cutaneous mastocytosis are most frequently observed in the form of large mast cell aggregates of solitary or multiple mastocytomas commonly in infants and children. Clinically, it is characterized with a single or several, red to reddish-brown minimally infiltrated nodule, or plaque. Definitive diagnosis requires histopathologic examination of the lesional skin specimen obtained by a skin biopsy. SSS when stained with toluidine blue or Giemsa stain, shows mast cells that have metachromatic granules in their cytoplasm. Hence may prove to be a rapid, noninvasive technique to support the diagnosis.[4]

Cutaneous Leishmaniasis

Post-kala-azar dermal leishmaniasis (PKDL) develops as a sequel to kala-azar after apparent complete treatment. The diagnosis of PKDL rests on the demonstration of the parasite in tissue smears, immune diagnosis by detection of parasite antigen or antibody in blood, or detection and quantitation of parasite DNA in tissue specimens. SSS is an old and reliable technique for the diagnosis of PKDL that shows *Leishmania donovani* bodies either as extracellular structures or intracellularly within mononuclear macrophages.[5]

Chronic Ulcerative Lesion

Any chronic ulcerative lesion resistant to healing and carrying a potential risk of malignant transformation.[6]

Leprosy

Sites

- Routine sites are one-right earlobe, two-forehead, three-chin, and four-left buttock in men and left upper thigh in women.[6]
- It is recommended to take smear from two sites under aseptic conditions, i.e., earlobe and active (erythematous or infiltrated) lesion.[3]
- The smears from forehead, cheek, chin, buttocks, or nasal mucosa are no longer recommended for cosmetic and practical reasons.[3] The same sites are used for follow-up smears and in relapsed cases along with new relapse lesions

EQUIPMENT, MATERIALS, AND STAINS

Equipment, materials, and stains required for slit-skin smear tray are given in **Table 1**.

Technique of Smear Taking, Staining, and Reading

- The procedure is explained to the patient and consent is obtained.
- Strict aseptic precautions are maintained.

Preparation of Slide

- Just before taking the smear, clean the skin site using sterile cotton wool soaked in methyl alcohol. Let it dry **(Fig. 1)**.
- Pinch the fold of skin tightly using the thumb and index finger till it blanches. Using a chalazion clamp, curved artery forceps or sponge holding forceps can help overcome this difficulty **(Fig. 2)**.[7]
- Using a surgical scalpel with a detachable sterile blade (Bard-Parker No. 15), make a cut on the skinfold 5 mm long and

TABLE 1: Equipment, materials, and stains required for slit-skin smear tray.

Equipment and materials	Stains	Others
• Gloves	• 1% carbol fuchsin	• Light microscope
• Swabs and spirit	• 5% sulfuric acid or 1% acid alcohol (1% hydrochloric acid in absolute ethyl alcohol)	• Immersion oil and blotting papers
• Bard-Parker scalpel handle and new blades (No. 15)		• Slide box
• Medicated dressing strips		• Sink with running water, staining rods
• Spirit lamp	• 1% methylene blue	• Safe disposals bins
• Microscope glass slides		
• Marking pencils		
• Record register		

2 mm deep just to expose the subepithelial tissue. The blade is then turned 90°. Scrape the bottom and sides of the slit to obtain sufficient material for smear. Ordinarily, there should be no bleeding as this may interfere with staining and reading. If bleeding is noted, wipe the blood away with cotton **(Fig. 3)**.

- Place the material thus obtained on the clean slide and spread evenly to make a smear about 8–10 mm in diameter. Tissue is collected from all the required sites on the same slide **(Fig. 4)**.
- Press the cut surface of the skin with a piece of cotton wool to stop bleeding and seal the part with tincture benzene.

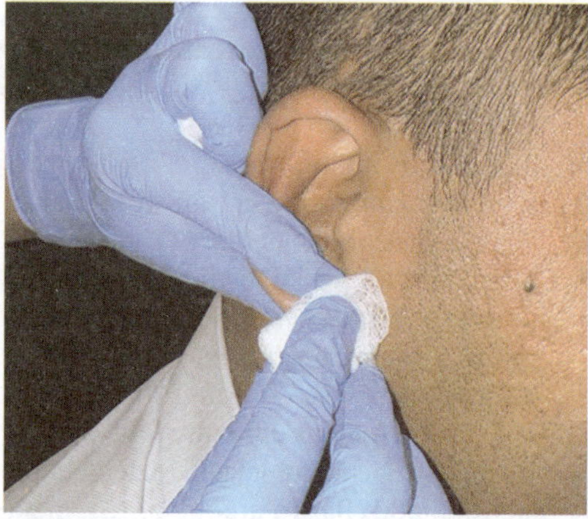

FIG. 1: First step: Clean the skin site using sterile cotton wool.

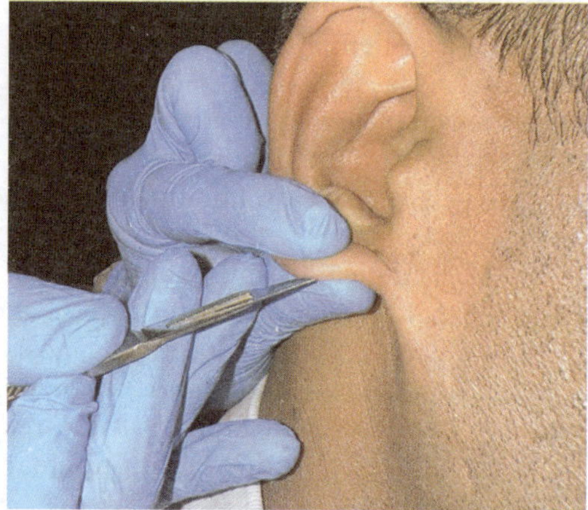

FIG. 3: Using a surgical scalpel with a detachable sterile blade (Bard-Parker No. 15), make a cut on the skinfold 5 mm long and 2 mm deep just to expose the subepithelial tissue.

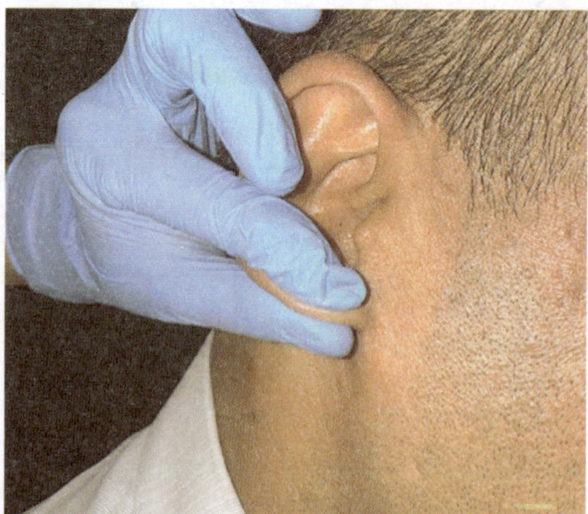

FIG. 2: Pinch the fold of skin tightly using the thumb and index finger till it blanches.

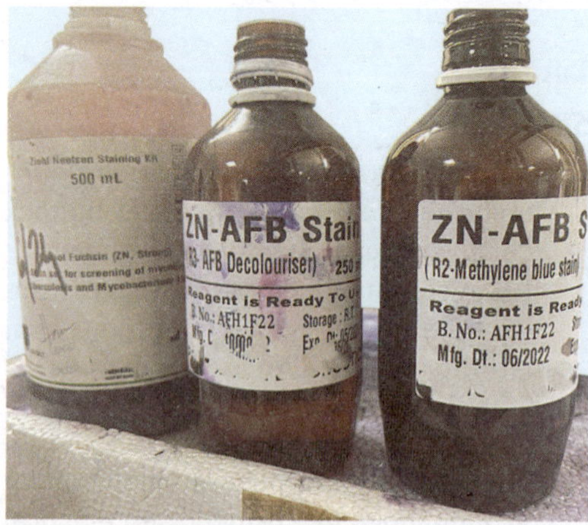

FIG. 4: Place the material thus obtained on the clean slide and spread evenly to make a smear about 8–10 mm in diameter.

- Let the smear air-dry and achieve fixation by passing the slide over a flame 2–3 times. Ensure sufficient heating, insufficient heat may result in an unfixed smear prone to washing out, while excessive heat can cause charring and cracking of the smear.

Staining of Slides: Ziehl–Neelsen Method

Chemicals required (Fig. 5):
- Basic fuchsin
- Decolorizing agent
- Methylene blue (counterstain)

Preparation of Reagents

Carbol fuchsin (to make 200 mL):
- *Basic fuchsin*: 2 g
- *Melted phenol*: 10 mL
- *Absolute alcohol (95%)*: 20 mL
- *Distilled water*: 170 mL

In a large conical flask put 2 g of basic fuchsin and then mix it with 10 mL of melted phenol. Add 20 mL of 95% absolute alcohol and mix well. Finally, pour in 170 mL of distilled water and shake until the dye is dissolved. Before using it, each time filter the solution (using Whatman filter paper No. 40)

Decolorizing Agent

Sulfuric acid (5%) (to make 200 mL):
- *1-N concentrated sulfuric acid*: 10 mL
- *Distilled water*: 190 mL

Pour 190 mL of distilled water into a large conical flask. Gently add 10 mL of concentrated sulfuric acid down the side of the flask. Rotate and shake the flask while pouring the acid.

Caution: Always add acid to water; never pour water into the acid.

Hydrochloric acid (1%) in 70% absolute alcohol (to make 100 mL):
- *Concentrated hydrochloric acid*: 1 mL
- *Absolute alcohol (70%)*: 99 mL

Counterstain

Methylene blue (0.2%) (to make 200 mL):
- *Methylene blue powder*: 0.4 g
- *Distilled water*: 200 mL

Method of Staining

The slides with the fixed smears are stained individually.

They are placed separately on staining rods over a sink.

- *Primary staining*: Flood the slide with freshly prepared and filtered 1% carbol fuchsin stain **(Fig. 6)** and gently heat it till slight fuming occurs **(Fig. 7)**. Do not let the stain boil. Keep the stain for 10–15 minutes without any further heating. Wash the slides gently in running water **(Fig. 8)**.

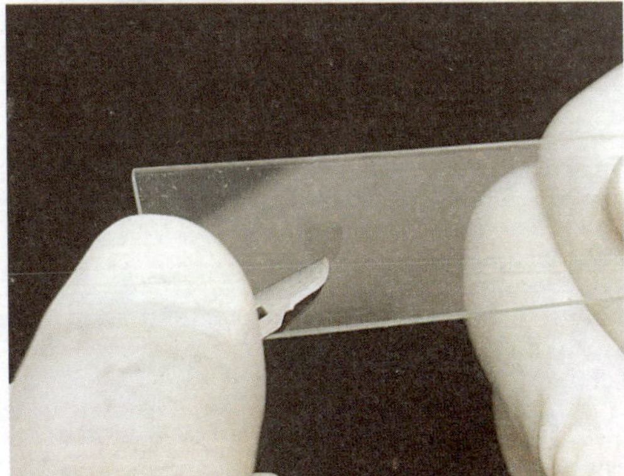

FIG. 5: Chemicals required for Ziehl–Neelsen (ZN) stain.

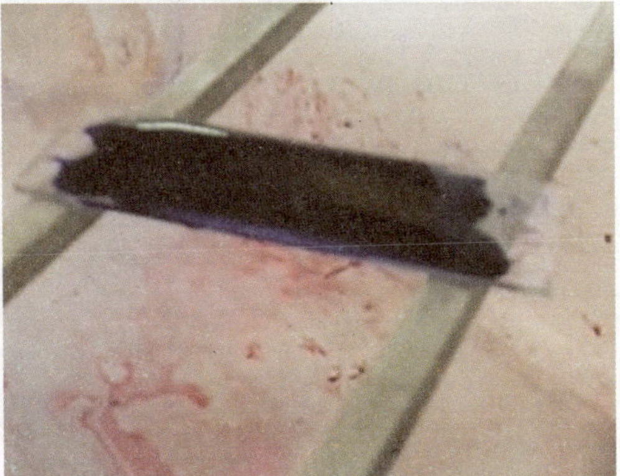

FIG. 6: Primary staining: Flood the slide with freshly prepared and filtered 1% carbol fuchsin stain.

- *Decolorizing*: Destain the slide by using either 5% sulfuric acid for 10 minutes or by using 1% hydrochloric acid in 70% absolute alcohol for 3–5 seconds, followed by rinsing.
- *Counterstaining*: Flood the slides with counterstain 0.2% methylene blue and keep it for 1 minute. Wash it gently under running water and let it dry **(Figs. 9 and 10)**.
- Now examine 100 fields of slide under 100× oil immersion lens

Interpretation of Smear

- Bacilli appear as red dots on a blue background
- Viable bacilli appear as uniformly stained rods (solid staining) and dead bacilli appear irregularly stained (fragmented bacilli) or as granules (granular bacilli)[8]
- The bacilli can be observed singly in small groups or closely packed bunches called globi

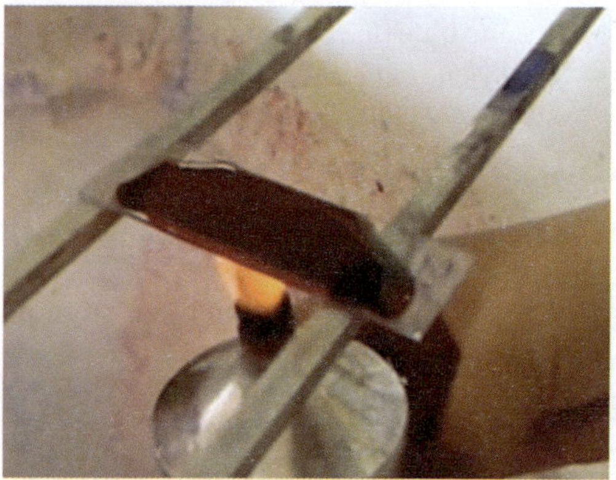

FIG. 7: Gently heat stained slide till slight fuming occurs. Do not let the stain boil. Keep the stain for 10–15 minutes without any further heating.

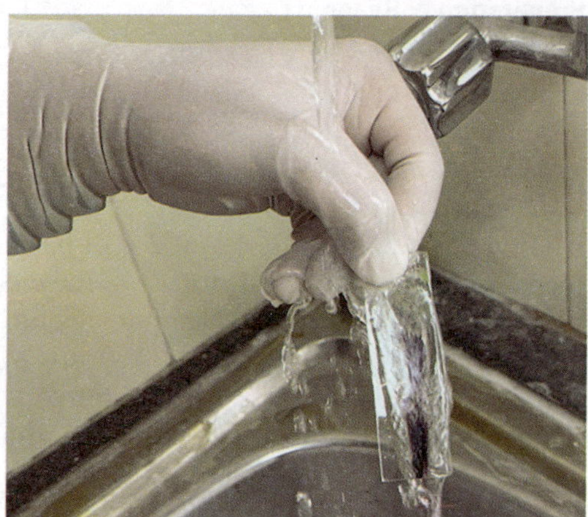

FIG. 8: Wash the slides gently in running water.

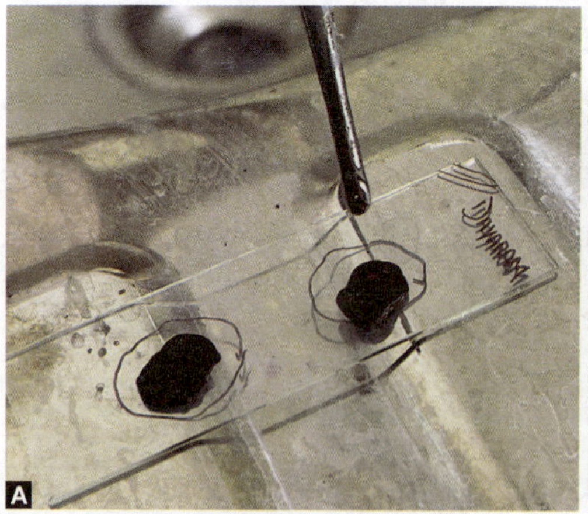

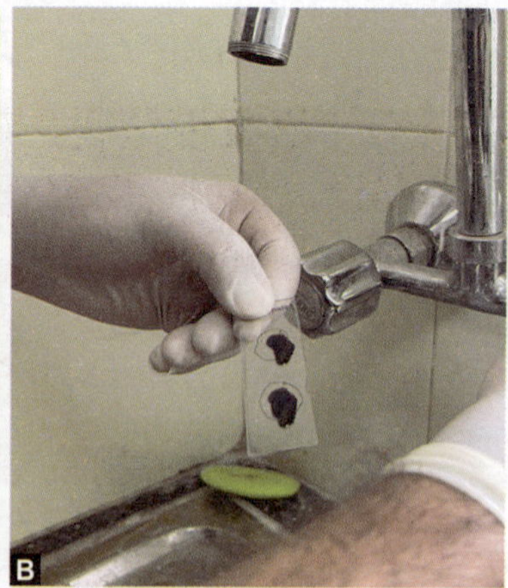

FIGS. 9A AND B: Counterstaining: (A) Flood the slides with counterstain 0.2% methylene blue; and (B) Keep it for 1 minute.

Bacteriological Index

The density of bacilli in a smear is the BI and it includes both living and dead bacilli.
Ridley's logarithmic scale for BI:

- 6+: Over 1,000 bacilli and globi in an average microscopic field **(Fig. 11)**
- 5+: Over 100 bacilli but <1,000 in an average microscopic field **(Fig. 12)**
- 4+: Over 10 bacilli but <100 in an average microscopic field **(Fig. 13)**
- 3+: 1–10 bacilli in an average field
- 2+: 1–10 bacilli in 10 microscopic fields
- 1+: 1–10 bacilli in 100 microscopic fields

- *Zero*: No bacilli observed after searching at least 100 microscopic fields
- BI is based on the number of bacilli seen in an average microscopic field using oil immersion objective. If several smears are taken, mean index is calculated
- BI is a function of cellular immunity as scavenging cells of the host eliminate deceased bacilli from the site. In skin smears, the BI starts to decline approximately one year into MDT, decreasing at a rate of around 0.6–1.0 log per year. This decline persists even after treatment cessation, forming the rationale for fixed-duration MDT.[7]

Morphological Index

Morphological index (MI) represents the percentage of solid-staining bacilli (living bacilli) among the total bacilli (solid + nonsolid). Bacilli are classified as solid-staining if:

- The entire organism is uniformly stained.
- The longitudinal sides are parallel.
- Both ends are rounded.
- The length is five times its width.
- It serves as an indicator of whether a patient's leprosy is currently active or inactive. By meticulously counting 200 individual bacterial elements and

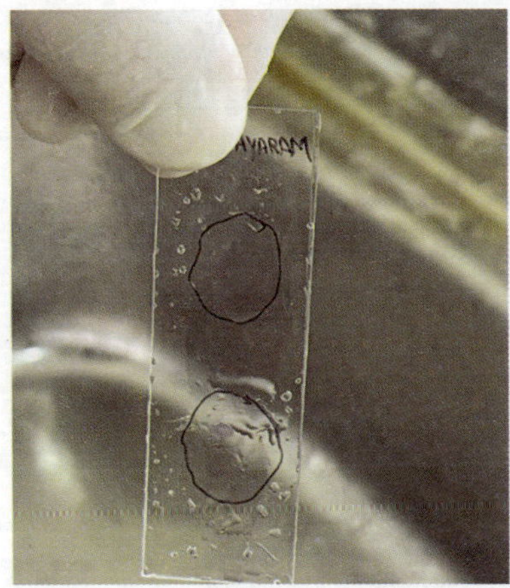

FIG. 10: Wash it gently under running water and let it dry.

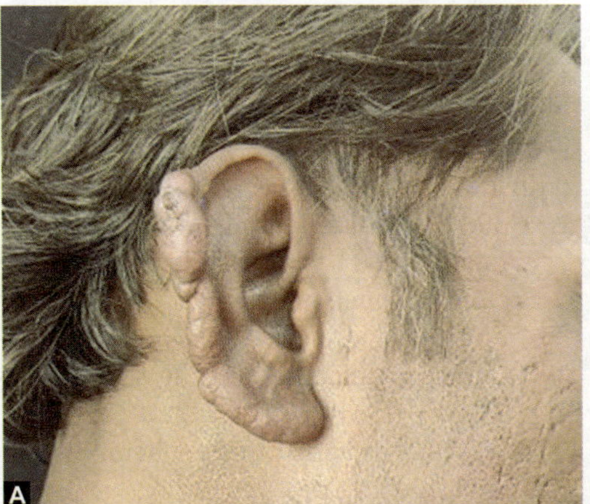

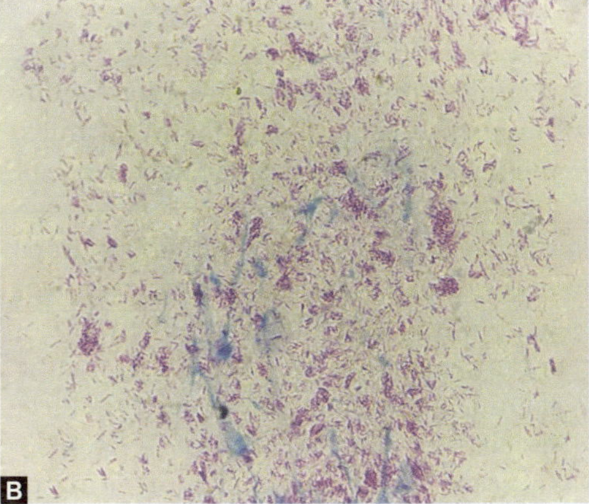

FIGS. 11A AND B: (A) Lepromatous leprosy patient and (B) 6+: Over 1,000 bacilli and globi in an average microscopic field.

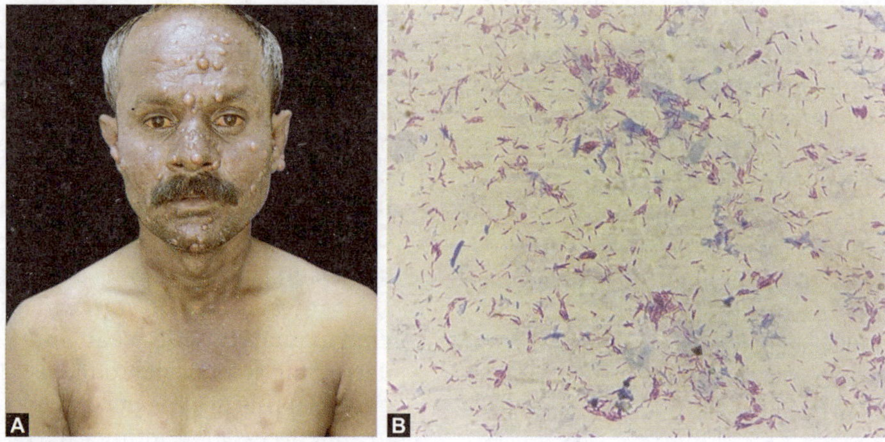

FIGS. 12A AND B: (A) Histoid leprosy patient and (B) 5+: Over 100 bacilli but <1,000 in an average microscopic field.

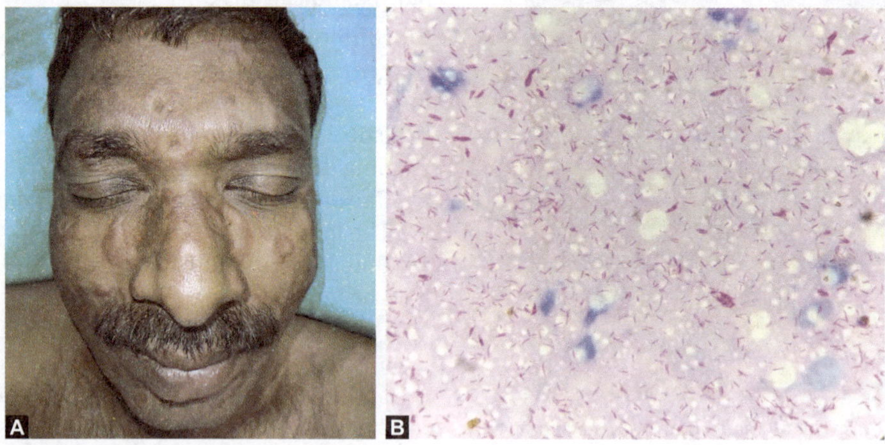

FIGS. 13A AND B: (A) Borderline lepromatous patient and (B) 4+: Over 10 bacilli but <100 in an average microscopic field.

distinguishing between regular solid-staining, fragmented, or granular ones, the MI is determined as the percentage of solid-staining rods.[1]

- Changes in the MI are rapid and it drops to 0 within 5 weeks following treatment with MTD-containing rifampicin. It is a more sensitive parameter of therapeutic failure, noncompliance, drug resistance, or relapse.[8]
- Increase in MI indicates worsening of patient's condition and decrease indicates improvement

Ridley's Solid, Fragmented, and Granular Index (Figs. 14 and 15)

It divides bacilli into three classes:

1. Solid (S)—solid staining unbroken rods
2. Fragmented (F), i.e., bacilli in which the acid-fast substance is interrupted at one or more points.
3. Round granules either in line or in clumps (G)

A value is assigned to the bacilli of each class in a smear:

- 2 if bacilli are numerous (over 20% of all bacilli)

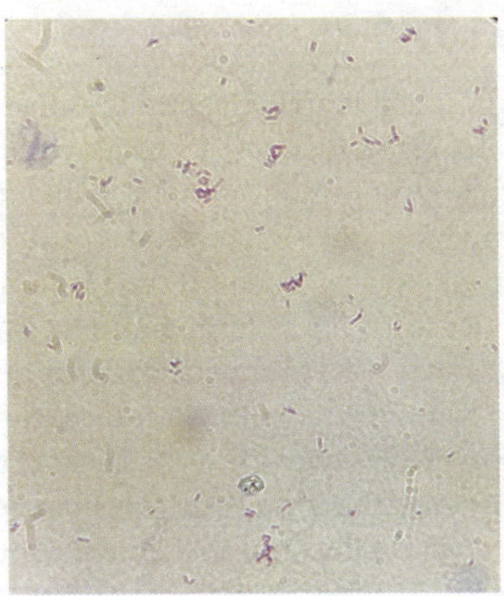

FIG. 14: Appearance of fragmented and granular bacilli on smear.

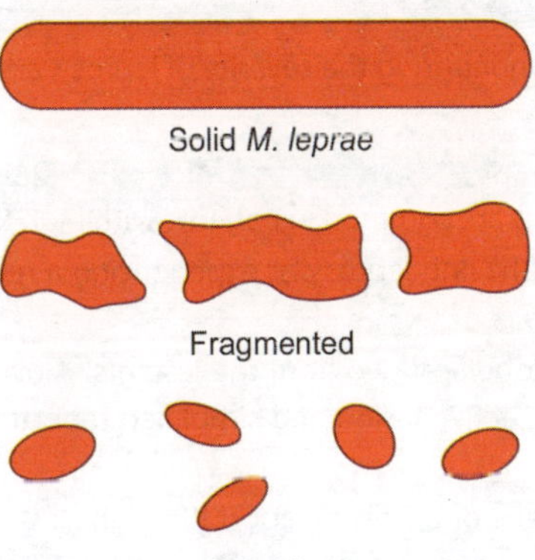

FIG. 15: Solid, fragmented, and granular index (SFG) diagrammatic representation.

- 1 if few bacilli (1–20%)
- 0 if <1%

Hence, the relative distribution of bacilli in the three categories SFG (in this sequence) is expressed as one of the arrangements of 2-1-0. The SFG index ranges from 0 (indicating no solid organisms) to 10.

Among the three indices discussed, BI is employed routinely due to its simplicity and ease of use.[3] MI and SFG indices, however, demand stringent standards in fixation, staining, and microscopy. Consequently, they are exclusively reserved for research purposes.

SENSITIVITY AND SPECIFICITY OF SLIT-SKIN SMEAR

- SSS has high specificity of 100% and low sensitivity (10–50%)[3]
- It is very sensitive in the diagnosis of lepromatous, borderline lepromatous, and histoid leprosy because it is dependent on the bacterial load; however, its sensitivity is low at the tuberculoid end (TT and BT).[8]

LIMITATIONS OF SLIT-SKIN SMEAR

- While SSS is a valuable diagnostic tool, it has limitations including potential false-negative results, especially in PB forms of leprosy where *M. leprae* are scantly present.[9]
- Clinical correlation is essential for accurate diagnosis.
- Since it requires a minimum of 10,000 bacilli/g of tissue for reliable detection by Ziehl–Neelsen (ZN) staining. Negative smear does not exclude leprosy.[3]
- Steps should be taken to improve the work by offering periodic refresher courses to technicians, strict supervision of laboratories, and introducing quality control measures.

INFERENCES

A positive SSS is not only the third cardinal sign and confirms the diagnosis of leprosy. Additionally, a bacteriological examination is a crucial screening procedure for individuals suspected of having leprosy. It is useful to study distribution of *M. leprae* in skin for assessing the infectivity and severity of leprosy. In MB leprosy patients, the bacteria are typically found in substantial numbers in the dermis, with as many as 7,000 to 4 million leprosy bacilli/g of skin tissue. However, detecting the bacilli through ZN staining requires at least 10,000 bacilli/g of tissue, making smears potentially negative in PB leprosy lesions where *M. leprae* is sparsely present. It is important to note that a negative smear does not automatically rule out the possibility of leprosy.

Negative smears or low BI figures should always be interpreted in relation to the history and clinical findings, bearing in mind that patients frequently conceal the truth with regards to previous treatment. Smears will never become negative in a new lepromatous leprosy (LL) patient during MDT but will become granular (dead) after relatively short time. Granular bacilli decrease in numbers at a rate of about 1 log per year and disappear 5 or 6 years after stopping MDT.

CONCLUSION

Slit-skin smear is an indispensable tool in the dermatologist's diagnostic armamentarium, particularly for mycobacterial skin infections. Its simplicity, cost-effectiveness, and diagnostic accuracy make it an invaluable asset. Despite its several limitations, the significance of SSS cannot be underestimated and it remains a gold standard for the diagnosis of leprosy until newer and more sensitive diagnostic tools such as polymerase chain reaction become available for routine testing.

Key Messages

- Slit-skin smear is valuable for diagnosis, classification, and monitoring the severity of leprosy, and it is crucial in ensuring appropriate treatment.
- Classify and treat all smears positive patients as MB leprosy.
- SSS also helps determine the prognosis (e.g., lepra reactions are common in patients with high BI).
- Conduct SSS examinations for all individuals suspected of having leprosy or experiencing a relapse before initiating MDT.
- Make smears from three sites including one from the earlobe and two from the lesion(s). However, remember a single SSS examination from the single most active lesion and simplified reporting of smears as "positive" or "negative" will be more practical.
- Record the BI for each smear separately and calculate average or best is to report the highest BI. MI is more sensitive parameter of therapeutic follow-up.
- Emphasize that the SSS remains the most valuable diagnostic method.
- Highlight that negative smears do not automatically rule out leprosy. Developing expertise in obtaining quality smears is essential and involves leadership, concern, and quality control.

REFERENCES

1. Sehgal VN, Joginder. Slit-skin smear in leprosy. Int J Dermatol. 1990;29(1):9-16.
2. Sukanya G, Manoharan K, Logeswari PT, Naidu DKI. Leprosy and broken bacilli on slit skin smear. QJM. 2023;116(7):545-6.
3. Gautam M, Jaiswal A. Forgetting the Cardinal Sign is a Cardinal Sin: Slit-skin Smear. Indian J Paediatr Dermatol. 2019;20(4):341-4.
4. Harman M, Akdeniz S, Mizrak B. Slit-skin smear in diagnosis of cutaneous mastocytomas. Indian J Dermatol Venereol Leprol. 2010;76(2):187-9.
5. Bhargava A, Ramesh V, Verma S, Salotra P, Bala M. Revisiting the role of the slit-skin smear in the diagnosis of Indian post-kala-azar dermal leishmaniasis. Indian J Dermatol Venereol Leprol. 2018;84:690-5.
6. Kumar B, Kar HK. IAL Textbook of Leprosy. New Delhi: Jaypee Brothers Medical Publishers; 2017.
7. Deshmukh KM, Sharma YK, Kumar A. The use of forceps for creating sustained pressure for slit skin smear. J Am Acad Dermatol. 2020;82(3):e77-8.

8. Mahajan VK. Slit-skin smear in leprosy: lest we forget it! Indian J Lepr. 2013;85(4):177-83.

9. Banerjee S, Biswas N, Kanti Das N, Sil A, Ghosh P, Hasanoor Raja AH, et al. Diagnosing leprosy: revisiting the role of the slit-skin smear with critical analysis of the applicability of polymerase chain reaction in diagnosis. Int J Dermatol. 2011;50(12):1522-7.

Tissue Smear and Giemsa Stain in Dermatology

Santhosh Battula, Senkadhir Vendhan, Nitin Kumar Sharma, Smriti Sharma

INTRODUCTION

In the intricate tapestry of dermatological diagnostics, the microscopic examination of tissue smears, adorned by the vivid hues of Giemsa stain, unveils a realm of cellular details that transcends the visible surface of the skin. This chapter delves into the art and science of tissue smear and Giemsa stain, illuminating the invaluable role they play in the elucidation of dermatological mysteries.

Tissue smear, a technique that involves the meticulous spread of a thin layer of tissue onto a glass slide, serves as a portal to the microscopic landscape of skin pathology. The subsequent marriage with Giemsa stain, a versatile dye renowned for its affinity to cellular structures, transforms this landscape into a vibrant canvas where cellular elements reveal their intricate tales.

As we embark on this exploration, we shall traverse the procedural intricacies from the delicate collection of tissue samples to the precise application of Giemsa stain. The amalgamation of these steps forms a symphony of laboratory techniques that not only preserves the cellular architecture but also embellishes it with hues that bring forth subtleties otherwise unseen.

The indications for employing tissue smear and Giemsa stain in dermatology are multifaceted, ranging from the identification of infectious agents like bacteria and parasites to unraveling the complexities of inflammatory responses within the skin. Furthermore, these techniques offer a discerning eye in the realm of tumor diagnosis, aiding in the differentiation of benign and malignant lesions.

Beyond the laboratory bench, the clinical significance of tissue smear and Giemsa stain reverberates in the precision of dermatological diagnoses. The applications extend to monitoring treatment responses and serve as indispensable tools in the pursuit of scientific understanding, contributing to the evolving tapestry of dermatological research.

In essence, tissue smear and Giemsa stain stand as essential chapters in the dermatological narrative, enriching our understanding of skin disorders at the microscopic level. As we traverse through this chapter, we invite the reader to embrace the magnified universe beneath the skin, where Giemsa-stained cells whisper the secrets of dermatological conditions, painting a more detailed portrait of skin health and pathology.[1]

PROCEDURE (FIGS. 1A TO C)

Step 1: Sample Collection

Purpose: Obtain a representative tissue sample.

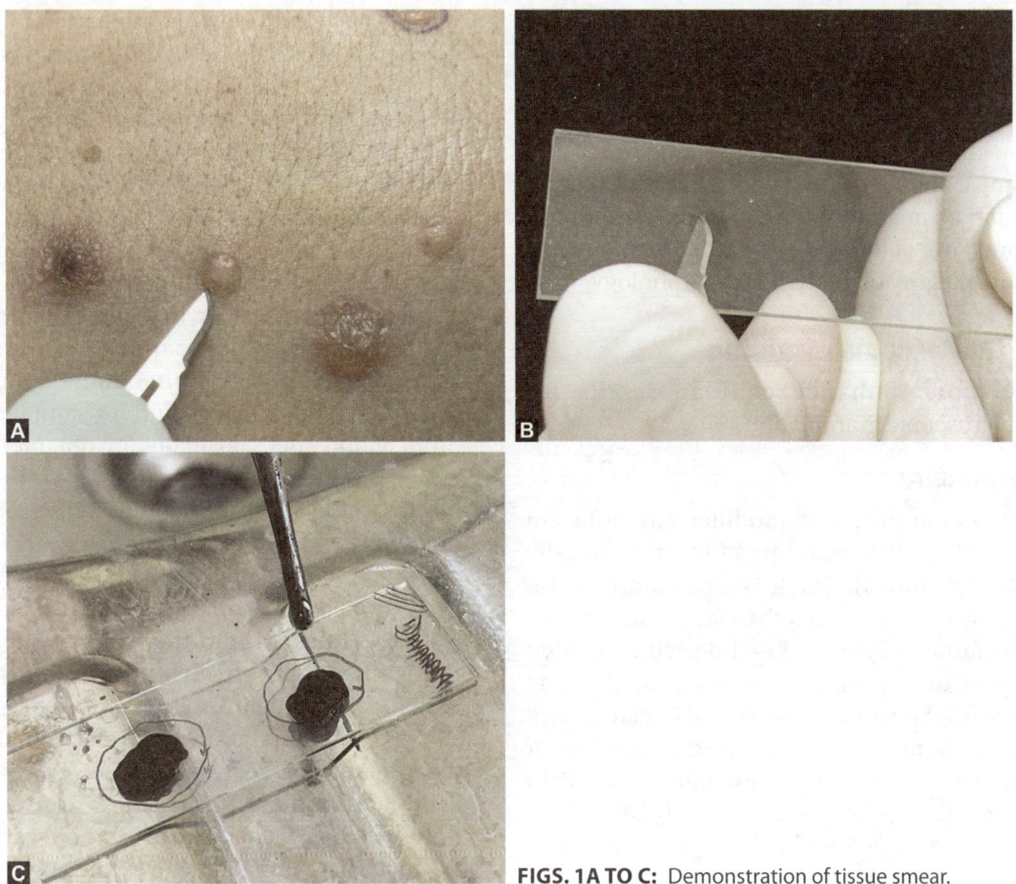

FIGS. 1A TO C: Demonstration of tissue smear.

Procedure

Use a sterile technique to collect the tissue sample. The representative lesion is incised superficially, avoiding any bleeding; with a No. 15 surgical blade.[2] The sample can be obtained by gently scraping with the blunt edge of the scalpel or a curette.[3] For open exuding lesions and freshly derived biopsy specimens, an impression/touch smear can be prepared.[4]

Step 2: Preparation of Smear

Purpose: Create a thin, even layer of tissue on a glass slide.

Procedure

Gently spread the tissue on a glass slide using a clean spatula or similar instrument.

For touch smears, the glass slide is simply pressed (not streaked) onto the moist lesions repeatedly. Aim for a thin and uniform layer to facilitate proper staining and microscopy. Allow the smear to air-dry completely to prevent artifacts.[2]

Step 3: Fixation

Purpose: Preserve cellular structures during staining process.

Procedure

The most commonly used fixation methods in dermatocytology are air-drying and alcohol fixation. For Romanowsky stains, such as Giemsa stain, air-drying is preferred. Since, longer air-drying time can alter cytological properties and cause cell shrinkage, and can lead to formation of artifacts, drying should be done quickly by handshaking or hot-air blowing. A thin even layer of tissue should be obtained on the slide to an aid faster air-drying. In case of longer time to air-dry, smear should be fixed with a fixation solution such as methanol for 2–3 minutes. Fixation prevents cellular degradation and ensures the integrity of the cellular morphology.[2]

Step 4: Giemsa Staining

Purpose: Enhance cellular details for microscopic examination.

Procedure

Flood the slide with modified Giemsa stain (1:10) for the recommended time (usually 8–10 minutes). For a Giemsa stain of 1:5 dilution in tap water, the stain is kept on for 20 minutes. Rinse the slide with distilled water to remove excess stain. The washing process must be done gently because hard and fast movements can lead to cell loss. A sufficient washing process must be done to view the cell boundaries clearly. Allow the slide to air-dry completely before microscopic examination.[2,5]

Step 5: Microscopic Examination

Purpose: Analyze stained cells to identify pathological features.

Procedure

Examine the stained slide under a microscope using appropriate magnification. Identify cellular elements, morphological changes, and any pathological features.[6]

INDICATIONS

Bacterial Infections

- *Syphilis*: Identification of spirochetes in tissue smears from suspected lesions or regional lymph nodes, on dark-field microscopy, provides the only absolute diagnosis of syphilis. The test is useful in primary, secondary, relapsing infectious, and early prenatal syphilis and is the test of choice for the diagnosis of primary syphilis, as it is highly sensitive, specific, and provides an immediate diagnosis. After cleaning the sore with normal saline, the ulcer is squeezed between the index finger and thumb to produce a serous exudate. For dry and crusted lesions, scraping and scarification with an open scarifier is required to be done to produce the exudate, and for samples from lymph nodes, exudates are obtained after puncturing the regional lymph nodes. After infiltrating the skin over the lymph node with 1% lignocaine, the overlying skin is stretched and the lymph node is held firmly. 0.2 mL sterile normal saline is injected into the lymph node. After massaging the lymph node, the fluid is aspirated and collected on a glass slide. Contamination with blood should be avoided as it decreases the sensitivity. Upon examination on a dark ground microscope, *Treponema pallidum* can be identified as a white glistening spiral-shaped organism with a characteristic corkscrew rotatory movement. The specimen should be immediately examined on dark-field microscopy as delays decrease the motility of the *Treponemes*. When samples cannot be examined immediately, direct fluorescent antibody staining of *Treponema pallidum* (DFA-TP) can be done instead.[7]
- *Donovanosis*: Tissue smear is more sensitive than biopsy in the diagnosis of donovanosis. It shows Greenblatt/Pund cells which are large macrophage/epithelioid cell with cystic spaces, nuclei pushed to one side and darkly staining inclusions called Donovan bodies. Donovan bodies are blue-black bipolar condensations with a safety pin appearance.

Parasitic Infestations

Leishmaniasis: Cytodiagnosis of leishmaniasis can be made by gentle scarification along the margins of newer cutaneous lesions. The protozoa can be identified as numerous small blue ovoid, ellipsoid, or pyriform bodies with a deeply basophilic cytoplasm, a trophonucleus, a paranucleus or kinetoplast, and a minute endocytoplasmic flagellum, in a swarm of bee arrangement as Leishman–Donovan (LD) bodies with histiocytes known as Wright cells. The test is of little significance in older lesions **(Fig. 2)**.[3]

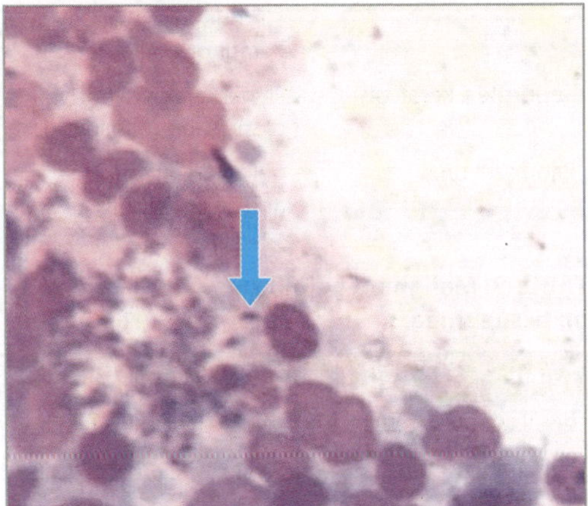

FIG. 2: *Leishmania* parasites in tissue smear.

Viral Infections

Molluscum contagiosum: Identification of characteristic basophilic intracytoplasmic Henderson–Patterson/molluscum inclusion bodies within large altered keratinocytes **(Figs. 3A and B)**.

Granulomatous Conditions

Infectious and noninfectious granulomatous conditions can be identified on tissue smears **(Table 1)**.

Tumors and neoplasms: Cellular atypia can be appreciated on representative tissue smears though histopathological diagnosis is needed in most cases. Cellular atypia in the form of anisocytosis (variation in cell size), poikilocytosis (variation in nucleus size), poikilokaryosis (atypical nuclear morphology and nuclear molding), variation in nucleoli number and size (anisonucleolus and meganucleoli), cytoplasmic granules, and tadpole cells can be appreciated.

Benign Tumors (Table 2)

Malignant Conditions (Table 3)

- *Basal cell carcinoma:* Employed for the identification of malignant cellular

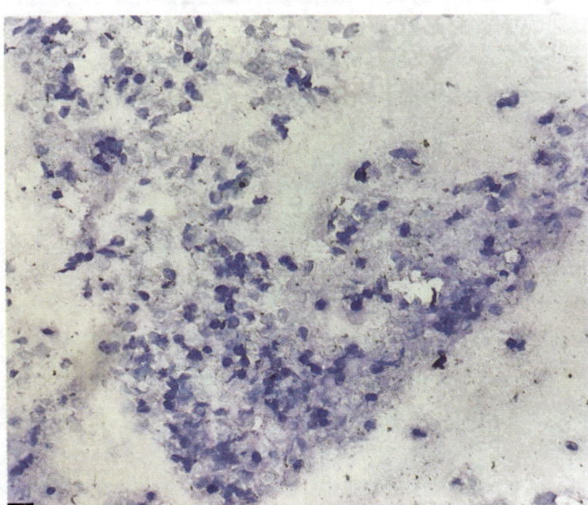

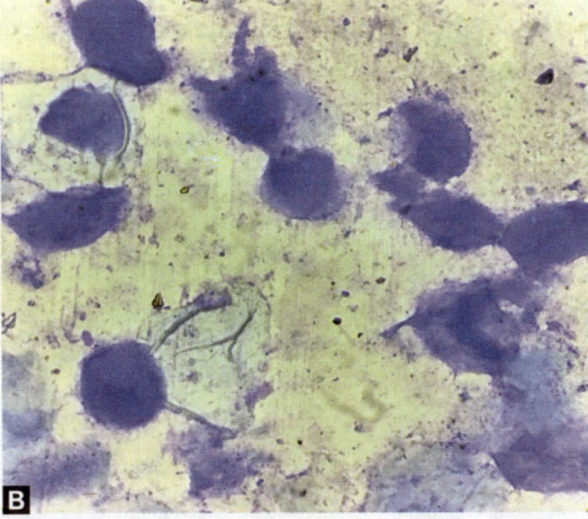

FIGS. 3A AND B: (A) Tissue smear of enucleated molluscum body showing numerous intracytoplasmic inclusion body (low power 10×); and (B) Tissue smear showing intracytoplasmic inclusion body—molluscum bodies (100×).

TABLE 1: Cytodiagnosis of cutaneous granulomatous conditions.

Infectious	Findings
Botryomycosis	Bacterial balls
Cutaneous leishmaniasis	Leishman–Donovan (LD) bodies
Mucormycosis	Nonseptate branching hyphae with variable width
Aspergillosis	Hyphae with acute 45° branching
Candidal granuloma	Pseudohyphae and spores
Majocchi granuloma	Hyphae and spores
Cryptococcosis	Narrow-based budding yeast
Blastomycosis	Broad-based budding yeast forms
Mycobacterial infections	Acid-fast bacilli
Demodicosis	Demodex parasites
Noninfectious	**Findings**
Juvenile xanthogranuloma	Foamy histiocytes and Touton giant cells
Granuloma annulare	Mucin structures and palisade-shaped granulomas
Necrobiosis lipoidica	Necrobiotic granulomas
Foreign body granuloma	Foreign body

TABLE 2: Benign neoplasms that can be identified on tissue smear.

Benign neoplasias	Findings
Melanocytic nevi	Epidermal and dermal nevoid cells
Clear cell acanthoma	Keratinocytes with periodic acid–Schiff (PAS) positive material
Sebaceous hyperplasia	Cluster of sebocytes
Juvenile xanthogranuloma	Touton type giant cells and foamy histiocytes
Dermatofibroma	Fibroblasts, histiocytes, and collagen stroma
Syringoma	Basaloid cells surrounding hyaline and keratinous material
Seborrheic keratosis	Hyperkeratosis, horny cysts, and basaloid cells
Pilomatrixoma	Calcification, ghost cells, and basaloid cells

TABLE 3: Malignant neoplasms cytodiagnosis on tissue smears.

Tumor	Findings
Basal cell carcinoma	Clusters of basaloid cells
Squamous cell carcinoma	Atypical keratinocytes
Sebaceous cancer	Atypical sebocytes
Langerhans cell histiocytosis	Atypical epithelial histiocytes
Eccrine porocarcinoma	Clusters of atypical basaloid cells and hyaline materials
Melanoma	Atypical melanocytes
Kaposi sarcoma	Cigar-shaped spindle cells
Plasmacytoma	Atypical plasma cells
Lymphoma	Atypical lymphocytes
Paget's disease	Paget cells
Metastatic carcinoma	Atypical cells of unknown origin

features to achieve a precise diagnosis. Smears reveal clusters of basaloid cells with some of them showing retention of peripheral palisading, as seen on histology. Basaloid cells appear similar to basal keratinocytes but are larger, more deeply basophilic, uniform in size, elongated with a central oval, intensely basophilic nucleus occupying four-fifths of the cells.

- *Squamous cell carcinoma:* Utilized to assess cellular atypia indicative of malignancy. Cytology is helpful in the diagnoses of nonkeratotic varieties of squamous cell carcinoma (SCC). The two characteristic features of SCC are the absence of cluster formation by cells and pleomorphism. Abnormal nuclear changes such as hypertrophic, hyperchromatic, or multilobated nuclei with abnormal mitoses, and bizarre changes in cytoplasm staining such as basophilic in some eosinophilic in others are seen.

- *Melanoma:* Applied to differentiate between benign and malignant melanocytic lesions.
- *Erythroplasia of Queyrat:* Stained smears show atypical spindle-shaped, polyhedral, and round cells with pleomorphic nuclei.
- *Paget's disease*: Paget's cells can be seen, which are round to oval cells with a weakly eosinophilic or amphophilic vacuolated cytoplasm, and a hypertrophic nucleolated nucleus and are larger than the normal keratinocytes. These Paget's cells can be seen singly or in small clusters and stain with special stains for epithelial mucin such as mucicarmine, Alcian blue, and periodic acid–Schiff stain.[3]

Lymphoproliferative Disorders

- *Cutaneous T-cell lymphoma:* Employed to contribute to the identification of malignant T-cell infiltrates.
- *Mycosis fungoides*: Utilized to aid in the diagnosis of early-stage malignant T-cell lymphoma.
- *Langerhans cell histiocytosis:* Smears show multinucleate atypical 12–15 mm sized pale, weakly eosinophilic or amphophilic Langerhans cells with a granular cytoplasm and large lobulated, convoluted, reniform, or centrally grooved nuclei. A histological and immunophenotypic examination should be performed to confirm the diagnosis.
- *Bullous mastocytosis*: A Tzanck smear from bullous lesions is stained with 1% methylene blue for 1 minute, which shows plenty of mast cells, identified by their irregular shape and metachromatic staining of granules as purple. This is especially useful in pediatric cases where biopsies may be difficult to perform.[3]

Metastatic Lesions

Metastatic carcinoma: Applied to assist in identifying metastatic and atypical pleomorphic cancer cells within the skin.

Unusual Presentations

Malignant hidradenitis suppurativa: Utilized to recognize malignant transformation in chronic suppurative conditions.

LIMITATIONS OF TISSUE SMEAR AND GIEMSA STAIN IN DERMATOLOGY

Artifacts

Artifacts may mimic or obscure genuine cellular features, leading to potential misinterpretations during microscopic examination.

Subjectivity in Interpretation

Variability in interpretation may occur, affecting diagnostic accuracy, especially in less-experienced hands.

Limited Specificity

Giemsa stain may be challenging to precisely identify and differentiate specific microorganisms or cellular structures in some cases.

Inability to Provide Real-time Information

Immediate insights into dynamic processes or evolving conditions may be limited, affecting the timeliness of diagnosis in certain situations.

Cellular Detail Dependency

In cases where obtaining a high-quality cellular sample is challenging, the diagnostic yield may be compromised.

Interference from Background Structures

Giemsa stain may interact with background structures, affecting the contrast between cellular elements and the surrounding tissue. This interference may hinder the clear visualization of specific cellular features.

Skill Dependent Technique

Inadequate technique or lack of expertise may lead to suboptimal staining and interpretation, affecting the reliability of results.

Difficulty in Quantification

Quantifying specific parameters, such as the extent of inflammation or the number of microorganisms, may be challenging.

CONCLUSION

In conclusion, the integration of tissue smear methodologies and Giemsa stain stands as a cornerstone in the meticulous delineation of dermatopathological landscapes. This synergistic approach, marked by precision and scientific finesse, unravels the intricate cellular narratives defining diverse derma-tological conditions. From microbial identi-fications to inflammatory responses and tumor pathologies, tissue smear and Giemsa stain offer unparalleled insights into the microscopic intricacies of cutaneous pathology.

The clinical significance of these techniques extends beyond mere diagnostic utility, encompassing therapeutic moni-toring and substantive contributions to dermatopathological research. As we navigate the nuanced interplay between tissue smear and Giemsa stain, it becomes evident that this scientific marriage illuminates microscopic shadows, enriching our comprehension and refining our therapeutic approach in the dynamic realm of dermatology. Yet, with the brilliance of Giemsa-stained cells comes the imperative for judicious interpretation, mindful of the inherent limitations.

This chapter serves as an invitation to delve into the microscopic subtleties, distinguishing benign from malignant, inflammatory from infectious, and ordinary from extraordinary. The combined insights of tissue smear and Giemsa stain provide a meticulous and nuanced lens, empowering clinicians to navigate the complex terrain of dermatopathology with acumen and precision.

Key Messages

- Tissue smears and Giemsa stain collaborate to reveal cellular details beyond the visible skin surface.
- Following step-by-step procedure, from meticulous tissue sample collection to Giemsa stain application preserves cellular architecture and unveil subtle details.
- It can aid significantly in providing precision to dermatological diagnoses, therapeutic monitoring, and contributing substantively to dermatopathological research.

REFERENCES

1. Barcia JJ. The Giemsa stain: its history and applications. Int J Surg Pathol. 2007;15(3):292-6.
2. Durdu M. Cutaneous Cytology and Tzanck Smear Test. Cham, Switzerland: Springer Nature; 2019.
3. Shana B, Ambooken B, Asokan N. Cytodiagnosis in dermatology. J Skin Sex Transm Dis. 2019;1(2):112-6.
4. Allen M, Schoen MS. (2011). World Small Animal Veterinary Association World Congress

Proceedings, 2011. [online] Available from https://www.vin.com/doc/?id=6698876 [Last accessed February, 2024].

5. ScienceDirect. Giemsa Stain—an overview. [online] Available from https://www.sciencedirect.com/topics/medicine-and-dentistry/giemsa-stain [Last accessed February, 2024].

6. Dolan M. The role of the Giemsa stain in cytogenetics. Biotech Histochem Off Publ Biol Stain Comm. 2011;86(2):94-7.

7. Kumar B. IADVL's Concise Textbook of Dermatology. Indian J Dermatol Venereol Leprol 2013;79: 138-9.

Tzanck Smear

Senkadhir Vendhan, Nidhi Sharma, Sreechithra Menon

INTRODUCTION

In the realm of dermatology, the Tzanck smear stands as a valuable diagnostic tool, aiding clinicians in the rapid assessment of various skin conditions. Named after the French dermatologist Arnault Tzanck, this straightforward yet insightful procedure plays a pivotal role in the initial evaluation of cutaneous lesions.

The Tzanck smear technique involves the microscopic examination of cells obtained from skin vesicles, bullae, or ulcers. It serves as a swift and cost-effective method, providing immediate insights into certain viral, bacterial, or parasitic dermatoses. By analyzing cells obtained from skin lesions, dermatologists can promptly identify characteristic cellular features, facilitating the preliminary diagnosis of several dermatological conditions.

This procedure's utility extends across a spectrum of dermatoses including herpes simplex infections, varicella–zoster virus (VZV) infections, and certain blistering disorders. The Tzanck smear's simplicity, speed, and reliability make it an invaluable aid in the dermatologist's diagnostic arsenal, guiding the early management and treatment decisions for numerous skin disorders.[1]

As we delve deeper into the technique, its applications, and the diverse conditions, it helps to identify the significance of the Tzanck smear in expediting diagnoses and guiding prompt therapeutic interventions and becomes increasingly apparent in the field of dermatology. A detailed explanation on the methodology and application of Tzanck smear in dermatology will be discussed in this chapter.

MATERIALS REQUIRED

- *Glass slides*: Clean and grease-free glass slides suitable for microscopy.
- *Vesicular fluid sample*: It is obtained from an intact vesicle or blister.
- *Sterile swabs or needles*: It is used for collecting vesicular fluid.
- *Giemsa stain*: It is available as a ready-to-use solution or as a powder that needs to be diluted according to the manufacturer's instructions.
- *Methanol or absolute ethanol*: It is used as a fixative.
- *Staining dish or slide rack*: It is used to hold the slides during staining.

METHODOLOGY (FIGS. 1A TO C)

Sample Collection

The sample collection process in a Tzanck smear is a crucial step that determines the quality of the specimen and subsequently impacts the accuracy of the diagnostic findings. Here is a detailed explanation of the various steps in sample collection process:

- *Preparation*:
    - Sterility: Ensure the area and equipment used for the procedure are sterile to prevent contamination.
    - Patient comfort: Inform and reassure the patient about the procedure to minimize discomfort and anxiety.
- *Identifying the lesion*:
    - Selection of lesion: Locate an intact vesicle or blister that appears to contain clear or cloudy fluid. This could be present in various dermatological conditions, such as herpes simplex, herpes zoster, or other vesicular eruptions.
- *Unroofing the vesicle*:
    - Cleaning the area: Clean the skin around the lesion with an antiseptic solution to reduce the risk of contamination.
    - Unroofing the vesicle: Use a sterile needle or scalpel blade to gently unroof the vesicle. Create a small incision or puncture to access the fluid inside while minimizing trauma to the surrounding tissue **(Figs. 1A and B)**.
    - Caution: Exercise caution to avoid excessive pressure or squeezing that might introduce blood into the sample, potentially interfering with diagnostic accuracy.

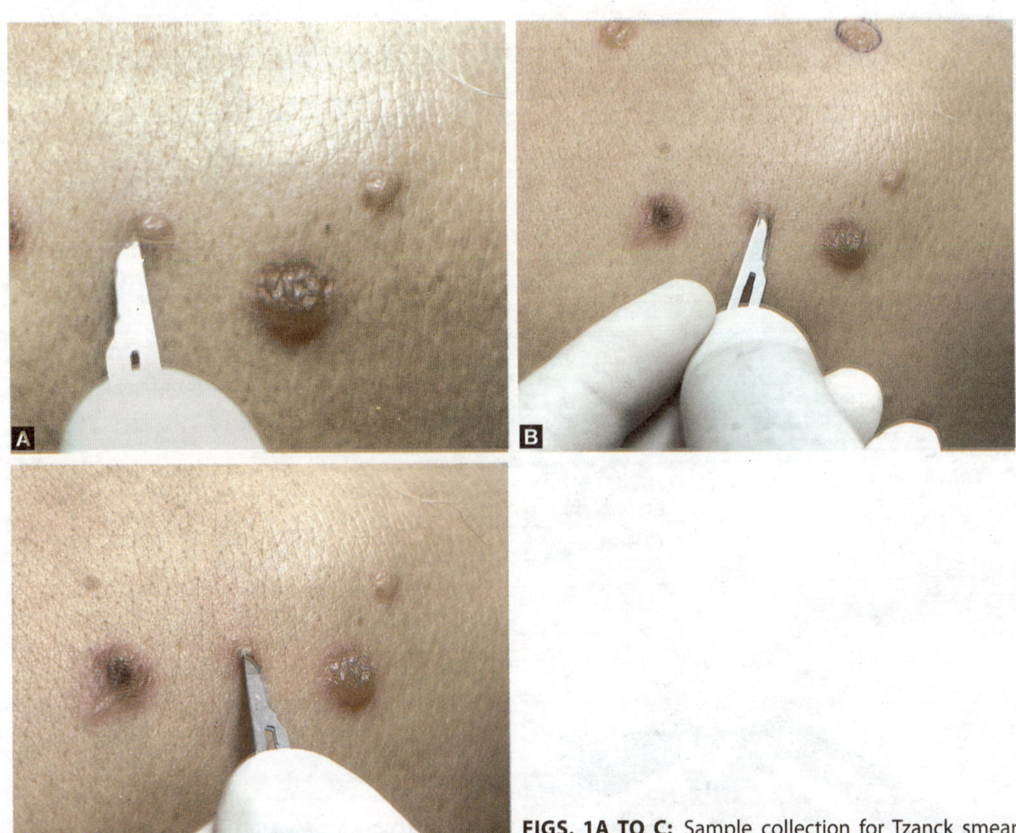

FIGS. 1A TO C: Sample collection for Tzanck smear procedure—(A) Unroofing the vesicle; (B) Collection of fluid; and (C) Placing the smear on the slide.

- *Collection of fluid*:
  - Collection technique: Touch the needle or blade to the base of the vesicle to allow the fluid to flow onto the slide **(Fig. 1C)**.
  - Multiple samples: Collect multiple samples from different vesicles, if present, to increase the likelihood of obtaining representative cells for examination.
  - Maintaining integrity: Ensure the collected fluid remains unaltered and uncontaminated during the transfer onto the glass slide.[2]

Key Considerations

- *Gentle handling*: Handle the vesicle delicately to prevent rupture or damage to the surrounding tissue, which could compromise the quality of the sample.
- *Avoiding contamination*: Minimize contact with nonsterile surfaces or materials to prevent contamination of the collected fluid.
- *Adequate quantity*: Collect sufficient fluid to create a thin, even smear on the glass slide for optimal microscopic examination.
- *Timeliness*: Perform the smear promptly after sample collection to maintain sample integrity and accuracy of findings.

PROCEDURE (FIGS. 2A TO C)

Preparation of Smear

- *Sample collection*: Collect vesicular fluid from an intact vesicle or blister using

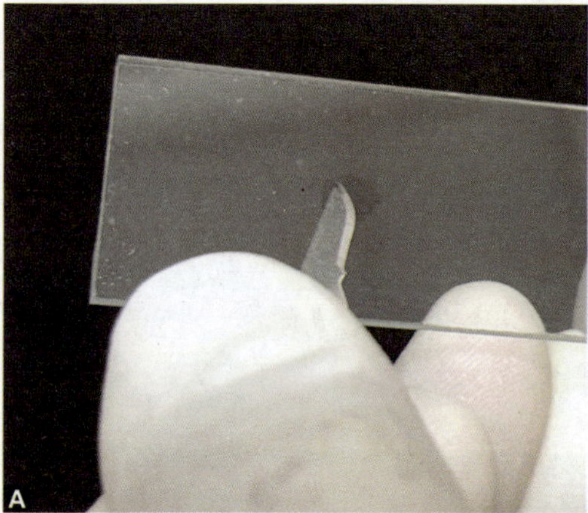

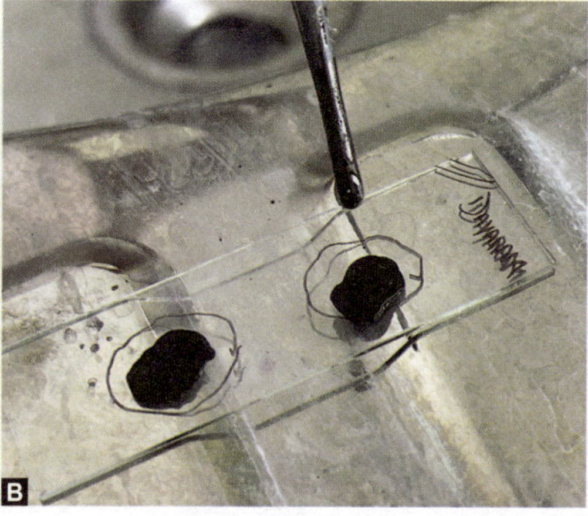

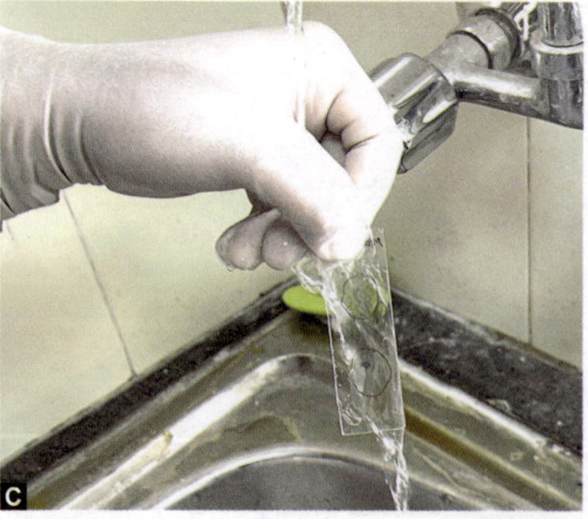

FIGS. 2A TO C: (A) Procedure showing preparation of smear; (B) Giemsa staining of smear; and (C) Rinsing of smear.

a sterile swab or needle, as previously detailed for the Tzanck smear.

- *Application onto slides*: Gently spread the collected fluid onto clean glass slides to create thin and uniform smears. Avoid applying too much pressure to prevent cell distortion **(Fig. 2A)**.

Fixation

- *Air-drying*: Allow the prepared slides to air-dry completely at room temperature. This step helps in adhering the cellular components to the slide.
- *Fixation with methanol or ethanol*: Submerge the air-dried slides in methanol or absolute ethanol for 3–5 minutes to fix the cellular material. Ensure complete coverage of the slides with the fixative.

Giemsa Staining

- *Preparation of Giemsa stain*: Follow the manufacturer's instructions for preparing the Giemsa stain solution or diluting the Giemsa powder with the recommended solvent.
- *Staining process*:
  - Submerge the fixed slides in the prepared Giemsa stain solution for the specified staining duration (typically 10 minutes) **(Fig. 2B)**.
  - Use staining dishes or slide racks to hold multiple slides during the staining process.
  - Ensure that the slides are fully immersed in the stain solution and avoid air bubbles.
- *Rinsing*: After the staining duration, rinse the slides thoroughly with distilled water or tap water to remove the excess stain.

Drying and Mounting

- *Air-drying*: Allow the slides to air-dry completely after rinsing.
- *Mounting*: Once dry, the stained slides can be mounted using a coverslip and an appropriate mounting medium for microscopic examination.[3]

Precautions

- Maintain sterility throughout the procedure to prevent contamination
- Adhere to recommended staining times to avoid over- or understaining
- Use appropriate personal protective equipment (PPE) to ensure safety when handling stains and fixatives

Preparing a smear for Giemsa staining involves precise steps, from sample collection to staining and mounting, to ensure optimal visualization of cellular details and viral inclusions. Following standardized procedures and protocols is crucial for obtaining accurate and reliable results for microscopic examination in dermatological diagnostics.

Microscopic Examination

The stained smear is examined under a microscope to identify characteristic cellular changes.

Examination Process

- *Microscope setup*:
  - Slide placement: Carefully place the Giemsa-stained slide onto the microscope's stage, ensuring its secure and centered for observation.
  - Initial magnification: Begin examination using the lowest magnification objective lens (typically 4× or 10×) to locate areas of interest and provide an overview of the cellular structures.
- *Observation and identification*:
  - Cellular details: Gradually increase the magnification (40×, 100×, or oil immersion at 1,000×) to focus on specific areas and observe cellular morphology.
  - Cellular structures: Look for cellular details, such as nuclei, cytoplasm, and any intracellular inclusions or

abnormalities present in the stained smear.

- ○ Pathogen identification: Scan for any identified pathogens, viral inclusions, or characteristic structures associated with certain infections, such as inclusion bodies or multinucleated giant cells in viral infections like herpes simplex virus (HSV) or VZV (**Fig. 3**).[4]
- *Systematic examination*:
  - ○ Grid or systematic approach: Consider using a systematic grid or pattern to ensure comprehensive examination of the entire slide, avoiding oversight of any critical areas.
- *Documentation*:
  - ○ Note-taking: Document any observed abnormalities, cellular changes, or pathogens seen during examination.
  - ○ Photography: Capture clear and focused images of significant findings for documentation and future reference, if possible.

Interpretation and Analysis

Identification of pathogens: Recognize specific cellular changes or inclusions indicative of certain infections, aiding in the diagnosis of viral or parasitic conditions.

Assessment of cellular abnormalities: Evaluate cellular morphology for any anomalies or atypical features that might indicate underlying dermatological disorders or infections.

Precautions

Ensure adequate lighting and focus adjustment for clear visualization.

- Handle slides carefully to avoid smudging or damaging the stained material
- Observe proper laboratory safety protocols and practices while using the microscope and handling specimens

DIAGNOSTIC APPLICATIONS

Viral Infections

Herpes Simplex Virus (Figs. 3 and 4)

Tzanck cells: Tissue smears from herpetic lesions often reveal Tzanck cells, which are multinucleated giant cells or individual multinucleated keratinocytes. These cells are indicative of herpetic infections, particularly caused by HSV-1 and HSV-2. Tzanck cells typically display a characteristic appearance with multinucleation and nuclear molding.

Herpetic cytopathic effect: Smears may exhibit a herpetic cytopathic effect characterized

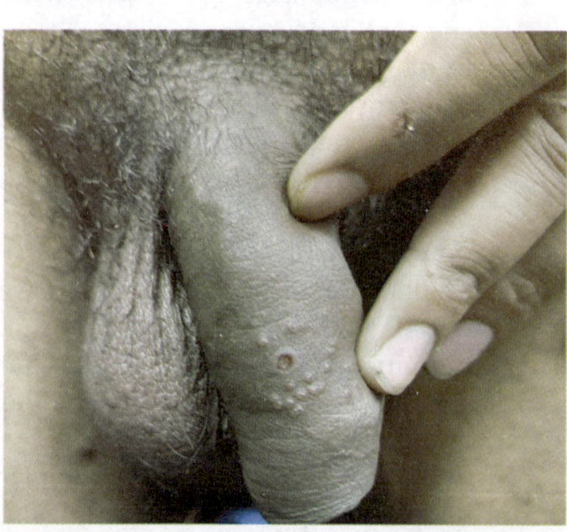

FIG. 3: Clinical image of herpes simplex patient.

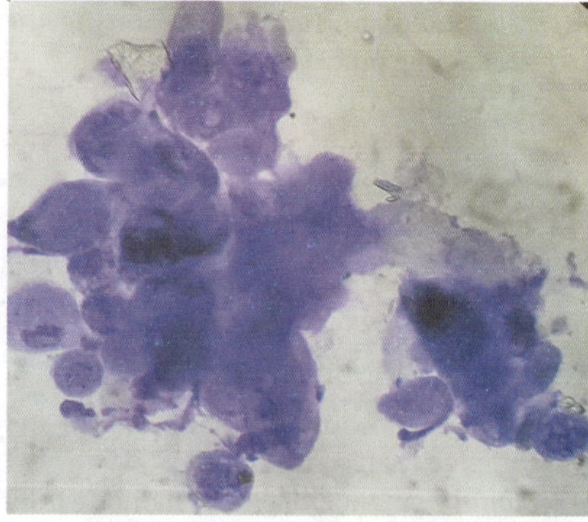

FIG. 4: Tzanck smear showing multinucleated giant cells.

by nuclear changes in infected cells. These changes include nuclear chromatin margination, multinucleation, and the presence of intranuclear inclusions (Cowdry type A inclusion bodies).

Inflammatory infiltrate: In tissue smears, an inflammatory infiltrate composed of lymphocytes and neutrophils surrounding the affected cells may be observed, indicating the immune response to the viral infection.

Eosinophilic intracytoplasmic inclusions (Cowdry type A inclusions): These intracytoplasmic inclusions can be visualized under microscopy in some cases of HSV infection.

Varicella–Zoster Virus (Figs. 5 and 6)

Multinucleated giant cells: Like HSV, VZV infections can also result in the formation of multinucleated giant cells or syncytia in tissue smears. These cells demonstrate nuclear molding and multinucleation, indicative of VZV infection.

Herpesvirus cytopathic effect: Smears may show characteristic cytopathic changes, such as nuclear enlargement, multinucleation, and the presence of intranuclear inclusions. These inclusions may be more prominent in cells derived from vesicular lesions.

Inflammatory response: The presence of an inflammatory infiltrate, including lymphocytes and macrophages, can be observed in tissue smears from VZV-infected lesions.

Clustering of infected cells: Tissue smears may reveal clusters of infected cells, particularly in vesicular lesions, demonstrating the characteristic viral replication and spread.

Hand-foot-and-mouth Disease (Caused by Coxsackievirus)

Multinucleated giant cells, characteristic of certain viral infections, can be identified in Tzanck smears, aiding in the diagnosis of hand-foot-and-mouth disease.

Autoimmune Vesiculobullous Conditions

Pemphigus Vulgaris and Pemphigus Foliaceus

Pemphigus vulgaris (PV) and pemphigus foliaceus (PF) are both characterized by the presence of autoantibodies targeting specific proteins within the skin, leading to intraepidermal blister formation. Under microscopic examination using Giemsa stain, distinct differences can be observed between these two conditions.[5]

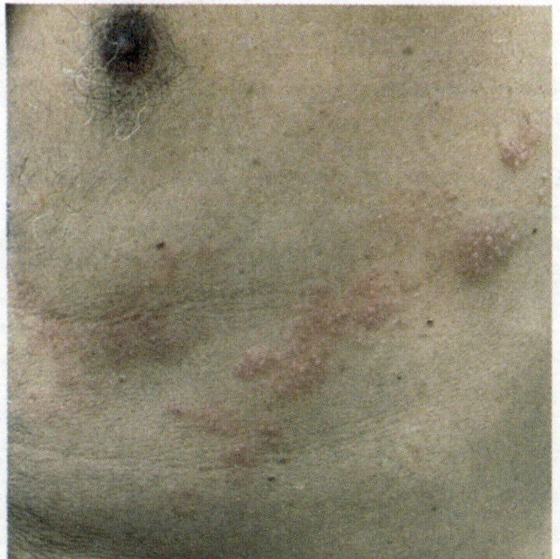

FIG. 5: Clinical image of herpes–zoster virus affected patient.

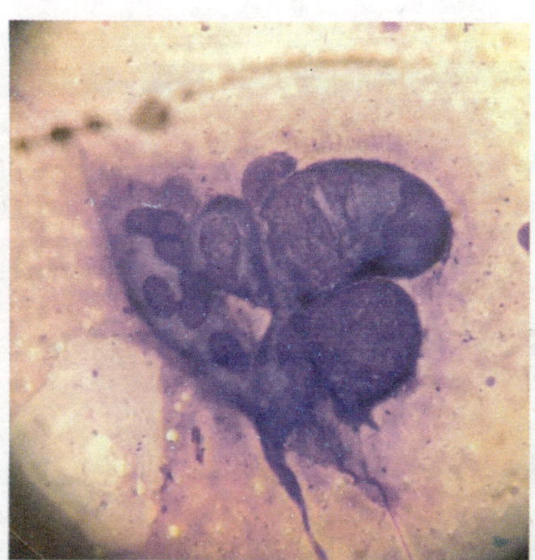

FIG. 6: Tzanck smear showing various multinucleated giant cells.

Pemphigus Vulgaris (Figs. 7 to 9)

Giemsa staining microscopic findings:

- *Acantholysis:* Giemsa stain highlights the characteristic finding of acantholysis, which is the detachment of epidermal cells (keratinocytes) from each other. This separation occurs due to the disruption of intercellular connections caused by autoantibodies against desmoglein 3, a protein crucial for cell adhesion in the epidermis.
- *Tzanck cells:* Giemsa staining reveals Tzanck cells, which are rounded, detached keratinocytes with a characteristic appearance under microscopy. These cells typically display a "fried egg" appearance due to a pyknotic nucleus surrounded by a clear halo resulting from the loss of cell-to-cell adhesion.
- *Inflammatory infiltrate:* It can also reveal an inflammatory infiltrate, predominantly comprising lymphocytes, which contributes to the destruction of keratinocytes.

Pemphigus Foliaceus (Figs. 10 and 11)

Giemsa staining microscopic findings:

- *Acantholysis:* Like PV, Giemsa stain also demonstrates acantholysis in PF.

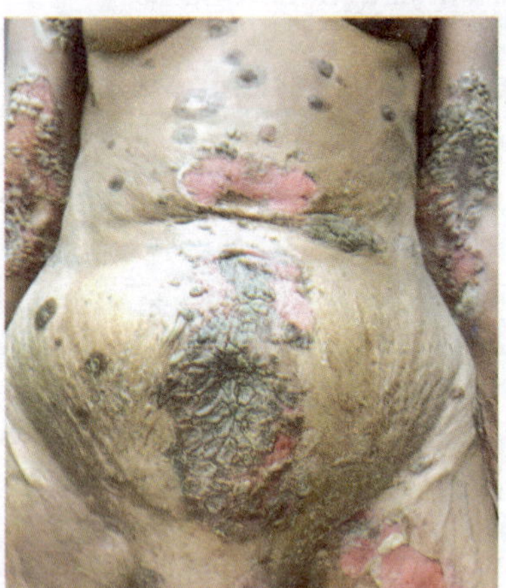

FIG. 7: Clinical image of a case of pemphigus vulgaris.

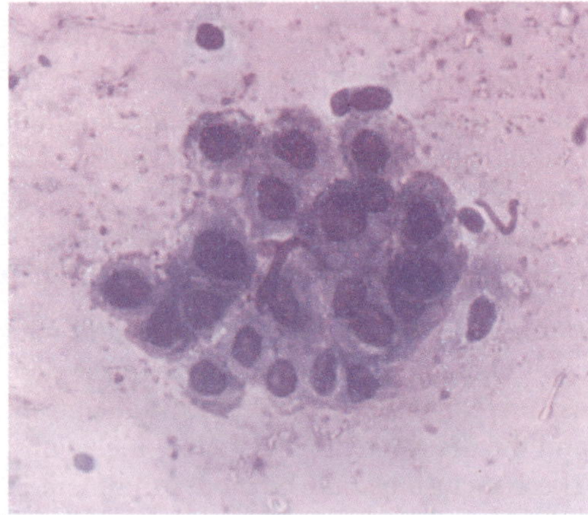

FIG. 9: Tzanck smear showing acantholytic cells in a patient with flaccid bullae suggestive of pemphigus.

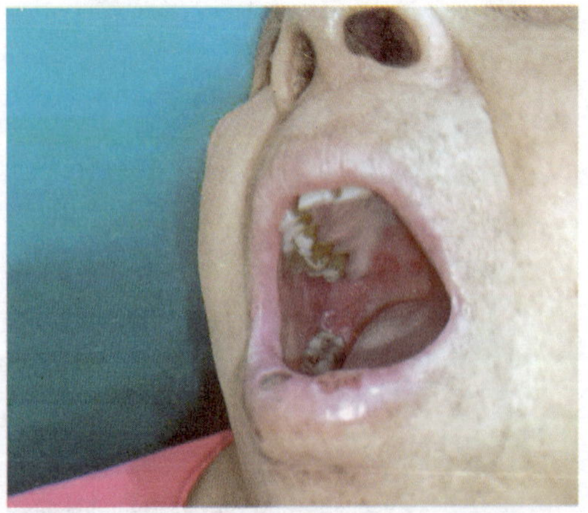

FIG. 8: Clinical image of a case of oral pemphigus.

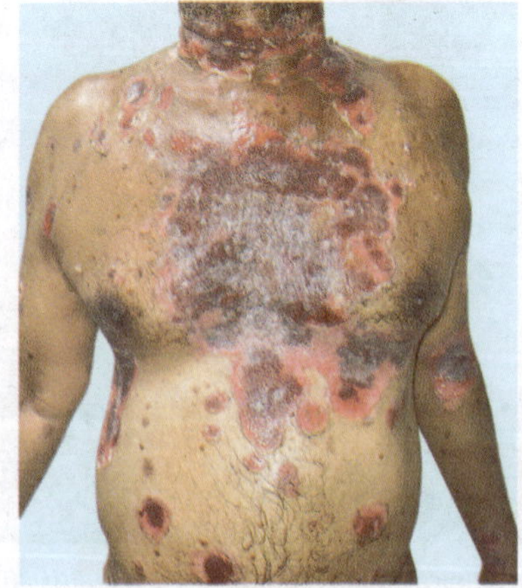

FIG. 10: Clinical image of a case of pemphigus foliaceus.

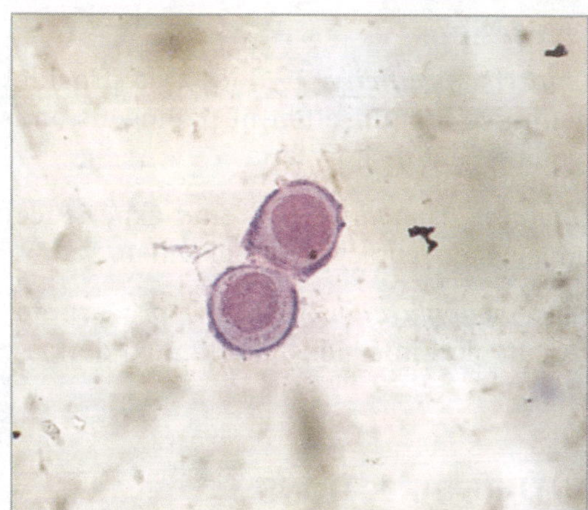

FIG. 11: Tzanck smear showing mourning edge cells in a patient with flaccid bullae suggestive of pemphigus.

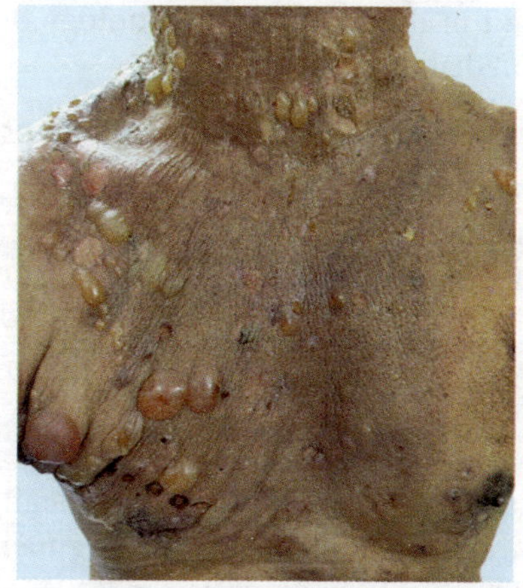

FIG. 12: Clinical image of a case of bullous pemphigoid.

- *Inflammatory infiltrate:* PF may present with an inflammatory infiltrate, but it is often less prominent compared to PV.
- *Absence of Tzanck cells:* Unlike PV, Tzanck cells are typically not observed in PF, reflecting the differences in the depth and nature of blister formation.

Understanding these microscopic findings under Giemsa stain is crucial for accurate diagnosis and differentiation between PV and PF, aiding in appropriate treatment strategies and management plans for patients with these conditions.

Bullous Pemphigoid

Smears often exhibit an abundance of inflammatory cells, predominantly eosinophils and neutrophils. Eosinophils are particularly notable and play a crucial role in the pathogenesis of bullous pemphigoid (BP) **(Figs. 12 and 13)**.

Linear Immunoglobulin A Disease

Smears show numerous inflammatory cells, predominantly neutrophils and occasional lymphocytes.

Other Bullous Disorders

Other bullous disorders, such as dermatitis herpetiformis (DH), epidermolysis bullosa

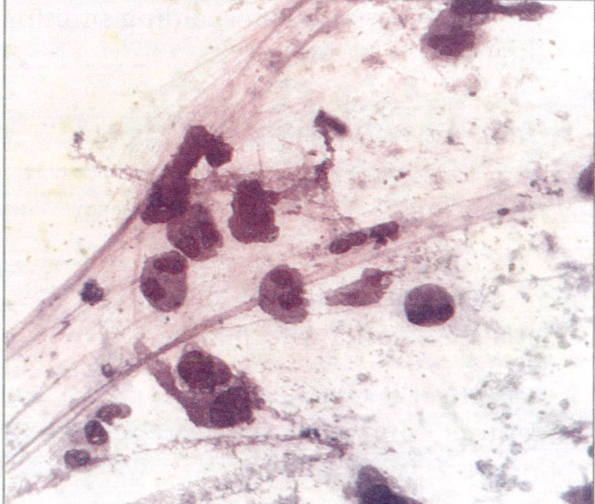

FIG. 13: Giemsa stain from tense bullae showing neutrophils and eosinophils.

acquisita (EBA), and Stevens–Johnson syndrome/toxic epidermal necrolysis (SJS/TEN)

Tzanck smear: Acantholytic cells or specific inflammatory patterns observed through Tzanck smear analysis may offer supportive evidence in differentiating between various bullous disorders.

Diabetic Bulla

Tzanck smear may reveal inflammatory cells, bacterial presence, or other cellular elements that aid in determining the etiology of the bulla in diabetic individuals.

Sepsis with Cutaneous Manifestations

Skin manifestations in sepsis, such as purpura or rash, can be sampled via Tzanck smear to detect signs of infection or inflammatory cells, contributing to a broader diagnostic approach.

Miscellaneous

- *Cutaneous leishmaniasis*: Examination may reveal amastigotes (intracellular parasites), aiding in the diagnosis of cutaneous leishmaniasis.
- *Scabies in Sarcoptes scabiei var. hominis (SCPD)*: Identification of mites, eggs, or fecal matter in skin scrapings supports the diagnosis of scabies, aiding prompt initiation of treatment.

ADVANTAGES AND LIMITATIONS

Advantages

Rapid analysis: Quick assessment allowing for immediate insights into certain viral, bacterial, or parasitic infections.

Cost-effective: It is a relatively inexpensive procedure compared to more complex laboratory tests.

Point-of-care diagnosis: It can be performed at the bedside or in outpatient settings for prompt evaluation.

Limitations

Limited specificity: It does not provide definitive identification of pathogens and requires confirmatory tests.

Operator dependent: Skill and experience impact the accuracy of interpretation.

Scope of application: Applicable primarily to certain viral infections and limited dermatoses.

FUTURE DIRECTIONS

Continued advancements in diagnostic techniques, including molecular diagnostics and immunohistochemistry, are augmenting traditional methods like the Tzanck smear. Integrating these advancements may enhance diagnostic accuracy and expand the utility of viral skin condition diagnosis.

CONCLUSION

The Tzanck smear remains a valuable tool in dermatology for diagnosing specific viral infections characterized by vesicular eruptions. While it has limitations, its simplicity, speed, and ability to provide immediate insights into certain viral skin conditions make it a useful adjunct in dermatological practice, aiding in effective patient management and treatment decisions.

Key Messages

- Tzanck smear is an easy-to-perform, simple, swift procedure and has a high sensitivity for clinical diagnosis of various diseases in dermatology.
- It involves the microscopic examination of cells obtained from skin vesicles, bullae, or ulcers.
- However, it has certain limitations like limited specificity and is operator dependent.

REFERENCES

1. Yaeen A, Ahmad QM, Farhana A, Shah P, Hassan I. Diagnostic value of Tzanck smear in various erosive, vesicular, and bullous skin lesions. Indian Dermatol Online J. 2015;6(6):381-6.
2. Nath P, Kabir MA, Doust SK, Ray A. Diagnosis of Herpes Simplex Virus: Laboratory and Point-of-Care Techniques. Infect Dis Rep. 2021;13(2):518-39.
3. Barcia JJ. The Giemsa stain: its history and applications. Int J Surg Pathol. 2007;15(3):292-6.
4. Mueller NH, Gilden DH, Cohrs RJ, Mahalingam R, Nagel MA. Varicella zoster virus infection: clinical features, molecular pathogenesis of disease, and latency. Neurol Clin. 2008;26(3):675-97, viii.
5. Noyan MA, Durdu M, Eskiocak AH. TzanckNet: a convolutional neural network to identify cells in the cytology of erosive-vesiculobullous diseases. Sci Rep. 2020;10(1):18314.

Gram Stain

Vinay Gera, Abhinav Kumar Verma, Biju Vasudevan

INTRODUCTION

The Gram stain was first used in 1884 by Danish bacteriologist Hans Christian Gram.[1] It is a differential staining procedure used to categorize bacteria as gram-positive or gram-negative depending upon the chemical and physical properties of their cell walls. Gram-positive cells impart purple while gram-negative cells impart pink color.

Crystal violet dye is used in the first step of Gram stain for staining the slide. Thereafter, the dye is fixed by using iodine which forms crystal violet-iodine complex. This complex prevents easy removal of dye. A decolorizing agent in the form of combined solvent of ethanol and acetone is then used to remove the dye.

The basic principle of Gram staining involves the ability of the bacterial cell wall to retain the crystal violet dye during solvent treatment.[2] Peptidoglycan content is higher in gram-positive microorganisms as compared to gram-negative, which have higher lipid content.[3] So gram-positive bacteria retain the dye.

In the final step of Gram staining, basic fuchsin stain is used so as to give the decolorized gram-negative bacteria a pink color. It is called as counterstain. Safranin can also be used as a counterstain. However, basic fuchsin stains gram-negative organisms more intensely than safranin.

In dermatological practice, Gram stain has been proved to be a very useful test, which can be done at bedside. It is inexpensive and an easy test to perform as it has very simple steps. However, because of its simplicity, the usefulness of this test should not be underestimated, as patient can be started empirically on antibiotic therapy while other investigations reports are still awaited. Cutaneous infections may arise due to break in the continuity of the skin or may be secondary to systemic infections. *Staphylococcus aureus* accounts for 30–50% of skin and soft tissue infections. Other organisms include Enterobacteriaceae, nonfermenters, streptococci including β-hemolytic group A and anaerobes.[4]

SPECIMEN COLLECTION

Commonly used specimens for Gram stain are:
- Pus swab from cutaneous bacterial infections
- Urethral discharge and genital ulcers swab to rule out sexually transmitted diseases
- Swabs from nostrils, throat, rectum, wound, and cervix
- Sputum and blood
- Cerebrospinal fluid, ascitic fluid, synovial fluid, and pleural fluid

Specimens should always be collected in sterile containers.

PROCEDURE

Required Equipment

- Personal protective equipment
- Bunsen burner
- Clean glass slide
- Slide rack
- Microscope
- Timer

Reagents

- *Primary stain*: Crystal violet/methylene blue **(Fig. 1A)**[5]
- *Mordant*: Gram's iodine solution **(Fig. 1B)**
- *Decolorizer*: Acetone/ethanol (50:50 v:v) **(Fig. 1C)**
- *Counterstain*: 0.1% basic carbol fuchsin/safranin solution **(Fig. 1D)**
- Water

Preparation of Glass Slide and Smear

- Clean glass slide is required to carry out this procedure. Wash the glass slide with soap and water, thereafter wipe with spirit or alcohol. Dry and keep the slides over sterile gauze or towel.
- Label the slides with glassware marking pen either on the edge or the undersurface to avoid staining of wrong side of the slides. Be cautious not to mix the ink of pen with stains.

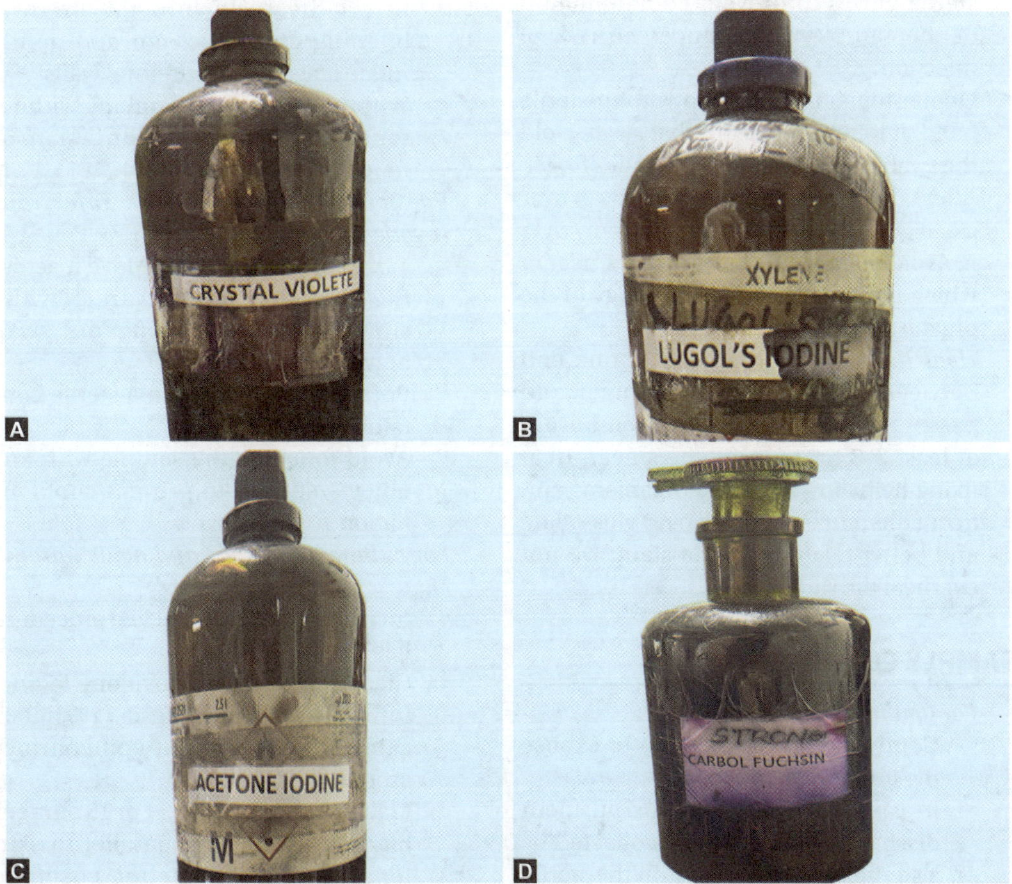

FIGS. 1A TO D: (A) Crystal violet stain; (B) Gram's iodine; (C) Acetone; and (D) Carbol fuchsin.

Preparation of the Smear

Smear can be made from swab sample, culture plate, and bacterial broth suspension. However, on bedside, only swab sample can be taken.

GENERAL INSTRUCTIONS BEFORE COLLECTION OF SAMPLES

- *Explain the procedure*: Before collection of samples, explain the procedure and its purpose to the patient. Take verbal consent. While taking the sample maintain the privacy of the patient especially in case of sampling from genital areas.
- *Hand hygiene and gloving*: Clean the hands with soap and water and wear sterile gloves to prevent contamination of the sample and reduce the risk of infection.
- Do not touch the swab tip with unsterile hand. If touched, discard that swab. Hold the swab between thumb and index finger.
- After taking the sample, roll the swab over clean glass slide and spread it evenly over it. Avoid making thick and dense smear in which identifying the morphology of the organisms will be difficult.
- *Heat fixing*: Hold the slide at one end between thumb and index finger and pass it over the flame of Bunsen burner at least 2–3 times to fix the smear. Heat fixing helps in killing the organisms and firm adherence of smear over glass slide and better taker up of the stain. Do not overheat the slide.

SAMPLE COLLECTION

- *For urethral smear in males*:
  - Gently retract the foreskin to expose the urethral opening
  - In case if there is copious purulent discharge, then it can be collected by a sterile swab or directly on the sterile container or glass slides.
  - If discharge is scanty, milking of the penile shaft can be done which will make discharge per urethra easily available for collection.
  - However, if discharge is very scanty and not visible at the time of examination, a sterile swab or collection device can be inserted into the urethral opening about 2–3 cm and sample can be collected by gentle rotation against the urethral walls. Avoid touching with skin.
- *For urethral smear in females*:
  - Spread the labia to expose the urethral opening. Copious purulent discharge can easily be collected on a sterile swab or directly on the sterile container or glass slides.
  - Insert the swab into the urethral opening about 1–2 cm and gently rotate it against the urethral walls.
  - Withdraw the swab carefully without touching the surrounding skin or mucosa.
- *For cutaneous bacterial infections (pyodermas)*:
  - Take a dry sterile swab. Move it across the pus discharging area, while simultaneously rotating the swab between fingers.
  - Put the sample swab in a sterile container
  - Avoid touching the sample with any objects/surface to prevent contamination
- *For cutaneous abscess and acute paronychia*:
  - Incision and drainage (I&D) procedure has to be done.
  - Clean the area with povidone iodine. Infiltrate local anesthesia (2% lignocaine with or without epinephrine) around the abscess
  - Make an incision with 11 or 15 number blade over the skin parallel to skin tension lines for better cosmetic outcome and to prevent the scar.

- ○ For acute paronychia **(Fig. 2A)** which is most commonly caused by bacterial infection especially staphylococci **(Fig. 2B)** use a flat probe or 11 number blade to elevate eponychial fold or incise the area of higher fluctuation in lateral nail fold with tip of blade.
- ○ Express the entire purulent materials and break up all the loculations. Take swab smear and roll it over a clean glass slide for Gram staining.
- ○ Dress the wound with sterile gauze and tape. Do not apply suture.

STAINING STEPS

Fixation of Specimen

Fix the specimen over a clean glass slide and allow it to air dry and keep on the slide rack.[6]

Primary Stain

- Flood the slide with crystal violet stain
- Keep the stain for 30–60 seconds, then pour it off, and the excess stain is rinsed with water.

Mordant

Flood the slide with Gram's iodine solution. This process is called "fixing the dye." After 30–60 seconds, rinse the slide with running tap water.

Decolorization

Add a few drops of decolorizer to the slide. This step is known as "solvent treatment." The slide is rinsed with water in 5–15 seconds.

Counterstaining

- Counterstain the slide with basic fuchsin solution for 30–60 seconds. The fuchsin solution is then washed off with water.
- Blot the slide with absorbent paper. Take care not to wipe the cells off the slide. Keep the slide for air dry
  Procedure of Gram stain steps is shown in **Flowchart 1**.

MICROSCOPIC EXAMINATION

- Examine the slide under a microscope, initially under 40× and then under 100× oil immersion
- All areas of the slide should be examined. Areas that are only one cell thick should be examined. Thick areas in slides often give variable and incorrect results.
- White blood cells and macrophages stain gram-negative
- Squamous epithelial cells stain gram-positive

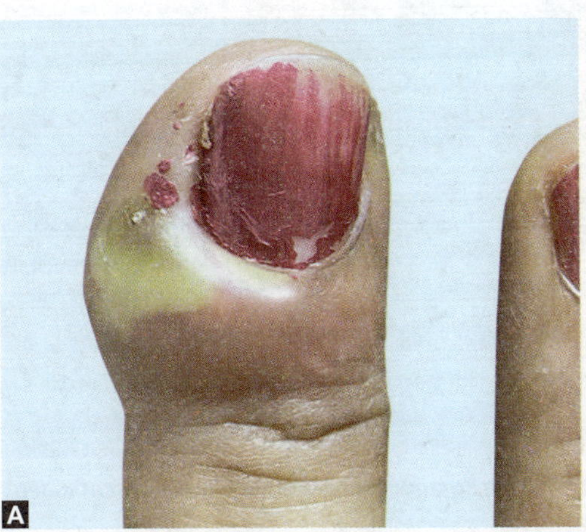

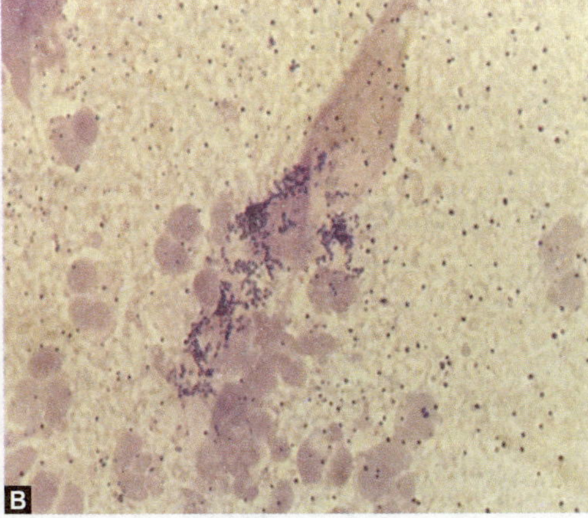

FIGS. 2A AND B: (A) Acute paronychia and (B) Gram stain shows gram-positive purpled colored staphylococci arranged in clusters, 100× oil immersion objective.

INTERPRETATION OF THE RESULTS

- Gram-positive organisms appear purple or blue and gram-negative organisms appear pink or red
- In adequate specimens, sheets of polymorphonuclear leukocytes will be seen along with interspersed bacteria.
- Morphological appearance of bacilli is rod-shaped and cocci are spherical in Gram stain.

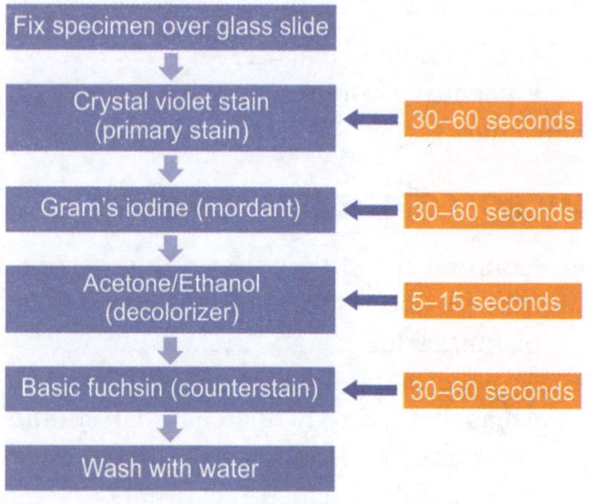

FLOWCHART 1: Steps of Gram stain procedure.

INDICATIONS

Gram stain is usually done if there is suspicion of bacterial infections such as:

- *Pyodermas*: Folliculitis **(Fig. 3A)**, furunculosis, impetigo, botryomycosis, etc. Folliculitis when caused by *S. aureus*, a gram-positive coccus, is seen on Gram stain as coccus arranged in clusters and appears purple in color **(Fig. 3B)**.
- Sexually transmitted disease with genital ulcer or urethral discharge **(Fig. 4A)** such as gonorrhea, chlamydia, candidiasis, bacterial vaginosis, syphilis, chancroid, lymphogranuloma venereum, genital herpes. Gonorrhea is caused by *Neisseria gonorrhoeae*, a gram-negative kidney-shaped intracellular diplococcus which is seen inside polymorphonuclear leukocytes **(Fig. 4B)**.
- Cutaneous abscess can be mainly caused by *Streptococcus pyogenes*, *Staphylococcus*, *Escherichia coli*, and *Klebsiella* species **(Fig. 5A)**. *Klebsiella* is a gram-negative bacillus, which appears as pink colored rods on Gram stain **(Fig. 5B)**.
- Erythrasma **(Figs. 6A and B)** is caused by *Corynebacterium minutissimum*, which

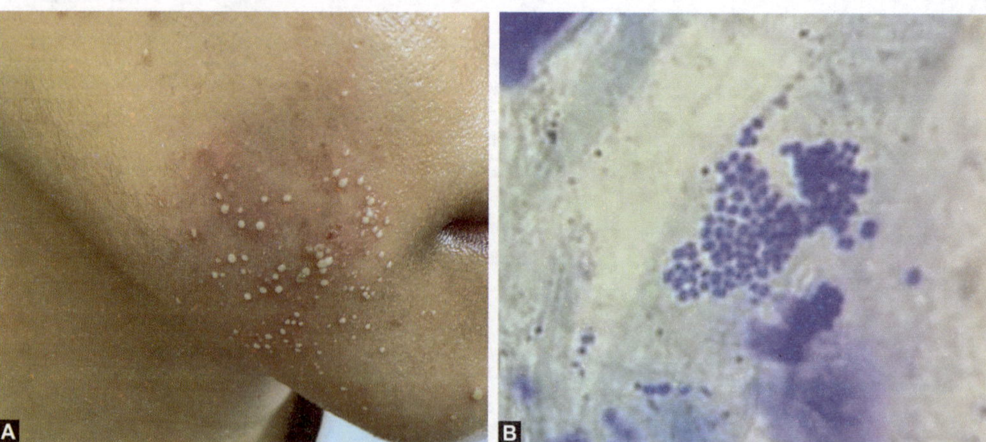

FIGS. 3A AND B: (A) Facial folliculitis and (B) Gram stain shows gram-positive cocci, *Staphylococcus aureus* arranged in cluster, 100× oil immersion objective.

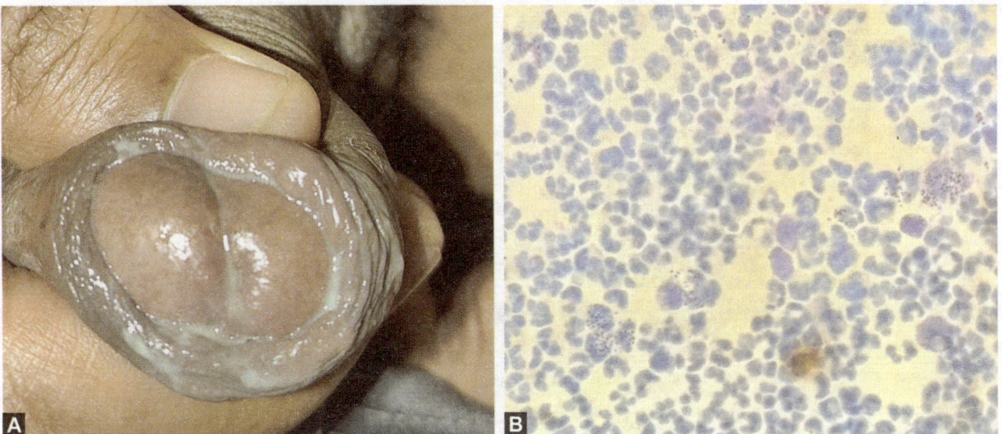

FIGS. 4A AND B: (A) Urethral discharge and (B) Gram stain shows gram-negative intracellular diplococci, *Neisseria gonorrhoeae*, 100× oil immersion objective.

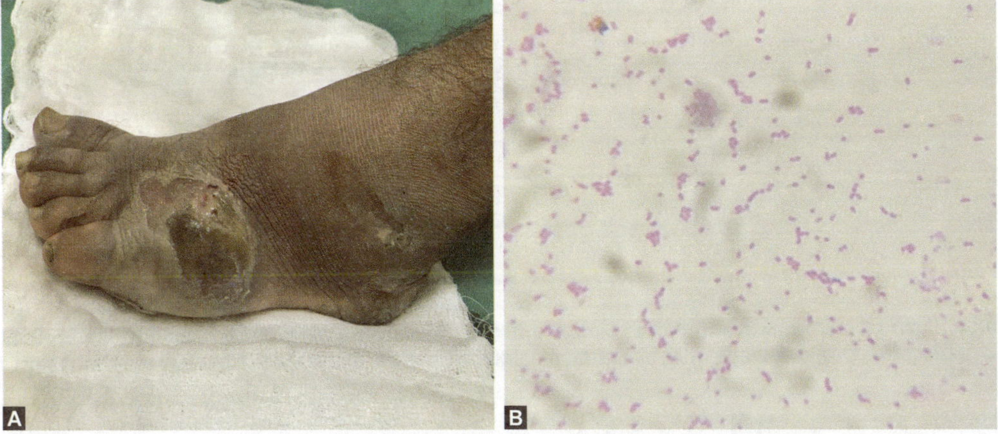

FIGS. 5A AND B: (A) Cutaneous abscess over foot and (B) Gram stain shows gram-negative rod-shaped bacilli, *Klebsiella pneumoniae*, 100× oil immersion objective.

is a gram-positive bacillus and appears purple colored on Gram stain **(Fig. 6C)**.

- Ecthyma gangrenosum **(Figs. 7A and B)** mainly caused by *Pseudomonas aeruginosa*, which is a gram-negative rod-shaped bacterium and appears pink colored on Gram stain **(Fig. 7C)**.
- Acute ulcers **(Fig. 8A)** mainly caused by *Staphylococcus, Streptococcus*, and *E. coli. E. coli* is a gram-negative rod-shaped bacillus, which appears pink colored on Gram stain **(Fig. 8B)**.

- Necrotizing fasciitis **(Fig. 9A)** caused by *Staphylococcus, Streptococcus*, and *Acinetobacter. Acinetobacter* is a gram-negative bacillus, which appears pink colored on Gram stain **(Fig. 9B)**
- Cellulitis and erysipelas **(Fig. 10A)** caused by *Streptococcus* and *Staphylococcus. Streptococcus* is a gram-positive coccus,

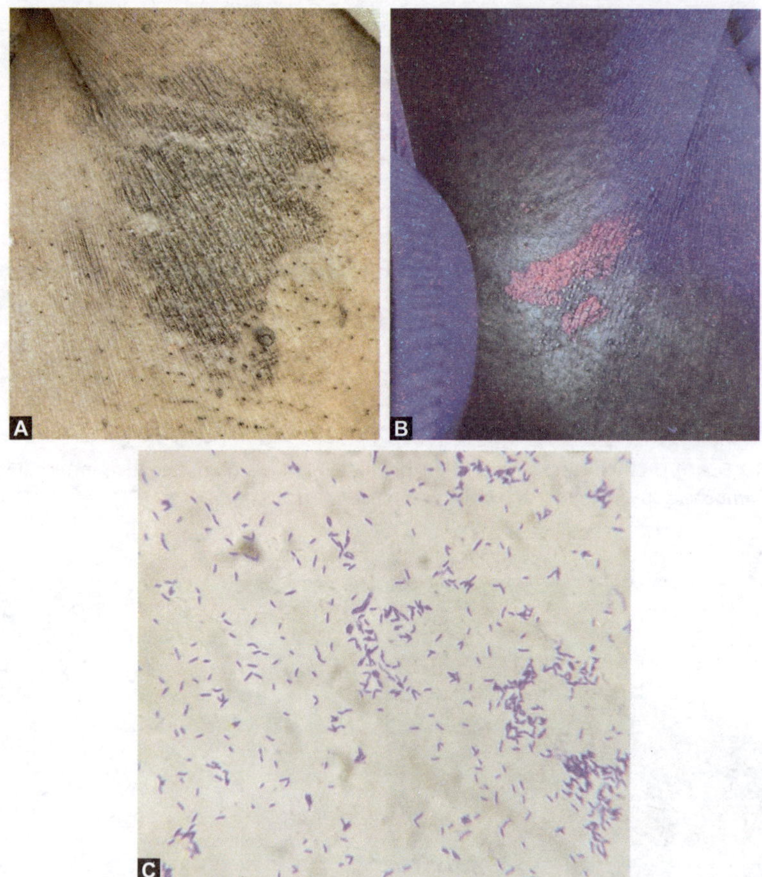

FIGS. 6A TO C: (A) Erythrasma; (B) Wood's lamp showing coral red fluorescence; and (C) Gram stain shows gram-positive coccobacilli, *Corynebacterium minutissimum*, 100× oil immersion objective.

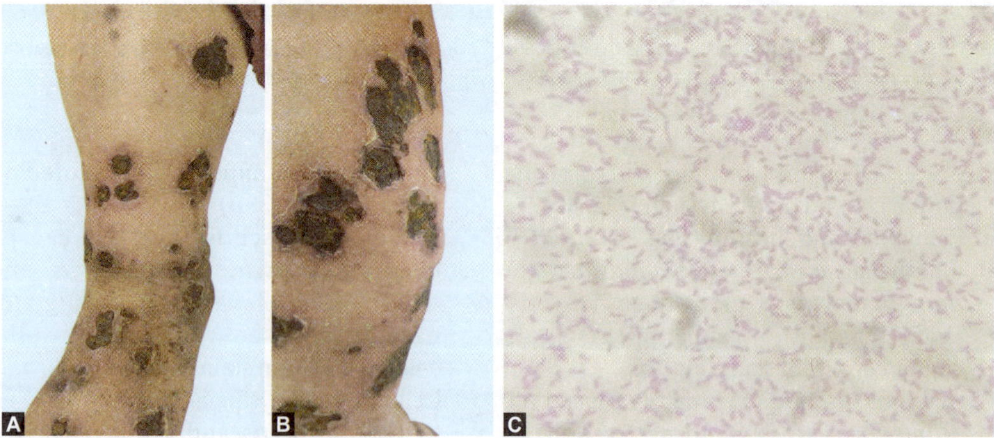

FIGS. 7A TO C: (A and B) Ecthyma gangrenosum and (C) Gram stain shows gram-negative rods, *Pseudomonas aeruginosa*, 100× oil immersion objective.

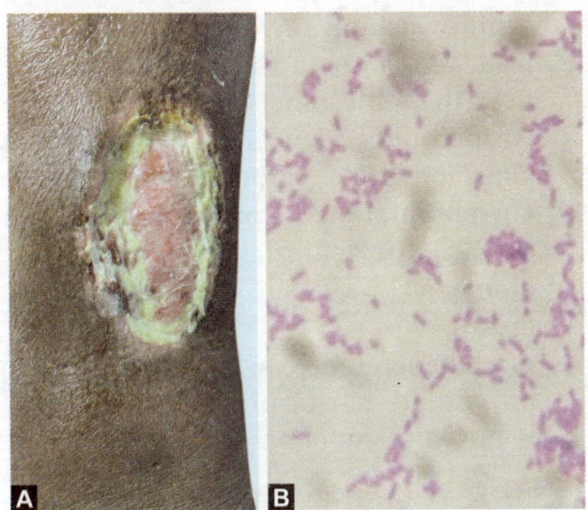

FIGS. 8A AND B: (A) Acute ulcer over leg and (B) Gram stain shows gram-negative rods, *Escherichia coli*, 100× oil immersion objective.

arranged in chains, and appears purple colored on Gram stain (**Fig. 10B**).

- Scalp pustulosis
- Pustular acne vulgaris
- Acute paronychia

Examples of gram-positive bacteria are:
- *Cocci*: *Staphylococcus* and *Streptococcus* species
- *Bacilli*: *Corynebacterium*, *Clostridium*, and *Listeria* species

Examples of gram-negative bacteria are:
- *Cocci*: *Neisseria gonorrhoeae*, *Neisseria meningitidis*, and *Moraxella* species
- *Bacilli*: *E. coli*, *Proteus*, *Klebsiella*, and *Pseudomonas* species

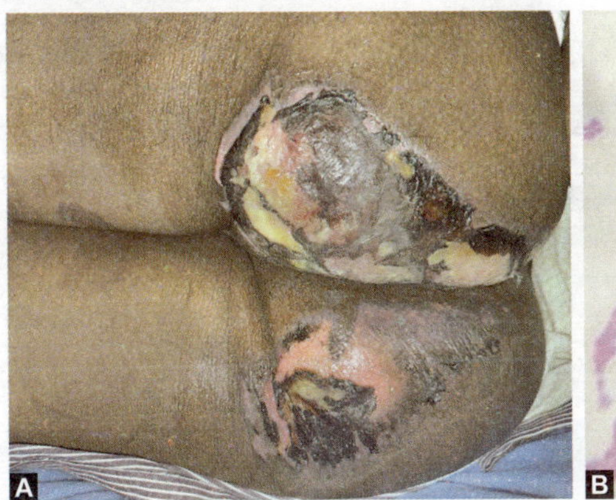

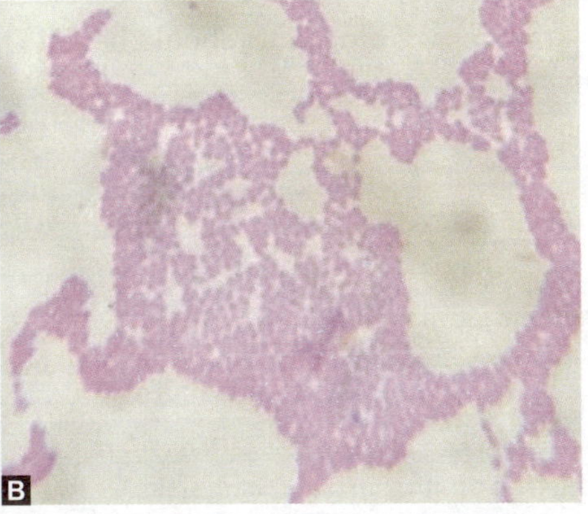

FIGS. 9A AND B: (A) Necrotizing fasciitis and (B) Gram stain shows gram-negative bacilli *Acinetobacter*, 100× oil immersion objective.

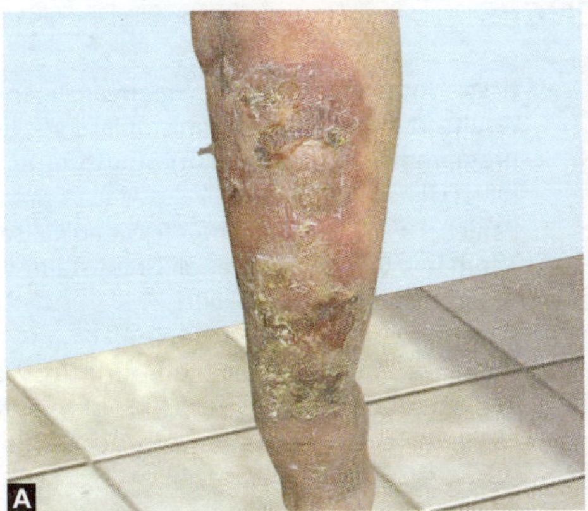

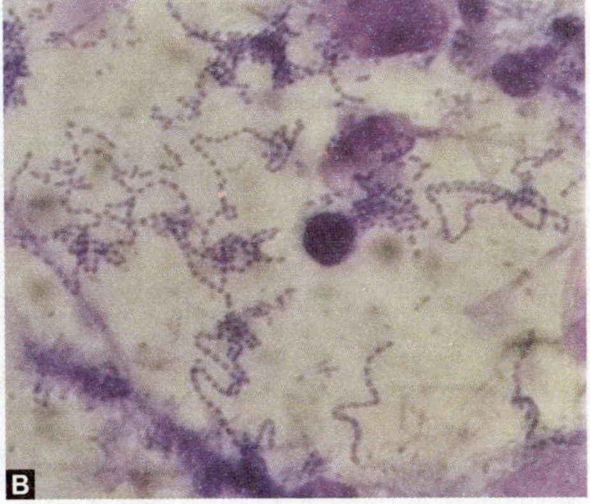

FIGS. 10A AND B: (A) Erysipelas over leg and (B) Gram stain shows gram-positive cocci arranged in chain suggestive of *Streptococcus*, 100× oil immersion objective.

GENERAL PRECAUTIONS WHILE PERFORMING GRAM STAIN

- Collect all the required materials beforehand
- Always wear gloves and laboratory coat to avoid risk of infections
- Collection of specimens should be sterile, as multiple organisms can contaminate the specimen.
- Adequate specimen collection is of utmost importance.
- If antibiotics have been taken by patient prior to specimen collection, it can interfere with the growth of organisms.
- Try to make a thin layer of smear (single cell layer)
- Do not overheat the slides
- All the steps of procedure should be time bound.

- While washing the stained slide with water, do not pour water stream directly over the slide otherwise stain may be washed out. Allow water to fall slowly along the surface of slide.
- On completion of procedure, always discard the materials in appropriate biomedical waste bin. Disinfect the work area.
- Wash hand properly with soap and water on completion of procedure. Sterilize hand with alcohol-based sanitizer.

CONCLUSION

Gram stain is rapid and initial bedside diagnostic test for the evaluation of bacterial infections. It gives quick result, on the basis of which patient can be initiated antibiotic therapy.

Key Messages

- Gram stain is a staining method used to classify bacterial species broadly into gram-positive and gram-negative.
- In dermatological practices, it is an important bedside test which is simple and easy to perform and provide quick result.
- While awaiting other investigation report, patient can be started empirically on antibiotic treatment based on positive result of Gram stain.

REFERENCES

1. Bartholomew JW, Mittwer T. The Gram stain. Bacteriol Rev. 1952;16(1):1-29.
2. LIBENSON L, McILROY AP. On the mechanism of the gram stain. J Infect Dis. 1955;97(1):22-6.
3. Shugar D, Baranowska J. Studies on the gram stain; the importance of proteins in the Gram reaction. Acta Microbiol Pol. (1952). 1954;3(1):11-20.
4. Gales AC, Jones RN, Pfaller MA, Gordon KA, Sader HS. Two year assessment of pathogen frequency and antimicrobial resistance pattern among organisms isolated from skin and soft tissue infections in Latin American hospitals: results from the sentry antimicrobial surveillance programme, 1997-98, SENTRY study group. Int J Infect Dis. 2000;4:75-84.
5. Panicker V, Nayak P, Krishna R, Sreenivaasan N, Thomas J, Sreedevan V, et al. Gram stain. J Skin Sex Transm Dis. 2022;5(1):60-1.
6. Smith AC, Hussey MA. (2005). Gram Stain Protocols. [online] Available from https://asm.org/getattachment/5c95a063-326b-4b2f-98ce-001de9a5ece3/gram-stain-protocol-2886.pdf [Last accessed February, 2024].

Bedside Tests in Sexually Transmitted Diseases

Nishu Bala, Senkadhir Vendhan, Sushmita Mishra

INTRODUCTION

In the realm of dermatology and venereology, the evolution of diagnostic modalities has been instrumental in addressing the complexities of sexually transmitted diseases (STDs). The integration of bedside tests has emerged as a transformative approach, offering immediate and convenient diagnostic solutions at the point of care. These rapid diagnostic tools play a pivotal role in the timely identification, management, and control of STDs, presenting a paradigm shift in clinical practice.

This chapter aims to explore the scientific underpinnings and clinical applications of bedside tests for STDs in dermatology and venereology. Understanding the nuances and limitations of each bedside test equips dermatologists and venereologists with the knowledge necessary to make informed decisions and optimize patient care in the challenging landscape of STD management. Through this exploration, we aim to provide a comprehensive understanding of bedside testing, accentuating its role as an invaluable asset in the arsenal against STDs.

In this chapter we will be elaborating on the following bedside tests:

- Urethral smear for Gram's stain
- Two glass, three glass, and four glass urine tests
- Lymph node aspiration in dermatology
- Prostatic massage in STDs
- Tests for syphilis—dark ground microscopy (DGM)
- Tissue smear for donovanosis
- Signs in STDs—groove sign, dory flop sign, and fluctuation in bubo
- Wet mount examination

URETHRAL SMEAR

Discharge from the urethra either of male or female may be very alarming symptoms that often bring the patients to the clinician, healthcare setup, or even quacks in rural areas. If a correct diagnosis is not made at an early-stage patients are likely to get exposed to multiple nonspecific antibiotics, antifungals, and antivirals which not only increase the financial burden to the concerned but even pose un-necessary risk of building resistance against critical anti-infective drugs and developing acute or long-term complications. Presumptive diagnosis based upon the history of sexual exposure, trauma, operation, examination findings like purulent discharge, copious mucoid discharge, scanty mucoid discharge, and regional lymphadenopathies is essential but simple bedside of urethral smear added in the approach of management of urethral discharge. The urethral smear, a diagnostic procedure commonly employed in various medical fields including dermatology and venereology, plays a pivotal role in identifying infections, particularly those related to STDs and dermatological conditions affecting the genital region.[1] According to the current Centers for Disease Control and Prevention (CDC) guidelines, urethritis can be documented based on any of the following signs or laboratory test results: (1) mucoid, mucopurulent, or purulent discharge on examination; (2) Gram stain of urethral secretions demonstrating ≥2 white blood cell (WBC) per oil immersion field on microscopy; (3) the microscopy diagnostic cutoff might vary, depending on background prevalence [≥2 WBCs/high-power field (HPF) in high-prevalence settings (STI clinics) or ≥5 WBCs/HPF in lower-prevalence settings]; (4) positive leukocyte esterase test from first-void urine; and (5) microscopic examination of sediment from a spun first-void urine demonstrating ≥10 WBC/HPF.[2]

Methodology

Procedure for Taking Urethral Smear

- *Preparation*:
  - Explain the procedure: Inform the individual about the procedure, its purpose, and what to expect to ensure cooperation and minimize discomfort.
  - Gather supplies: Gather the necessary equipment including a sterile swab or collection device, gloves, lubricant (if needed), and a suitable container for sample storage.
- *Patient positioning*:
  - Positioning: The patient typically lies down on an examination table or bed with their knees bent and feet placed flat, allowing access to the genital area.
- *Sterile technique*:
  - Hand hygiene and gloving: Perform hand hygiene and wear sterile gloves to prevent contamination of the sample and reduce the risk of infection.

- *Sample collection*:
  - Male urethral smear:
    - Gently retract the foreskin (if applicable) to expose the urethral opening (meatus). Copious purulent discharge can easily be collected on a sterile swab or directly on the sterile container or glass slides. At times milking of the penile shaft makes discharge per urethra easily available for collection.
    - If discharge is very scanty and not visible at the time of examination, we can use a sterile swab or collection device, to insert it into the urethral opening about 2–3 cm and rotate it gently against the urethral walls.[3]
  - Female urethral smear:
    - Using a sterile swab, spread the labia to expose the urethral opening. Copious purulent discharge can easily be collected on a sterile swab or directly on the sterile container or glass slides.
    - Insert the swab into the urethral opening about 1–2 cm and gently rotate it against the urethral walls
    - Withdraw the swab carefully without touching the surrounding skin or mucosa
- *Sample handling*:
  - Sample transfer: Place the swab or collection device with the obtained sample into a suitable transport medium (Amies transport medium) or container recommended for the specific laboratory test.
  - Labeling: Properly label the container with the patient's identification information and other required details.
- *Postprocedure*:
  - Patient comfort: Ensure patient comfort and provide any necessary instructions or postprocedure care.

○ Sample transport: Transport the sample to the laboratory promptly, following appropriate storage and transportation guidelines.

Considerations

- *Sterility*: Maintaining a sterile technique during sample collection is crucial to prevent contamination and ensure accurate test results.
- *Patient comfort*: Although the procedure may cause mild discomfort, efforts should be made to minimize pain or anxiety through clear communication and gentle technique.
- *Safety measures*: Adherence to standard precautions and safety protocols is essential to prevent transmission of infections between healthcare providers and patients.

Laboratory Analysis

Microscopic examination: The sample is examined under a microscope to observe cellular elements, microorganisms, or any pathological changes present. This examination can provide immediate insights into the presence of infectious agents or inflammatory cells.

Gram staining: This staining technique helps differentiate and classify bacteria based on their cell wall characteristics. The presence of gram-negative intracellular diplococci indicates gonorrhea infection caused by *Neisseria gonorrhoeae* (**Fig. 1**).

Overview of the Gram Stain Procedure

- *Preparation of smear and fixation*:
  ○ Preparation: A small amount of the collected sample is evenly spread and air-dried on a clean glass slide.
  ○ Fixation: Heat fixation is applied by passing the slide through a flame a few times to ensure the sample adheres to the slide and prevents washing off during staining.

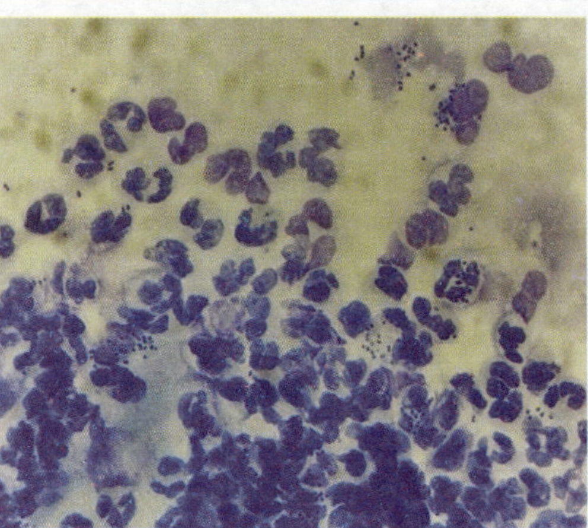

FIG. 1: Gram stain showing numerous neutrophils and gram-negative intracellular diplococci arranged in pairs.

- *Staining steps*:
  ○ Crystal violet (primary stain): The fixed smear is flooded with crystal violet solution for approximately 30 seconds. This stains all bacterial cells purple.
  ○ Iodine (mordant): Iodine solution is added to the slide, allowing it to stand for about a minute. Iodine serves as a mordant, forming a crystal-violet-iodine complex that enhances staining and prevents the primary stain from washing off.
- *Decolorization*:
  ○ Alcohol or acetone wash: The slide is washed with alcohol or acetone for a brief moment (3–5 seconds). This step differentiates between gram-positive and gram-negative bacteria based on their cell wall properties.
- *Counterstaining*:
  ○ Safranin (counterstain): The slide is stained with safranin solution for about a minute. This step counterstains the decolorized gram-negative bacteria, imparting a pink or red color to them.
- *Microscopic examination*:
  ○ The prepared slide is then observed under a light microscope using oil

immersion at high magnification (typically 1,000×). The examiner examines the stained bacteria to classify them as either gram-positive or gram-negative based on their coloration and morphology.[4,5]

Interpretation of Results

- *Gram-positive bacteria*:
  - Retain the crystal violet-iodine complex and appear purple or blue under the microscope.
  - Have a thicker peptidoglycan layer in their cell wall, which retains the crystal violet stain.
- *Gram-negative bacteria*:
  - Lose the crystal violet-iodine complex during decolorization and are counterstained with safranin, appearing pink or red.
  - Have thinner peptidoglycan layers, making them more susceptible to decolorization.
  - A standardization of urethral smear microscopy seems to be impossible. The cutoff value should discriminate between low and high prevalence of chlamydia, mycoplasma, and gonorrhea to include as many as possible with a specific infection in syndromic treatment, without overtreating those with few poly-morphonuclear leukocyte (PMNL)/HPF and high possibility of having nonspecific or no urethritis.

Characteristics of Neisseria Gonorrhoeae under Microscope

- *Morphology*:
  - Gram-negative diplococci: These bacteria appear as pairs of round or oval-shaped cells (cocci) when observed under a microscope **(Fig. 1)**.
  - Arrangement: They typically arrange themselves in pairs, resembling two adjacent kidney beans or coffee beans.

- *Size*:
  - Small size: *Neisseria gonorrhoeae* are relatively small bacteria, measuring about 0.6–1.0 µm in diameter.
- *Staining*:
  - Gram staining reaction: *Neisseria gonorrhoeae* stains pink or reddish-pink when using the Gram staining technique, indicating a gram-negative nature.
- *Intracellular and extracellular presence*:
  - Location: These bacteria may be found inside the cytoplasm of neutrophils (intracellularly) or as extracellular diplococci.
- *Cellular arrangement*:
  - Pairs within cells: When present intra-cellularly, they are often observed within phagocytic cells, particularly neutrophils.[6]

Significance of Urethral Smear Analysis

Treatment planning: The Gram stain results guide clinicians in selecting appropriate antibiotic therapies based on the identification of gram-positive or gram-negative bacteria and their susceptibility patterns.

Limitations and Considerations

- *Variable sensitivity*: The sensitivity of the Gram stain method can vary based on the quality of the sample and the presence of certain bacterial species.
- *Supplemental tests*: In some cases, additional tests, such as culture and sensitivity testing, may be required to confirm and further characterize bacterial infections identified through the Gram stain.

The Gram stain procedure of urethral smears remains a cornerstone in diagnosing bacterial infections in the urogenital tract, aiding in prompt and targeted therapeutic interventions based on accurate bacterial identification and characterization. Alternatively, Giemsa stain can also be used for visualization of the diplococci **(Fig. 2)**.

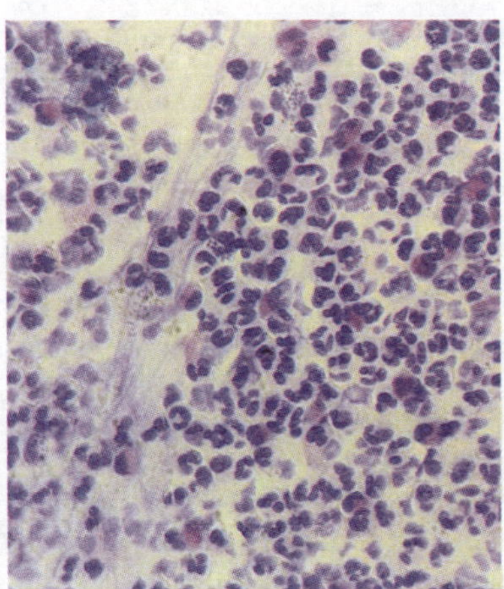

FIG. 2: Giemsa stain showing numerous neutrophils and intracellular diplococci.

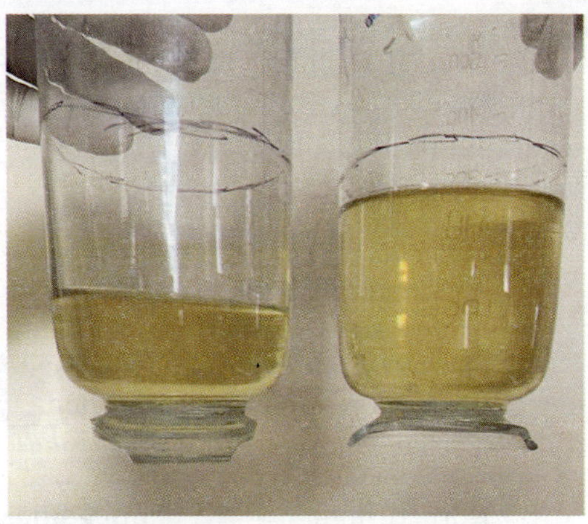

FIG. 3: Glass urine tests.

Significance in Dermatology

Diagnostic tool: Urethral smear analysis is instrumental in diagnosing infections and dermatological conditions affecting the genital area. It helps in identifying pathogens, cellular changes, and inflammatory responses, aiding in accurate diagnosis and subsequent treatment planning.

GLASS URINE TESTS

Two-glass Urine Test (Fig. 3)

Objective: The two-glass urine test aims to distinguish between urethral and bladder sources of inflammation or infection.

Methodology

Sample collection: Patient voids urine into two separate containers.
1. *First sample (G1)*: It represents the initial urethral urine, capturing the initial stream.
2. *Second sample (G2)*: It collects urine after voiding has commenced, representing bladder urine.

Application: Helps differentiate urethritis (urethral inflammation) from cystitis (bladder inflammation), aiding in diagnosing urogenital conditions

Three-glass Urine Test

Objective: The three-glass urine test assists in localizing the origin of inflammation or infection in the urogenital tract.

Methodology

Sample collection: Patient voids urine into three separate containers at different phases of urination.
1. *First sample (G1)*: It represents initial urethral urine.
2. *Second sample (G2)*: It collects midstream urine.
3. *Third sample (G3)*: It represents final urine stream.

Application: Facilitates the differentiation between urethritis, prostatitis, and cystitis.

Four-glass Urine Test

Objective: The four-glass urine test helps differentiate urethral, prostate, and bladder sources of inflammation or infection.[7]

Methodology

Sample collection: Patient voids urine into four separate containers at specific intervals during urination.

1. *First sample (G1—initial urethral urine)*:
   - Normal findings: The initial urine sample (G1) predominantly represents the initial urethral flow, which should ideally show minimal to no cloudiness or significant sedimentation.
   - Abnormal findings: Cloudiness, blood, or any signs of significant inflammation or infection may indicate urethritis or urethral inflammation.
2. *Second sample (G2—expressed prostatic secretion)*:
   - Normal findings: The sample after prostatic massage (G2) may show prostatic fluid with minimal cells and no significant turbidity.
   - Abnormal findings: Presence of pus cells, bacteria, or significant cloudiness may suggest prostatitis or inflammation within the prostate.
3. *Third sample (G3—midstream urine)*:
   - Normal findings: Midstream urine (G3) represents urine from the bladder and should typically be clear, without cloudiness or sedimentation.
   - Abnormal findings: Presence of pus cells, bacteria, or cloudiness may indicate cystitis or bladder inflammation.
4. *Fourth sample (G4—postprostatic massage urine)*:
   - Normal findings: Postprostatic massage urine (G4) might contain prostatic secretions and residual cells from the massage, similar to the second sample (G2).
   - Abnormal findings: Persistent presence of pus cells, bacteria, or significant cloudiness, particularly after vigorous massage, may further support prostatitis diagnosis.

LYMPH NODE ASPIRATION IN DERMATOLOGY

Lymph node aspiration serves as a crucial diagnostic procedure in dermatology, aiding in the evaluation of lymphadenopathy and associated conditions.

Preprocedure Preparation

Patient positioning: Place the patient in a comfortable position, exposing the area containing the enlarged lymph node(s). Ensure adequate lighting and patient relaxation.

Gather equipment: Prepare sterile gloves, an antiseptic solution, sterile drapes, a local anesthetic (if required), a syringe with an attached fine needle (22–25 gauge), and suitable specimen containers.

Procedure Steps

Patient consent and explanation: Explain the procedure to the patient, addressing any concerns, and obtain informed consent.

Preparation of the site: Clean the overlying skin with an antiseptic solution and drape the area, creating a sterile field around the lymph node.

Local anesthesia (if required): Administer a local anesthetic to minimize discomfort, especially if the procedure involves a sensitive area or deeper lymph nodes.

Needle insertion: With a firm yet gentle approach, insert the needle into the enlarged lymph node. Use a slow and controlled technique to avoid multiple attempts and patient discomfort.

Aspiration technique: Apply gentle negative pressure to the syringe plunger while redirecting the needle within the lymph node. Aspirate fluid or tissue material into the syringe. If resistance is encountered, reposition the needle slightly before attempting again.

Specimen collection: Carefully detach the syringe and expel the aspirated material into appropriate specimen containers for further analysis. Label the containers accurately.

Postprocedure care: Apply pressure to the site using a sterile gauze pad to prevent bleeding and assist in hemostasis. Provide appropriate wound care if necessary and advise the patient on postprocedure care instructions.

Postprocedure Considerations

Specimen handling: Label the collected specimen containers accurately and promptly send them to the laboratory for cytological, microbiological, or pathological evaluation.

Lymph node aspiration is a valuable diagnostic procedure in dermatology, aiding in the evaluation of lymphadenopathy and guiding the diagnosis of various dermatological conditions. Performing this procedure with proper technique, aseptic precautions, and adequate specimen handling ensures accurate diagnostic information and optimal patient care.[8]

PROSTATIC MASSAGE IN SEXUALLY TRANSMITTED DISEASES: A DERMATOLOGICAL APPROACH

Prostatic massage is occasionally employed in the dermatological realm for evaluating STDs that might affect the genitourinary system, particularly in cases involving suspected prostatic infections. Here is a comprehensive overview.

Purpose in Dermatology

Diagnostic aid: Prostatic massage serves as a means to obtain prostatic secretions or fluid for laboratory analysis, aiding in the assessment of prostatic infections associated with STDs.

Clinical assessment: A digital rectal examination (DRE) to assess the size, texture, tenderness, and presence of abnormalities in the prostate gland.

Massage technique: Using gentle, controlled motions, pressure is applied to the prostate gland through the rectal wall, facilitating the release of prostatic secretions.

Sample collection: Prostatic secretions obtained post-massage, usually through urination or via expressed fluid, are collected for laboratory analysis.

Diagnostic Significance

Laboratory analysis: The collected prostatic secretions undergo laboratory testing including leukocyte count, bacterial culture, and microscopic examination for pathogens.

Limitations: Prostatic massage may not consistently yield sufficient samples, necessitating supplementary tests for a comprehensive diagnosis.[9]

DARK GROUND MICROSCOPY

Dark ground microscopy is a specialized technique employed in the direct visualization of live microorganisms under dark-field illumination. This method enables the observation of specimens against a dark background, enhancing the contrast and visibility of microorganisms, including the delicate and spiral-shaped *Treponema pallidum*.

Principle and Procedure

Dark-field illumination: Utilizing a specialized condenser, the specimen is illuminated obliquely against a dark background, allowing only scattered light to reach the objective lens.

Visualization of Treponema pallidum: The spiral morphology and motility of *T. pallidum* are accentuated against the dark background, enabling their visualization **(Fig. 4)**.

Utility in Syphilis Diagnosis

Direct visualization of spirochetes: DGM facilitates the direct observation of live *T. pallidum*, confirming the presence of active infection.

Enhanced sensitivity: It provides higher sensitivity in primary and secondary syphilis stages, when spirochetes are more abundant and actively multiplying.

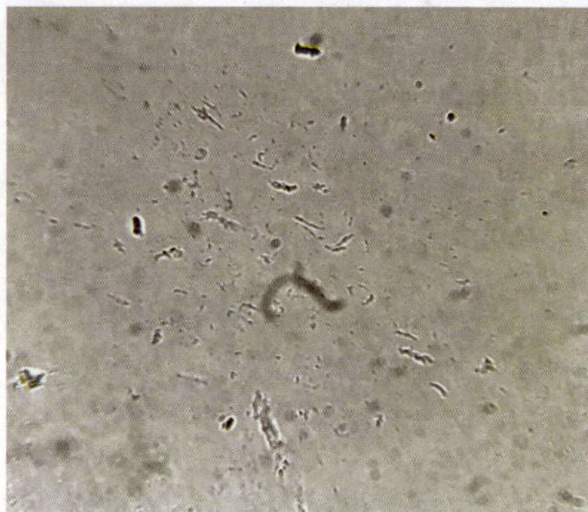

FIG. 4: Dark ground microscopy in syphilis.

Differentiating features: It helps distinguish *T. pallidum* from other microorganisms or cellular debris, aiding in accurate diagnosis.

Clinical Applications

Primary syphilis: DGM demonstrates the spiral-shaped *T. pallidum* in samples from chancre lesions, confirming the diagnosis.

Secondary syphilis: It is useful in diagnosing secondary lesions, such as skin rashes and mucous membrane lesions.

Follow-up and monitoring: Assessing treatment efficacy by monitoring the disappearance of *T. pallidum* after therapy.

Challenges and Limitations

Skill-dependent technique: It requires expertise in specimen collection and microscopy, impacting its availability and reliability.

Sensitivity in late stages: It reduced sensitivity in late stages of syphilis when spirochetes are less abundant.[10]

DONOVANOSIS—GIEMSA-STAINED TISSUE SMEAR

Donovanosis, caused by *Klebsiella granulomatis*, manifests as progressive, chronic genital ulcers. Here is how Giemsa-stained tissue smears can aid in diagnosing this condition.

Preparation of Tissue Smear

Sample collection: Obtain material from the base of the ulcer, ensuring adequate cellular material for examination.

Slide preparation: Spread the collected material evenly on a glass slide, allowing it to air-dry or fixate with methanol before staining.

Giemsa Staining Technique

Staining time: Incubate the slide with modified Giemsa stain for the specified duration (usually 8–10 minutes).

Rinse and drying: Rinse the slide gently with buffered water or distilled water, air-dry thoroughly.

Features of Donovanosis in Giemsa-stained Smears

Identification of Donovan Bodies (Klebsiella Granulomatis)

Appearance: Under microscopy, Donovan bodies appear as intracytoplasmic, oval-shaped, and bipolar staining organisms **(Fig. 5)**.

Color: Stained with Giemsa, these bodies present with a characteristic deep purplish-blue hue.

Histocytes: Often, there is an abundance of histiocytes or macrophages in the smear surrounding the Donovan bodies.

Presence within macrophages: Donovan bodies are primarily observed within the cytoplasm of histiocytes.

Diagnostic Significance

Confirmation of donovanosis: Identification of characteristic Donovan bodies within

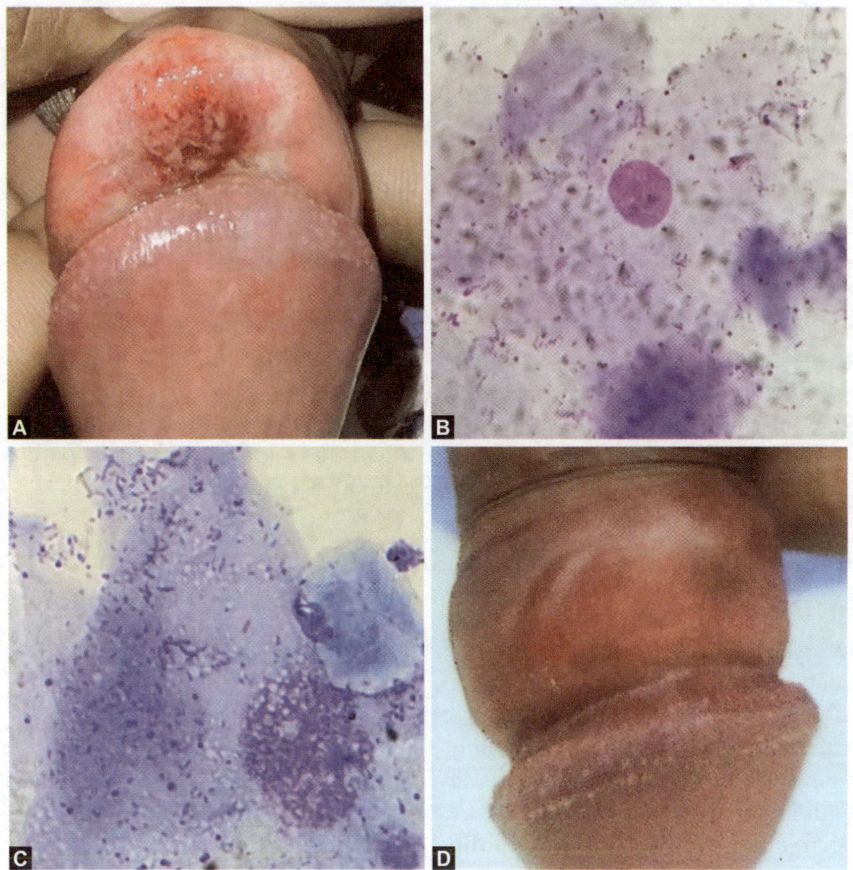

FIGS. 5A TO D: Giemsa-stained tissue smear in donovanosis.

histiocytes in Giemsa-stained smears strongly supports the diagnosis of donovanosis.

Differential diagnosis: It helps distinguish Donovan bodies from other intracellular inclusions or microorganisms seen in other conditions.[11]

DERMATOLOGICAL SIGNS IN SEXUALLY TRANSMITTED DISEASES

Groove Sign in Sexually Transmitted Diseases

Relevance: In STDs affecting the inguinal region, such as lymphogranuloma venereum (LGV), the Groove sign becomes significant.

Explanation: LGV, caused by *Chlamydia trachomatis* serotypes L1, L2, and L3, often leads to inguinal lymphadenopathy. Enlarged lymph nodes in the groin can cause palpable grooves along the lymphatic pathways due to inflammation and lymph node enlargement.

Dermatological implication: Recognition of the Groove sign aids in diagnosing LGV and assessing the extent of lymph node involvement, guiding appropriate management and treatment strategies for STD-related lymphadenopathy.[12]

Dory Flop Sign in Sexually Transmitted Diseases

Definition

The motion exhibited upon retraction of the prepuce, termed the dory flop sign, indicates a sudden flip akin to a dory, a flat-bottomed fishing boat overturning.

Named by John Stokes, this sign reflects the abrupt retraction due to induration around a syphilitic chancre, affecting the skin's elasticity.

Explanation of significance: The sudden flip during prepuce retraction highlights the decreased skin elasticity in the presence of a syphilitic chancre, suggesting induration.

While not solely diagnostic, the dory flop sign suggests syphilitic chancres, usually more indurated compared to other preputial ulcers.

Location adjacency to the frenulum, a common site for syphilitic chancres, further supports the diagnostic considerations.

Diagnostic Importance

Recognizing the dory flop sign aids in early detection and treatment of syphilitic chancres.

Early identification contributes to timely management, thereby supporting efforts in the prevention and control of syphilis.

This sign, elucidated by the sudden flip of the prepuce during retraction, denotes the decreased elasticity in the area of a syphilitic chancre, potentially aiding in prompt identification and treatment of this condition.[13]

Fluctuation in Bubo in Sexually Transmitted Diseases

Relevance: Fluctuation in a bubo is particularly significant in the context of bacterial STDs causing suppurative lymphadenitis.

Explanation: In STDs like chancroid or bubonic plague (rare but possible), infected inguinal lymph nodes can develop abscesses. The sensation of fluid movement within an enlarged lymph node upon palpation signifies abscess formation or pus accumulation.

Dermatological implication: Recognition of fluctuation in a bubo aid in diagnosing and distinguishing suppurative lymphadenitis associated with bacterial STDs, guiding appropriate antimicrobial therapy and management.[14]

WET MOUNT TECHNIQUES IN DERMATOLOGY

The wet mount technique is an invaluable tool in dermatology, allowing for the examination of skin samples under a microscope. This method provides a dynamic view of various skin conditions, aiding in the identification of microorganisms, parasites, and cellular structures.

Introduction to Wet Mount Technique

The wet mount involves preparing a slide with a small skin sample suspended in a liquid medium. By using this technique, dermatologists can observe live microorganisms or cellular elements in their natural state, enhancing the accuracy of diagnoses. The process requires precision and attention to detail to ensure a clear and reliable view under the microscope.

Materials Required

- *Microscope*: A compound light microscope with varying magnification capabilities is essential.
- *Glass slides and coverslips*: Clean and sterile slides provide a suitable surface for mounting the sample. Coverslips protect the sample and facilitate clearer observations.
- *Microscope immersion oil*: This oil aids in maximizing the resolution and clarity of high-power objectives.
- *Saline solution or other mounting media*: A liquid medium is necessary to suspend and observe the sample.

Procedure

- *Preparation of work area*:
  - Ensure a clean and sterile workspace

- ○ Wear gloves and other necessary personal protective equipment to prevent contamination
- *Sample collection*:
  - ○ Using a sterile cotton swab or another appropriate medical collection device, collect genital secretions from the affected area. Gently swab the area, ensuring minimal pressure to avoid discomfort or bleeding.
  - ○ Handle the swab carefully to prevent contamination and maintain the integrity of the sample
- *Preparation of slide*:
  - ○ Place a clean glass slide on a flat and clean surface
  - ○ Carefully transfer a small amount of the collected genital secretions from the swab onto the center of the slide. Be cautious not to touch the slide surface with the swab handle to prevent contamination.
- *Addition of mounting media*:
  - ○ Apply a few drops of sterile saline solution or suitable mounting media directly onto the genital secretion sample on the slide
  - ○ The mounting media helps to suspend the sample and facilitates observation under the microscope
  - ○ Ensure the drops cover the sample adequately without overflowing the edges of the slide
- *Cover slipping*:
  - ○ Gently place a coverslip over the sample on the slide. Hold the coverslip at a slight angle and carefully lower it onto the sample area to prevent trapping air bubbles.
  - ○ Apply light pressure using a finger or a slide presser to spread the mounting media evenly and ensure there are no bubbles.
- *Microscopic examination*:
  - ○ Place the prepared slide on the stage of a microscope
  - ○ Start with the lowest magnification objective lens to locate areas of interest or any structures present in the sample
  - ○ Gradually increase the magnification to observe cellular structures or microorganisms within the genital secretions **(Fig. 6)**
  - ○ Focus carefully by adjusting the microscope knobs to obtain a clear view and make detailed observations[15]

Precautions

- Maintain aseptic techniques throughout the process to prevent contamination
- Handle the genital secretion sample and equipment carefully to preserve the integrity of the sample
- Promptly examine the slide under the microscope as live samples may deteriorate over time
- Interpret findings based on the observed structures or organisms present in the sample

Significance in Genital Infections

- *Identification of causative agents*: Wet mounts assist in identifying the microorganisms responsible for genital

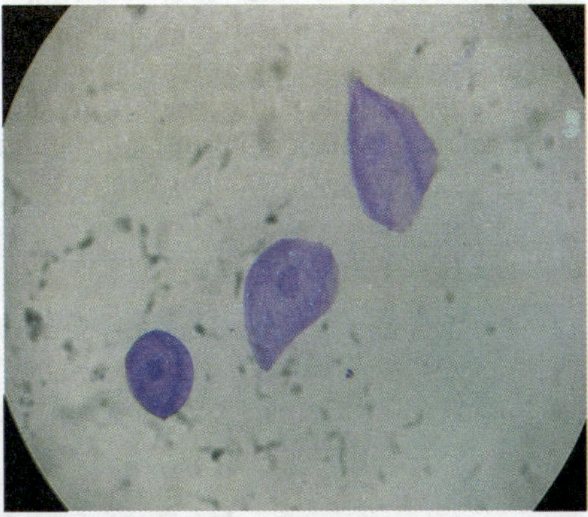

FIG. 6: Wet mount microscopy showing *Trichomonas vaginalis* species.

infections. For instance, observing yeast cells can indicate a yeast infection (such as candidiasis), while the presence of clue cells may suggest bacterial vaginosis.

- *Diagnosis of sexually transmitted infections (STIs)*: Wet mounts aid in diagnosing various STIs including trichomoniasis, gonorrhea, and genital candidiasis, by observing the characteristic microorganisms associated with these infections.
- *Assessment of inflammation*: The presence of inflammatory cells, such as neutrophils or eosinophils, in the wet mount can indicate an immune response to an infection or inflammation in the genital area.[16]

Challenges and Considerations

- *Time sensitivity*: Live samples may deteriorate quickly, requiring immediate examination to ensure accurate results.
- *Technical expertise*: Precision in sample preparation and microscopic handling is crucial for obtaining reliable observations.
- *Variability of findings*: Interpretation of wet mount findings requires experience and may vary based on the expertise of the observer.

The wet mount technique is an indispensable tool in dermatology, offering a dynamic view of skin samples that aid in diagnosing a wide array of dermatological conditions. Its ability to provide real-time observations of microorganisms and cellular elements makes it an invaluable asset in the clinical setting, enhancing diagnostic accuracy and patient care.

Clinical Significance

Sexually transmitted disease diagnosis: Urethral smears aid in diagnosing bacterial infections, such as gonorrhea, chlamydia, and nongonococcal urethritis.

Genital dermatoses identification: Beyond STDs, urethral smears can assist in identifying noninfectious dermatological and other inflammatory skin diseases.

Treatment monitoring: Urethral smears are valuable for monitoring the effectiveness of treatment. Follow-up smears post-treatment can indicate the presence or absence of the causative agent, aiding in determining treatment success.[17]

CONCLUSION

Urethral smear analysis and wet mount techniques stand as a fundamental diagnostic tool in dermatology, enabling the identification of infectious agents, inflammatory changes, and noninfectious dermatoses affecting the genital area. Its role in early diagnosis, targeted therapy, and treatment monitoring significantly contribute to effective patient management and public health efforts to control STDs and genital dermatological conditions.

Key Messages

- Bedside tests play an important role in diagnosis of STDs.
- Bedside urine tests can give a clue to urethritis.
- Smears from urethral discharge can help in diagnosing gonorrhea and chlamydial infection.
- Tzanck smear and tissue smear can help in diagnosing herpes genitalis and donovanosis respectively.

REFERENCES

1. World Health Organization. Guidelines for the management of symptomatic sexually transmitted infections: urethral discharge syndrome. Geneva: World Health Organization; 2021.

2. Centers for Disease Control and Prevention. (2021). Sexually Transmitted Infections Treatment Guidelines, 2021. [online] Available from https://www.cdc.gov/std/treatment-guidelines/urethritis-and-cervicitis.htm [Last accessed February, 2024].

3. Centers for Disease Control and Prevention. (2014). Recommendations for the Laboratory-Based Detection of *Chlamydia trachomatis* and Neisseria gonorrhoeae—2014. [online] Available from https://www.cdc.gov/std/laboratory/2014labrec/recommendations.htm [Last accessed February, 2024].

4. Moi H, Hartgill U, Skullerud KH, Reponen EJ, Syvertsen L, Moghaddam A. Microscopy of Stained Urethral Smear in Male Urethritis; Which Cutoff Should be Used? Sex Transm Dis. 2017;44(3):189-94.

5. Becerra SC, Roy DC, Sanchez CJ, Christy RJ, Burmeister DM. An optimized staining technique for the detection of Gram positive and Gram negative bacteria within tissue. BMC Res Notes. 2016;9:216.

6. Tripathi N, Sapra A. Gram Staining. Treasure Island (FL): StatPearls Publishing; 2023.

7. Seiler D, Zbinden R, Hauri D, John H. 4- oder 2-Gläserprobe bei der chronischen Prostatitis? [Four-glass or two glass test for chronic prostatitis]. Urologe A. 2003;42(2):238-42.

8. Gjurašin B, Lepej SŽ, Cole MJ, Pitt R, Begovac J. *Chlamydia trachomatis* in Cervical Lymph Node of Man with Lymphogranuloma Venereum, Croatia, 20141. Emerg Infect Dis. 2018;24(4):806-8.

9. Richens J. Main presentations of sexually transmitted infections in men. BMJ. 2004;328(7450):1251-3.

10. Dark ground microscopy and treponemal serology for diagnosis of early syphilis. J Clin Pathol. 2004;57(12):1263.

11. Richens J. Donovanosis (granuloma inguinale). Sex Transm Infect. 2006;82 Suppl 4(Suppl 4):iv21-2.

12. Ceovic R, Gulin SJ. Lymphogranuloma venereum: diagnostic and treatment challenges. Infect Drug Resist. 2015;8:39-47.

13. Raj C, Agarwal A. Dory Flop Sign in Primary Syphilis. J Cutan Med Surg. 2022;26(2):217.

14. Cunha Ramos M, Nicola MRC, Bezerra NTC, Sardinha JCG, Sampaio de Souza Morais J, Schettini AP. Genital ulcers caused by sexually transmitted agents. An Bras Dermatol. 2022;97(5):551-65.

15. Patil MJ, Nagamoti JM, Metgud SC. Diagnosis of Trichomonas Vaginalis from Vaginal Specimens by Wet Mount Microscopy, In Pouch TV Culture System, and PCR. J Glob Infect Dis. 2012;4(1):22-5.

16. Stoner KA, Rabe LK, Meyn LA, Hillier SL. Survival of Trichomonas vaginalis in wet preparation and on wet mount. Sex Transm Infect. 2013;89(6):485-8.

17. Madico G, Quinn TC, Rompalo A, McKee KT Jr, Gaydos CA. Diagnosis of Trichomonas vaginalis infection by PCR using vaginal swab samples. J Clin Microbiol. 1998;36(11):3205-10.

Dark-field Microscopy

AW Kashif, Aneez Ali, Lalita Kumari

INTRODUCTION

In the realm of dermatology, the use of advanced imaging techniques has revolutionized the way skin disorders are diagnosed and understood. Dark-field microscopy, a powerful tool in the armamentarium of pathologists, has emerged as a valuable method for observing microorganisms and structures that might otherwise go unnoticed. Dark-field microscopy is a specialized optical microscopy technique that allows the visualization of translucent specimens against a dark background.[1] This technique employs a specialized condenser that blocks direct light from entering the objective lens, illuminating the sample with oblique or angled light. The light that is scattered or refracted by the specimen is then collected by the objective lens, producing an image where the specimen appears bright against a dark background.

EVOLUTION OF DARK-FIELD MICROSCOPY

The history of dark-field microscopy dates back to the 17th century when early microscopists experimented with different illumination techniques to improve the visualization of microscopic specimens. However, it was in the 19th century that dark-field microscopy was more formally developed and used in scientific research. One of the pioneers in dark-field microscopy was Friedrich Reinitzer, an Austrian scientist who, in the late 19th century, developed a dark-field microscope to study colloidal solutions and microscopic particles.[2,3] His work laid the groundwork for the application of dark-field illumination in microscopy.

August Köhler, a German microscopist, further refined dark-field microscopy in the late 19th and early 20th centuries by developing a standardized method of illuminating specimens using specialized dark-field condensers and techniques to optimize the illumination angle.[4] Dark-field microscopy found extensive applications in various scientific fields, including biology, materials science, and medicine. It became particularly useful in observing live and unstained biological specimens, such as bacteria, cells, and small organisms, allowing researchers and pathologists to study their morphology, behavior, and interactions without the need for staining, which could alter the specimens.

In medicine, dark-field microscopy has been utilized in various areas, including the examination of blood samples for the visualization of live microorganisms like spirochetes, which cause diseases such as syphilis and Lyme disease. This technique enabled the observation of these organisms in their natural state without the need for fixation or staining. Over time, advancements in microscopy technology, including phase contrast and fluorescence microscopy, provided alternative methods for visualizing transparent or unstained specimens, contributing to the evolution of microscopy techniques beyond dark-field microscopy.[5]

Today, while dark-field microscopy remains a valuable tool in certain applications, newer microscopy techniques and imaging modalities continue to expand researchers and pathologists capabilities for observing and analyzing microscopic structures and processes. As a pathologist, understanding the history and principles of various microscopy techniques, including dark-field microscopy, can aid in the interpretation and analysis of microscopic samples and contribute to a comprehensive understanding of pathological conditions.

In the primary stage of syphilis, it is the most specific and sensitive technique to diagnose and can confirm it even before serological testing. This technique provides a presumptive diagnosis of syphilis even before the development of antibodies. Although ordinary light microscope can be used to visualize unstained living organisms, they are seen much more clearly and with a better resolution using a dark-field microscope which has an optical system that enhances the contrast of unstained bodies.

However, dark-field microscopes are quite expensive and not widely used. A simple modification to ordinary light microscope can be can be used in resource poor settings.[6] In this chapter, we emphasize on the principle and uses of bed side dark filed microscopy.

PRINCIPLE OF DARK-FIELD MICROSCOPY

The fundamental principle of dark-field microscopy lies in preventing direct light from entering the objective lens. Instead, light is directed around the specimen, and only scattered or refracted light rays enter the objective, resulting in the specimen appearing bright against a dark background **(Fig. 1)**. This method accentuates minute details and increases visibility, particularly for transparent or translucent structures, aiding in the visualization of live and unstained specimens.[7]

In the context of syphilis diagnosis, this technique leverages the unique morphology and motility of *Treponema pallidum*. The spiral-shaped bacteria are slender and highly motile, making them challenging to detect using conventional microscopy methods **(Fig. 1)**.

PARTS OF A DARK-FIELD MICROSCOPE

It consists of several key components that work together to create a specialized illumination technique for viewing translucent specimens against a dark background. Here is a brief description of the main parts of a dark-field microscope:

- *Light source*: This can be a halogen lamp or another light source that provides intense illumination. The light passes through the condenser and is directed toward the specimen.
- *Condenser*: The condenser is a critical component in dark-field microscopy. It is designed to block direct light from entering the objective lens. Instead, it allows only oblique or angled light to pass through. This angled light hits the specimen from the sides, creating a contrasting effect where the specimen appears bright against a dark background.
- *Specimen stage*: The stage is where the specimen is placed for observation. It holds the specimen slide securely in place and allows for precise movement and adjustments to focus on specific areas of interest.

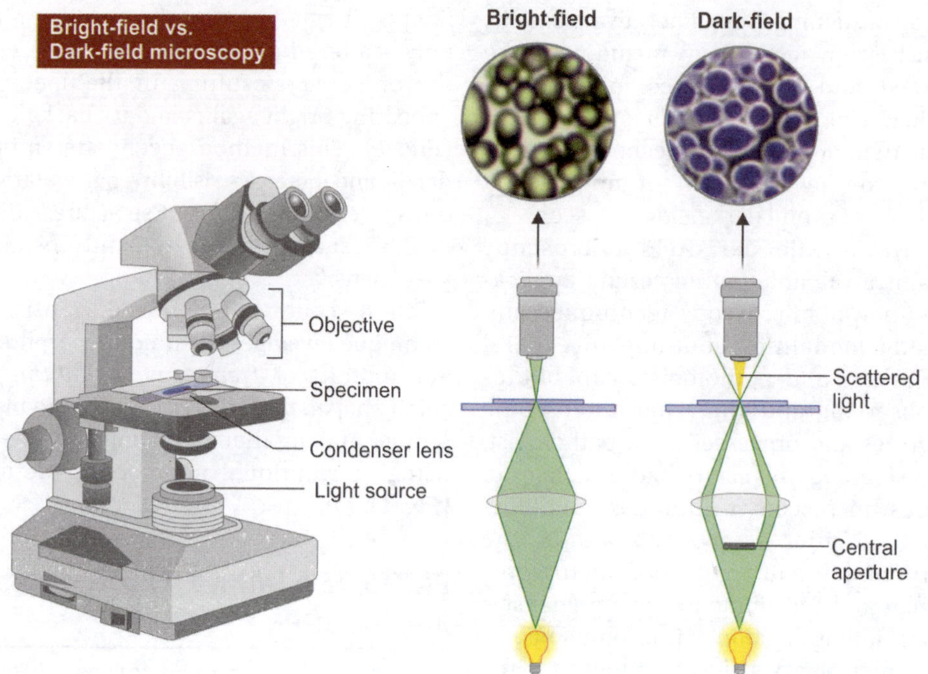

FIG. 1: Differences between a light-field and dark-field microscope.

- *Objective lens*: Similar to other types of microscopes, dark-field microscopes have various objective lenses with different magnification levels. The objective lens collects the light that has been scattered or refracted by the specimen, creating the magnified image that is observed by the user.
- *Eyepiece or ocular lens*: The eyepiece further magnifies the image produced by the objective lens, allowing the observer to see the specimen in greater detail.
- *Adjustment controls*: Dark-field microscopes have controls for adjusting the focus, stage positioning, and sometimes the angle of the light to optimize the illumination for the best image quality.

The dark-field microscope's unique design prevents direct light from entering the objective lens, resulting in a dark background and allowing only the light that is scattered or refracted by the specimen to be observed. This creates high contrast and enhances the visibility of the specimen's fine details, making it particularly useful for viewing live, unstained, or transparent specimens such as certain bacteria, cells, or small organisms.

Understanding these components and their functions is crucial for using a dark-field microscope effectively in observing and analyzing various specimens in fields such as biology, microbiology, and pathology.

PREREQUISITES FOR CREATING A DARK-FIELD MICROSCOPE

There is a cost-effective method for converting a light microscope into a dark ground microscope. It entails use of following:

- *A dark-field condenser*: Its purpose is to restrict the direct light from the lamp source and allows the focused oblique light onto the specimen.

- *A funnel stop*: This reduces the aperture size of the objective lens to <1.0.
- A high intensity lamp.

Steps to Convert a Light Microscope to Dark-field Microscopy

- *Adjustment of condenser*:
  - Begin by removing the standard bright field condenser from the microscope.
  - Replace it with a specialized dark-field condenser designed for this purpose. The dark-field condenser has an arrangement that blocks direct light from entering the objective lens.
- *Insertion of dark-field stop*: Place a dark-field stop or patch stop beneath the condenser. This stop blocks the central portion of the light beam, allowing only oblique or scattered light rays to pass through to the specimen.
- *Light source modification*: Modify the light source by incorporating a specialized annular or oblique lighting system that directs light at an angle onto the specimen. This ensures that only scattered light reaches the objective lens, creating the dark-field effect.
- *Sample preparation*: Prepare the specimen as usual on a clean glass slide, ensuring proper mounting and alignment for observation under dark-field conditions.
- *Microscope alignment*: Insert the prepared slide into the microscope stage and focus the objective lens carefully to obtain a clear view of the specimen against the dark background.
- *Observation and imaging*:
  - Observe the specimen under the modified dark-field conditions, where structures not visible in bright field microscopy become highlighted against the dark background.
  - Capture images or make observations as required for analysis and documentation.

Converting a light microscope to dark-field microscopy requires precision in adjustments and the incorporation of specialized components to manipulate the light path effectively. These modifications enhance the microscope's capabilities, enabling the visualization of translucent or transparent specimens with improved contrast and clarity **(Figs. 2A and B)**.

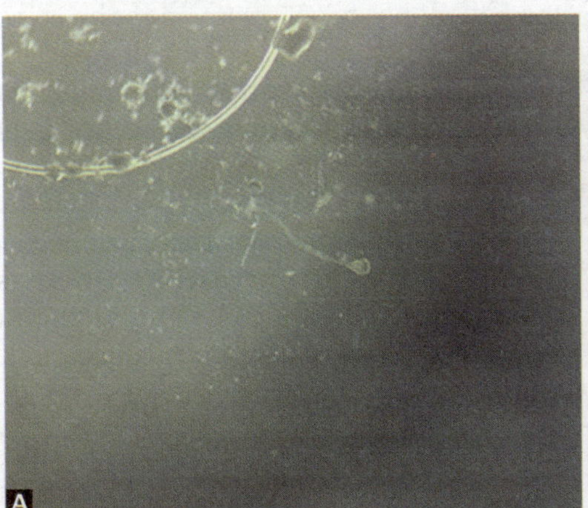
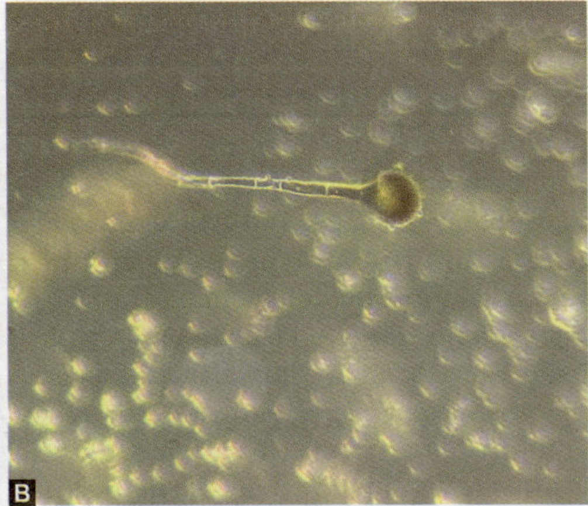

FIGS. 2A AND B: An image of a septate, acute angle branched fungal hyphae with terminal vesicle and conidia as visualized under a dark-field microscope (A—100×; B—400×). The dark-field microscope used in the imaging was converted from a light microscope as per the methodology explained earlier.

PROCEDURE FOR SAMPLE COLLECTION IN CASE OF SYPHILIS FOR DARK-FIELD MICROSCOPY

- *General*: The primary source for detecting *T. pallidum* using dark-field microscopy is the collection of samples from active syphilitic lesions.
  - Clear the wound site by removing any scab/crust and exudates with a piece of gauze or cotton.
  - Squeeze the base of the lesion to let collect tissue fluid on the surface.
  - Using a glass slide, gently touch it to the surface of the lesion.
  - Apply a glass coverslip on the slide specimen. Remove any air bubble by tapping the coverslip.
  - Quickly examine the slide under dark-field microscope.
- *In case of dry, papule-squamous lesions in the skin:*
  - Gently remove the superficial layers of the skin.
  - Compress the lesion to let fluid accumulate.
  - Touch a glass slide to the lesion.
  - Place a coverslip on the slide and examine under dark-field microscope.

INTERPRETATIONS OF DARK-FIELD MICROSCOPY IN CASE OF SYPHILIS

Treponema pallidum can be visualized as brightly illuminated objects against a dark background **(Figs. 2A and B)**. The two key features to identify treponemes are their morphology and unique motility. The size of *T. pallidum* varies from 6 to 16 µm in length and 0.25 to 0.3 µm in width. In addition, they typically have 8–14 regularly placed, tightly wound, deep spirals. The nonsyphilitic spirochaetes such as *T. pertenue* and *T. carateum* differ in them having irregular loose and thick coils. The motility of the two groups also differs. While the *T. pallidum*

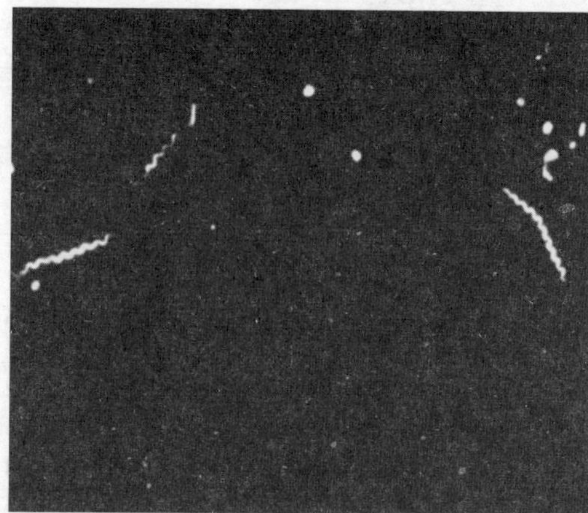

FIG. 3: *Treponema pallidum* visualized in dark-field microscopy.

have abrupt and quick movements (akin to corkscrew movement with bending and twisting), the nonsyphilitic treponemes have more writhing movement.

One must remain careful while interpreting the motility of the organism as false positive results may occur if the motility is mistaken or if there is no organism, especially in an oral sample. In fact, whenever one does find spirochaetes in oral cavity, it must be confirmed by various immunological methods. Likewise false-negative results may occur if there is insufficient exudate or the patient has taken treatment or he is in a natural remission phase of the disease. The delay in sample preparation and examination of slide may also lead to false-negative result **(Fig. 3)**.

Hence, it is always advisable to collect blood sample for serological tests irrespective of the dark-field microscopy findings. Ideally three consecutive samples should be examined before a lesion is labeled nonsyphilitic.

ADVANTAGES OF DARK-FIELD MICROSCOPY

The thin and fragile organism is difficult to be identified by light microscopy. The high resolution of a dark ground microscope allows easy recognition.

LIMITATIONS OF DARK-FIELD MICROSCOPY

- As the light passes around rather than through the organism, the internal anatomy/morphology of organisms cannot be studied.
- In cases of rectal or nongenital lesions, due to interference from the commensal spirochetes, dark-field microscopy may not be reliable.
- Transmission risk of human immuno-deficiency virus (HIV)/hepatitis C/ hepatitis B infection from contaminated specimens.

APPLICATIONS IN DERMATOLOGY

Dark-field microscopy, with its ability to highlight fine structures and details of translucent specimens against a dark background, finds several applications across various scientific fields, including dermatology.[8] In dermatology, dark-field microscopy can be employed for several purposes:

- *Observation of skin lesions*: Dark-field microscopy allows dermatologists to examine skin lesions, such as rashes, lesions, or ulcerations, in a noninvasive manner. It helps in observing microorganisms, such as bacteria or fungi, present on the skin's surface or within skin lesions.
- *Detection of microorganisms*: It enables the visualization and identification of various microorganisms that might be implicated in skin conditions, including bacteria such as *T. pallidum* (the causative agent of syphilis), *Demodex* mites, certain yeasts, and other parasites. For instance, in cases of suspected *Demodex* infestation contributing to skin disorders like rosacea or blepharitis, dark-field microscopy can help in detecting and observing these mites.
- *Diagnosis of infectious skin diseases*: Dark-field microscopy aids in diagnosing infectious skin diseases caused by specific microorganisms. For example, in syphilis diagnosis, the visualization of *T. pallidum* using dark-field microscopy from skin lesions or serous exudates can confirm the presence of the bacteria and help in diagnosing the disease.
- *Evaluation of wound infections*: For chronic wounds or ulcers, dark-field microscopy can be used to examine wound exudates to identify the presence of bacteria or other microorganisms contributing to the infection. This information can guide appropriate treatment strategies for wound management.
- *Monitoring treatment progress*: It can be useful in monitoring the effectiveness of treatment for certain skin conditions. By observing changes in the presence or concentration of microorganisms over time, dermatologists can assess treatment responses and adjust therapies accordingly.
- *Research and education*: Dark-field microscopy is valuable in research and educational settings within dermatology. It allows researchers to study the behavior, morphology, and interactions of microorganisms associated with various skin conditions, contributing to a deeper understanding of dermatological diseases.

While dark-field microscopy can provide valuable insights in dermatology, it is important to note that it may not be the primary diagnostic tool for all skin conditions. Its utility often complements other diagnostic techniques and clinical assessments performed by dermatologists to provide a comprehensive understanding of skin diseases and aid in appropriate patient management.[9]

CONCLUSION

Dark-field microscopy stands as a valuable, convenient adjunct in the diagnostic armamentarium of dermatologists and pathologists. Its ability to illuminate the unseen, uncover minute details, and provide real-time observations contributes significantly to the understanding and diagnosis of a myriad of dermatological conditions, mainly in the identification of *T. pallidum*, the causative agent of syphilis.[10] By capitalizing on the distinct morphology and motility of the spirochetes, this technique enables accurate and rapid diagnosis, especially in cases where other diagnostic methods may be inconclusive. A meticulous approach to sample collection, microscope preparation, and methodical observation are crucial for the successful application of dark-field microscopy in syphilis detection, aiding in timely intervention and disease management.

Key Messages

- The dark-field microscope's unique design prevents direct light from entering the objective lens, resulting in a dark background and allowing only the light that is scattered or refracted by the specimen to be observed. This creates high contrast and enhances the visibility of the specimen's fine details, making it particularly useful for viewing live, unstained, or transparent specimens such as certain bacteria, cells, or small organisms.
- Dark-field microscopy particularly useful in observing live and unstained biological specimens, such as bacteria, cells, and small organisms, allowing researchers and pathologists to study their morphology, behavior, and interactions without the need for staining, which could alter the specimens.
- Advancements in microscopy technology, including phase contrast and fluorescence microscopy, provided alternative methods for visualizing transparent or unstained specimens, contributing to the evolution of microscopy techniques beyond dark-field microscopy.
- In the primary stage of syphilis, dark-field microscopy is the most specific and sensitive technique to diagnose and can confirm it even before serological testing.
- In the context of syphilis diagnosis, this technique leverages the unique morphology and motility of *T. pallidum*. The spiral-shaped bacteria are slender and highly motile, making them challenging to detect using conventional microscopy methods.

REFERENCES

1. Motic Microscopes. (2021). Introduction to Dark-Field Microscopy. [online] Available from https://moticmicroscopes.com/blogs/articles/introduction-to-dark-field-microscopy. [Last accessed February, 2024].

2. ASM.org. (2020). A Brief History of Laboratory Diagnostics for Syphilis. [online] Available from https://asm.org:443/Articles/2020/January/A-Brief-History-of-Laboratory-Diagnostics-for-Syph. [Last accessed February, 2024].

3. Bai Y, Abbott NL. Recent Advances in Colloidal and Interfacial Phenomena Involving Liquid Crystals. Langmuir ACS J Surf Colloids. 2011;27(10):5719-38.

4. Bagnell CR. Dark field microscopy. In book: Pathology; 2012.

5. Weigel A, Sebesta A, Kukura P. Dark Field Microspectroscopy with Single Molecule Fluorescence Sensitivity. ACS Photonics. 2014;1(9):848-56.

6. Sriram CK, Sivakumar A. (2022). Cost-effective method of dark field microscopy in everyday

practice. [online] Available from https://cosmoderma.org/cost-effective-method-of-dark-field-microscopy-in-everyday-practice/. [Last accessed February, 2024].

7. Ambooken B, Binesh VG, Asokan N, Sarin A, Natarajan B, Subi CT. Dark ground microscopy for identification of Treponema pallidum. J Skin Sex Transm Dis. 2022.

8. Aryal S. (2022). Darkfield Microscope—Definition, Principle, Uses, Diagram. [online] Available from https://microbenotes.com/darkfield-microscopy/. [Last accessed February, 2024].

9. Mehta V, Saurav K, Balachandran C. Dark ground microscopy. Indian J Sex Transm Dis. 2008;29(2): 105-6.

10. Wheeler HL, Agarwal S, Goh BT. Dark ground microscopy and treponemal serological tests in the diagnosis of early syphilis. Sex Transm Infect. 2004;80(5):411-4.

Bedside Urine Tests

Vijayshankar Palaniappan, Ankan Gupta, Sunmeet Sandhu, Sreechithra Menon

INTRODUCTION

Medical tests are playing an increasingly vital role in the diagnosis and treatment of diseases. Blood tests, urine tests, and stool tests constitute the three major routine examinations of modern medicine. Modern laboratory practice in developing and developed nations has long moved beyond piecework manual procedures and primarily utilizes fully automated systems for the diagnosis of medical conditions. However, the availability of kits, high cost, and support from an expert technician for the interpretation of results are a few cons associated with advanced laboratory facilities.[1,2]

Urine is a body fluid rich in biological information, metabolized by the human body, and excreted through the urinary system. It is the easiest bodily fluid to obtain and can be studied in resource-poor settings where it is of great value in improving diagnostic and therapeutic pathways. Compared with using blood as a test sample, medical tests in urine samples have several advantages such as convenient collection, noninvasiveness, collection in large quantities, easy to store, handle, and transport, at times can be monitored macroscopically, and aids in the early diagnosis of diseases.[1-4] This chapter intends to provide an overview of bedside urine tests that can aid dermatologists.

INHERITED DISORDERS

Alkaptonuria

Alkaptonuria is characterized by congenital absence of homogentisate 1,2-dioxygenase resulting in defective tyrosine metabolism. Homogentisate accumulates in body fluids and is excreted in the urine which darkens on standing. The condition may be initially noticed in infancy when the napkins are stained black. In later life, most cartilage is stained black. This may have a bluish-grey tinge to the pinna of the ear and nose. The affected synovial cartilage is more easily damaged by the mechanical forces.[5]

Visualization of Urine

Principle: Homogentisic acid in an alkaline medium undergoes oxidative polymerization to quinone derivatives which are brown to black.

Reagents: Not needed

Procedure: Take 5–10 mL freshly voided urine sample in a clean test tube and keep it aside for 10–12 hours.

Interpretation: Fresh urine samples will be usually pale yellow, but on keeping aside for 12 hours, the top layer turns brown black **(Fig. 1)**.

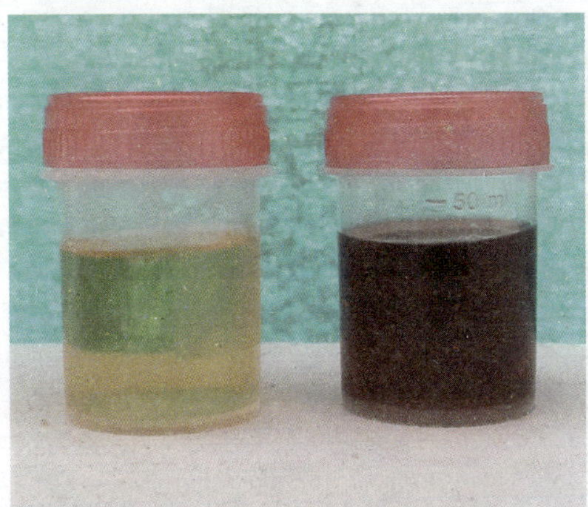

FIG. 1: Pale-yellow fresh urine sample and brown-black sample on keeping aside for 12 hours.

Ferric Chloride Test

Principle: Phenols of homogentisic acid form a violet complex with Fe (III), which is intensely colored.

Reagent: 10% ferric chloride solution: 2 g ferric chloride salt is dissolved in 100 mL distilled water. To this, add 1 mL 2N HCl.

Procedure: To 1 mL urine sample, add 2–4 drops of 10% ferric chloride solution. Mix gently and observe the color change.

Interpretation: A transient blue color that rapidly fades within 1 minute indicates a positive test.[4,6]

AMINO ACID DISORDERS

Phenylketonuria

Phenylketonuria is an autosomal recessive inherited amino acid metabolism disorder that occurs due to a defect in the phenylalanine hydroxylase enzyme, the enzyme that catalyzes the conversion of phenylalanine to tyrosine. It results in increased phenylalanine concentrations in the blood. In skin, untreated patients have an increased incidence of eczema (20–40%). They may also have reduced pigmentation of the skin, hair, and iris. The urine specimen can be useful in screening for phenylketonuria. However, it lacks sensitivity and specificity.[4,7]

Test-tube Test with Ferric Chloride

It is the oldest, best-known, and most widely used diagnostic urine test for phenylketonuria.

Reagents required: Ferric chloride solution and sulfuric acid

Procedure: Add 2 drops of ferric chloride solution (50 g/L water) to 1 mL urine.

Add sulfuric acid (50 mL/L in water) dropwise to dissolve any precipitate.

Interpretation: The presence of phenylpyruvic acid gives an immediate medium-dark blue-green to gray-green color response, which begins to fade in a matter of seconds or minutes depending on the concentration of phenylpyruvic acid in the urine and the strength of the ferric chloride solution being used.[4,8]

METABOLIC DISORDERS

Porphyria Cutanea Tarda

Porphyria cutanea tarda (PCT) is a metabolic disorder that occurs due to a deficiency of the enzyme uroporphyrinogen decarboxylase (UROD). It results in the accumulation of highly carboxylated porphyrinogens like uroporphyrinogen in the liver that eventually appear in the plasma and urine.[9] Although various methods have been developed for the estimation of increased porphyrin levels in the urine, Wood's lamp examination is a simple and rapid bedside screening test for PCT.[10,11]

Procedure: In a test tube, to a 5 mL fresh urine specimen, 1 mL glacial acetic acid, 5 mL of ethyl ether, and three drops of fresh 3% hydrogen peroxide are added in the sequence.

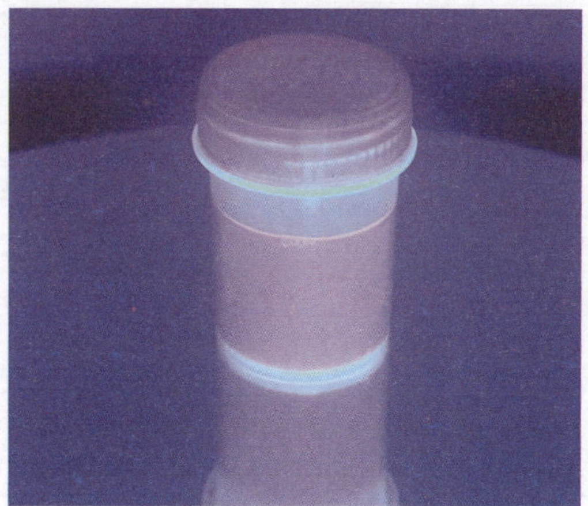

FIG. 2: Orange-pink fluorescence under Wood's lamp examination in a case of porphyria cutanea tarda.

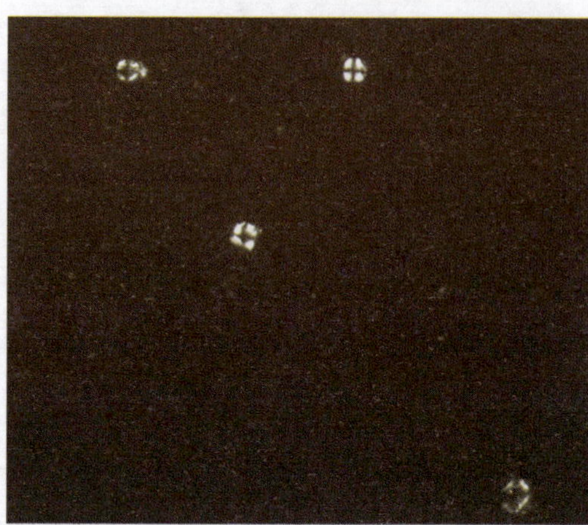

FIG. 3: Maltese cross appearance of mulberry cells under polarizing microscopy in a case of Fabry disease.

The test tube should be closed with a rubber stopper inverted a few times and allowed to stand for 10 minutes.

Examine the specimen under Wood's lamp.

Interpretation: Orange-pink fluorescence is indicative of the presence of porphyrinogens in the urine **(Fig. 2)**.[4,11]

Fabry Disease

Fabry disease is a deficiency of lysosomal enzyme alpha-galactosidase A, manifesting as an inherited neurological disorder. Absence of enzyme leads to inefficient breakdown of glycolipids, specifically, globotriaosylceramide (Gb3), which build up to harmful levels in the body's autonomic nervous system, eyes, kidneys, and cardiovascular system.[12]

Procedure: The first void sample is preferred and smeared on a slide and visualized under a 40K lens.

Interpretation: Mulberry cells, which are kidney-derived cells, with accumulated Gb3 can be seen. The presence of just proteinuria and albuminuria without the classical mulberry cells in the correct context is also suggestive of renal involvement in Fabry disease **(Fig. 3)**.[4]

LEPROSY

Urine Spot Test for Monitoring Dapsone Self-administration

History of the presence of orange-pink discoloration is a recognized marker of compliance with monthly rifampicin dosing in leprosy. Daily self-administration of dapsone is a vital part of multidrug regimens recommended by the World Health Organization. Several tests to monitor patient compliance have been described in the past. The late H Huikeshoven in the early research of de Castro in Brazil recommended the field use of the urine spot test for monitoring dapsone self-administration.

Reagent: 0.2 g p-Dimethylaminobenzaldehyde, 1.0 g oxalic acid, and 0.1 g sodium dodecylbenzene-sulfonate are dissolved in 100 mL of 50–70% (v/v) ethanol.

Procedure: Preparation of controls.

Solution (A): A negative control solution is prepared by adding 10 mL of 1 mol/L HCl to

90 mL of urine from an individual who has not taken dapsone or sulfonamides.

Solution (B): Dissolve 1 g dapsone in 100 mL of 1 mol/L HCl. Then 1 mL of this solution (B) is added to 49 mL of water to give solution (C).

Finally, 1 mL of solution (C) is added to 39 mL of solution (A) to give solution (D), the positive control, which contains approximately 5 mg/L dapsone in acidified urine.

Spot test: A drop of urine is placed on the impregnated filter paper.

After 1 minute, a yellow ring appears at the periphery, caused by urea, and an inner orange spot develops if dapsone is present.

The urine spots are best examined by viewing the paper against the light.

The urine is positive if it gives a central spot whose intensity is more than equals to that produced by the positive control test (D).

In a borderline case, a spot is taken to be positive, particularly if the solution is rather colorless.

Interpretation: A positive test corresponds to sulfone levels in the blood well above the minimum inhibitory concentration for the multiplication of *Mycobacterium leprae*.

A negative test indicates that dapsone was not taken according to the schedule of 100 mg/day and possibly, that the time since the last intake is sufficiently long for the level of dapsone in blood to have fallen below the minimum inhibitory concentration.[13,14]

INVESTIGATION OF URETHRITIS

Two-glass Test

This is a time-honored test, considered by some to be of debatable value. It can help to differentiate pure urethritis (usually sexually acquired) from urethritis in association with cystitis [i.e., a urinary tract infection (UTI), and not sexually acquired].

Procedure: The patient is asked to hold urine overnight and come in the morning without any active treatment. The patient is asked to pass urine in two glasses (approximately 50 mL each). Any remaining urine is passed into the urinal.

Interpretation: If both the glasses are clear, it is considered normal **(Fig. 4)**.

If the first specimen contains threads, and flakes, or is hazy with pus, and the second glass is clear, it indicates anterior urethritis.

If both specimens contain pus, it indicates posterior urethritis or cystitis.

The addition of acetic acid will clear when excess phosphates are causing haziness, as phosphaturia is a common cause of cloudy urine. If the haze remains, it indicates pyuria.

Three-glass Test

For greater accuracy, it is necessary to apply a three-glass test.

Procedure: The anterior urethra is irrigated with a colorless antiseptic solution (such as 1:8,000 oxy cyanide of mercury) until the washings contained in the glass seem to be

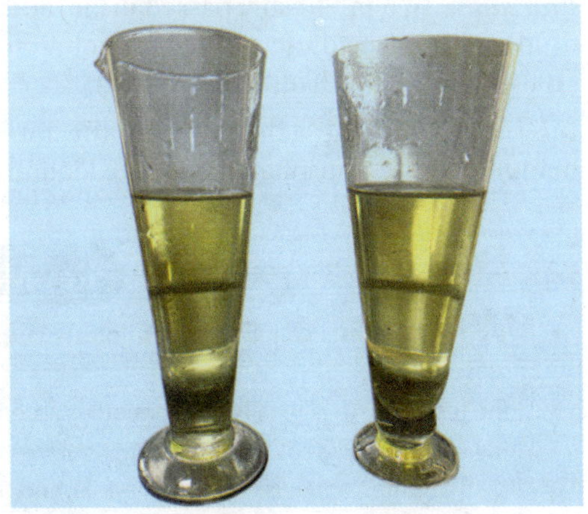

FIG. 4: Normal two-glass urine test showing clear urine in both first and second specimens.

clear. This is taken as the first glass. Then, the patient is asked to pass urine in two glasses.

Interpretation: If pus is present in the second glass, it indicates the posterior urethra is infected.

If pus is present in the third glass, it indicates bladder infection.

Another variation of this test, the glass test is done for diagnosing prostatic involvement, which is better done by urologists.[15,16]

SKIN TUMORS

Malignant Melanoma

Principle: Melanin can be found in the urine of patients with malignant melanoma, usually when there are secondaries in the liver. Freshly passed urines contain a colorless precursor, melanogen, which is oxidized to melanin when the urine is allowed to stand in contact with air. The urine slowly darkens to dark brown or black, from the surface downward, taking as long as 24 hours or more to become distinctly noticeable.

Ferric Chloride Test

Principle: It is based on the oxidation of melanogen to melanin by ferric chloride.

Procedure: To 5 mL freshly passed urine, add drop by drop an acidic ferric chloride solution (100 g/L in 3 mol/L hydrochloric acid).

Interpretation: The acid prevents the formation of ferric phosphate but the oxidation of melanogen results in a darkening in urine color from varying shades of brown to black according to the amount of melanin formed.

Nitroprusside Test of Thormählen

Procedure: Freshly prepare sodium nitroprusside solution by dissolving a few crystals in a few mL of water.

Add 3 or 4 drops of the nitroprusside solution to about 5 mL urine and make it strongly alkaline with about 0.5 mL sodium hydroxide.

Shake well to mix and add a few mL of acetic acid.

Interpretation: The presence of melanogen is characterized by the development of a blue to blue-black color.

The actual color depends on the color of the original urine. If the urine is deep yellow, a dark-green color will appear after the reaction. The less pigmented the urine, the bluer the color produced.[4]

CONCLUSION

Urine is a freely available noninvasive "substrate" of kidneys, which can guide a clinician to several pathogenetic mechanisms happening in the body. The presence of renal involvement in several skin diseases can sometimes guide a treatment modification, but it is these reagent-based special tests that prove extremely cost-effective in practice.

Key Messages

- Bedside urine tests can aid dermatologists in quick assessment of certain metabolic and infectious diseases.
- Urine tests help in clinically differentiating anterior urethritis, posterior urethritis, and cystitis.
- Urine samples have several advantages such as convenient collection, noninvasiveness, collection in large quantities, and ease to store, handle, and transport.
- Most of the urine tests involve macroscopical examination of samples, aiding in the early diagnosis of diseases.

REFERENCES

1. Zhang Z, Liu J, Cheng Y, Chen J, Zhao H, Ren X. Urine analysis has a very broad prospect in the future. Front Anal Sci. 2022;1:812301.

2. Lepowsky E, Ghaderinezhad F, Knowlton S, Tasoglu S. Paper-based assays for urine analysis. Biomicrofluidics. 2017;11(5):051501.

3. Dreyer G. Examining the urine–what can it tell us at the bed-side? Malawi Med J. 2010;22(4):126-8.

4. Gowenlock AH, Varley H, McMurray JR, McLauchlan M. Varley's Practical Clinical Biochemistry, 6th edition. London: Heinemann Professional Publishing Ltd.;1988.

5. Zatkova A, Ranganath L, Kadasi L. Alkaptonuria: Current perspectives. Appl Clin Genet. 2020;13: 37-47.

6. Jacomelli G, Micheli V, Bernardini G, Millucci L, Santucci A. Quick diagnosis of alkaptonuria by homogentisic acid determination in urine paper spots. JIMD Rep. 2017;31:51-6.

7. van Spronsen FJ, Blau N, Harding C, Burlina A, Longo N, Bosch AM. Phenylketonuria. Nat Rev Dis Primers. 2021;7(1):36.

8. Centerwall WR, Chinnock RF, Pusavat A. Phenylketonuria: Screening programs and testing methods. Am J Public Health Nations Health. 1960;50(11):1667-77.

9. Di Pierro E, De Canio M, Mercadante R, Savino M, Granata F, Tavazzi D, et al. Laboratory Diagnosis of Porphyria. Diagnostics (Basel). 2021;11(8): 1343.

10. Edel Y, Mamet R. Porphyria: What is it and who should be evaluated? Rambam Maimonides Med J. 2018;9(2):e0013.

11. Ponka D, Baddar F. Wood lamp examination. Can Fam Physician. 2012;58(9):976.

12. Lenders M, Brand E. Fabry Disease: The current treatment landscape. Drugs. 2021;81(6):635-45

13. Huikeshoven H. A simple urine spot test for monitoring dapsone self-administration in leprosy treatment. Bull World Health Organ. 1986;64(2):279-81.

14. Ellard GA, Gammon PT, Helmy HS, Rees RJ. Urine tests to monitor the self-administration of dapsone by leprosy patients. Am J Trop Med Hyg. 1974;23(3):464-70.

15. Seiler D, Zbinden R, Hauri D, John H. [Four-glass or two glass test for chronic prostatitis]. Urologe A. 2003;42(2):238-42.

16. Hussen SA (Ed). Sexually Transmitted Infections in Adolescence and Young Adulthood. A Practical Guide for Clinicians, 1st edition. Switzerland: Springer Cham; 2020.

Wood's Lamp

Bhabani Singh, Sonal Jain, Prince Malla

INTRODUCTION

While most skin diseases are diagnosed by clinical examination, technological advances have led dermatologists to take help from various sophisticated devices to refine their clinical and diagnostic skills. Since the discovery of the light spectrum, ultraviolet (UV) light has been used in the medical field for multiple purposes. As early as 1903, the world saw the invention of Wood's lamp, which has stood the test of time and is being used for various purposes in the medical field. Still, it was not until 1925 that Margaret and Deveze first used Wood's lamp for detecting fungal infections of hair and paved the way for the practical use of this device in dermatology.[1] Robert Williams Wood (Baltimore physicist) discovered this technology and instrument. Skin examination with Wood's lamp is easy, quick to perform, noninvasive, safe, accurate, and requires minimal training. Wood's lamp is a small, durable, readily available, inexpensive device with minimal maintenance **(Figs. 1A and B)**.

PRINCIPLE

Long-wave UV radiation, also called black light is emitted by Wood's lamp via a Wood's filter made up of a high-pressure mercury arc fitted with barium silicate with 9% nickel

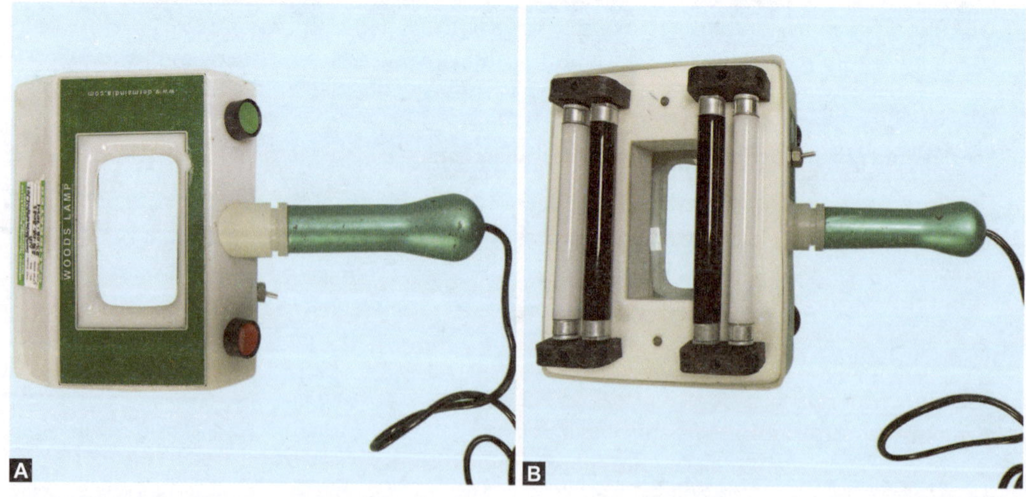

FIGS. 1A AND B: Wood's lamp instrument.

oxide. This filter blocks all light rays except the 320–400 nm band with a peak at 365 nm. It works on the principle of fluorescence or phosphorescence wherein a light of longer wavelength is produced by the tissue following irradiation with UV light as a result of photochemical response.

Skin comprises a myriad of fluorescent compounds, such as collagen, elastin, and coenzymes, which are responsive to ultraviolet A (UVA) light but because of the low concentrations of these compounds, their mutual fluorescence cannot be distinguished in broad daylight. In a dark room, normal skin emits bluish fluorescence. The fluorescence pattern and color change if the skin is diseased.

PREREQUISITE

Prior fulfilment of a few conditions is needed to increase its sensitivity and better results.
- Prior warming of the lamp for at least 1 minute.
- A dark examination room with no windows or black occlusive shades.
- The examiner should be dark and accommodated before the examination.
- The lamp should be kept at least 4–5 inches from the lesion.
- Before the examination, avoid washing the area because it may lead to false-negative results due to pigment dilution.
- Topical medicines, fibers, and soap particles should be removed from the examination site since these can emit fluorescent petrolatum emit bluish or purplish fluorescence, salicylic acid emits green fluorescence, and the examiner's white apron can produce blue fluorescence.
- The patient's eyes should be covered to prevent injury to the retina or conjunctiva.

APPLICATIONS

In dermatology, Wood's lamp is predominantly used to diagnose pigmentary disorders, infections, infestations, and porphyria. The various indications and science involved are briefly explained hereby.

Pigmentary Disorders (Table 1)

The intensity of the fluorescence signal is diminished by melanin on the absorption of Wood's light, thus making Wood's lamp quite helpful in diagnosing pigmentary disorders. However, Wood's lamp examination is unreliable in Fitzpatrick skin type VI individuals because of the requirement of low levels of endogenous melanin to make out subtle pigmentary changes increased by Wood's lamp. Hence, pigmented lesions in them are better apparent under visible light than UV light.

TABLE 1: Wood's lamp application in pigmentary disorders.

Disease	Chromophore	Fluorescence
Melasma	Epidermal/dermal melanin	Dark brown
Vitiligo	Absent melanin	Bluish-white (bright)
Nevus anemicus	Autofluorescence	–
Pityriasis alba	Autofluorescence	–
Tuberous sclerosis	Less melanin	White
Progressive macular hypomelanosis	• Absent melanin • Coproporphyrin III	Bluish-white and follicle bound coral red
Lentigo maligna	Melanin	Dark brown to black

Melasma

It is one of the common diseases of hyper-pigmentation. It occurs due to excess pigment production, with lesions mainly occurring on the face. It can be epidermal, dermal, or mixed. Confirmation of the diagnosis, as well as the level of pigment deposition, can be done by Wood's lamp examination, thereby helping in the management of melasma. Epidermal pigmentation is enhanced and becomes more visible under Wood's lamp **(Figs. 2A and B)**. At the same time, the contrast is less pronounced in dermal cases. Mixed cases show color enhancement in a few areas. Sanchez et al.[2] classified melasma into four subtypes, i.e., epidermal, dermal, mixed, and Wood's light inapparent.

Vitiligo

It is not easy to diagnose vitiligo in fair-skinned individuals or on palms and soles; less obvious vitiligo patches can be better visualized and delineated under UV light.

In disorders of hypopigmentation, the absence of epidermal melanin creates a window through which the fluorescence of dermal collagen can be seen. Abrupt cutoff in the visible emission from lesional skin leads to sharp demarcation of the margins of vitiligo lesions under Wood's light. Bright blue-white fluorescence is seen under the Wood's lamp examination in vitiligo patches **(Figs. 3A and B)**. Wood's light can do the earliest detection of follicular regimentation following therapy. Wood's lamp helps distinguish vitiligo from nevus anemicus, pityriasis versicolor, and pityriasis alba. Nevus anemicus (local dermal vasoconstriction), having normal epidermal pigment, is not visible under UV light. Yellow-gold fluorescence is characteristic of pityriasis versicolor. Pityriasis alba, on the other hand, cannot be seen under Wood's lamp.[3]

Tuberous Sclerosis

Early diagnosis of this entity warrants the identification of ash-leaf macules, which helps prevent the onset of seizures in these patients using prophylactic medicines. Wood's light is an essential tool in the location of these lesions, however, with less specificity.[3] Therefore, a careful family history, clinical findings, and Wood's lamp findings should be appropriately corelated to reduce the error in diagnosis.

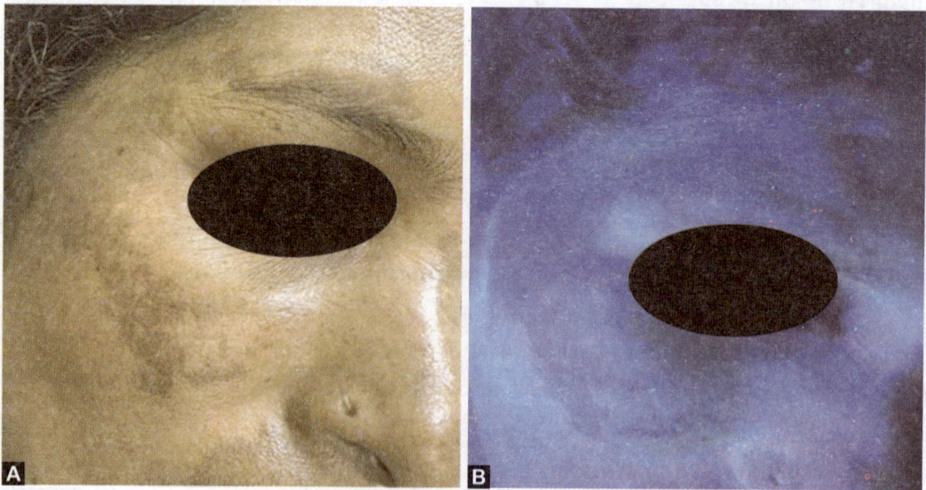

FIGS. 2A AND B: Enhanced pigmentation of epidermal melasma under Wood's lamp.

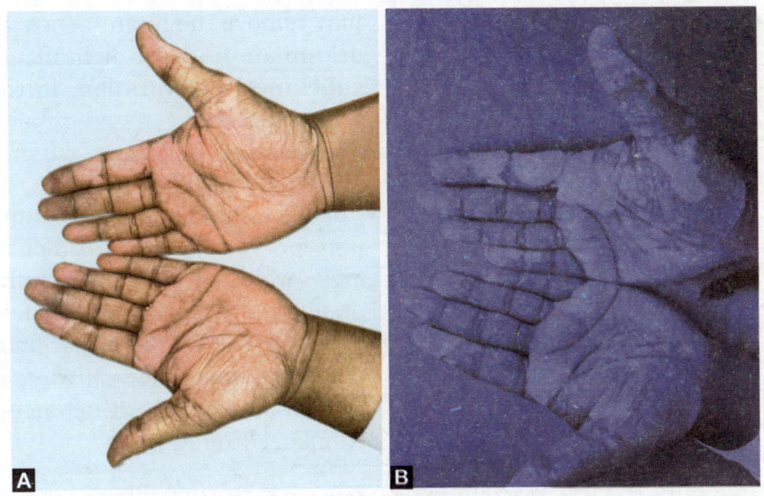

FIGS. 3A AND B: Bright bluish-white fluorescence under Wood's lamp in contrast to the naked eye appearance of vitiligo patches.

TABLE 2: Wood's lamp application in infections and infestations.

Disease	Chromophore	Fluorescence
Pseudomonas	Pyoverdine	Yellow-green
Erythrasma	Coproporphyrin III	Coral red
Propionibacterium acnes	Coproporphyrin III/protoporphyrin IX	Coral red
Microsporum species	Pteridine	Bright green
Microsporum gypseum		Dull yellow
Trichophyton schoenleinii		Blue
Pityriasis versicolor	Malassezia furfur	Chamois leather like
Pityrosporum folliculitis	Malassezia furfur	Follicle-bound bluish-white

Hypomelanosis of Ito

It presents with whorled or streaked hypopigmentation, with less visibility in fair-skinned individuals, wherein Wood's lamp comes handy for better delineation of subtle hypopigmentation. It is prudent to diagnose the systemic involvement in hypomelanosis of Ito early with Wood's lamp.

Progressive Macular Hypomelanosis

Progressive macular hypomelanosis (PMH) has been related to *Propionibacterium acnes* by Westerhof.[4] PMH lesions emit bright bluish-white fluorescence as a result of no melanin. At the same time, the presence of coproporphyrin III (chromophore produced by *P. acnes*) leads to follicle-bound coral-red fluorescence.

Infections and Infestations (Table 2)

Various bacterial and superficial fungal infections show varied fluorescence under Wood's lamp which may be helpful in diagnosis when in doubt.

Bacterial Infections

Pseudomonas

"Pyoverdine" or "fluorescein" is the pigment produced by *Pseudomonas*, which emits green fluorescence under UV light. A bacterial count of $10^5/cm^2$ is required to demonstrate fluorescence from the sample. Extensive erosions of burns, bullous disorders, and severe adverse drug reactions (SCARs) are commonly infected by *Pseudomonas*, which can be detected with Wood's lamp examination even earlier than the culture positivity. Ecthyma gangrenosum can be confirmed many hours ahead of confirmatory blood culture reports by examining withdrawn solution injected into the wound under Wood's light.[5] Hot tub folliculitis caused by *Pseudomonas* can also be diagnosed with Wood's lamp examination.

Erythrasma

Erythrasma is a superficial infection of the skin caused by *Corynebacterium minutissimum* with lesions occurring in groin and axilla that show characteristic coral-red fluorescence on Wood's lamp examination due to water-soluble coproporphyrin III produced by the organisms **(Figs. 4A and B)**. Hence, the area should not be washed as it may remove the fluorescence. Wood's lamp examination is also helpful in diagnosing subclinical colonization, in the toe webs, scalp, or trunk.

Propionibacterium acnes

Cornelius and Ludwig[6] demonstrated the presence of coproporphyrin production by *P. acnes* which is the cause of intracomedonal orange-red fluorescence. *P. acnes* populations correlate well with follicular fluorescence on the face. Often, yellowish-white fluorescence is seen associated with comedones due to compacted keratin.

Fungal Infections

Dermatophytosis

Wood's lamp examination is instrumental in the diagnosis of tinea capitis. Broken-off hairs and intrafollicular portions with plucked hair emit characteristic fluorescence. *Microsporum audouinii* and *M. canis* infections, *M. distortum*, *M. ferrugineum*, and *M. gypseum* show bright-green fluorescence. *Trichophyton schoenleinii* on the other hand emits faint blue color. *T. tonsurans* and *T. verrucosum* show negative fluorescence upon UV light examination. Generally, members of the *Microsporum* genus show

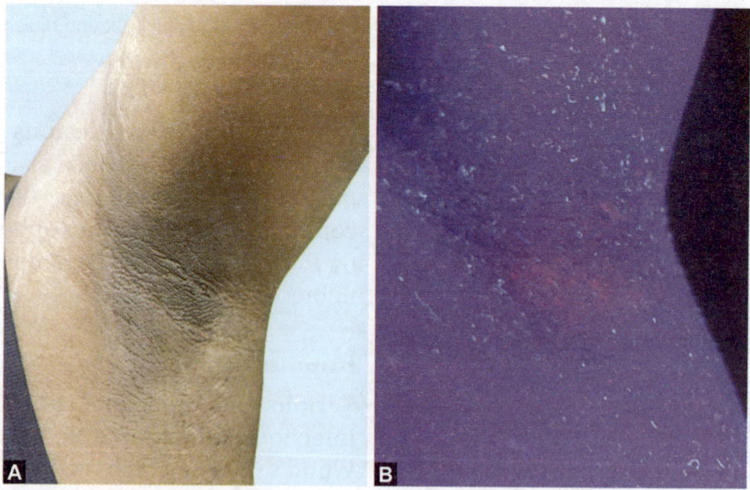

FIGS. 4A AND B: Characteristic coral-red fluorescence on Wood's lamp.

fluorescence. *T. schoenleinii* gives blue-green characteristic fluorescence **(Figs. 5A and B)**. Differentiation of the causative organisms is impossible with Wood's lamp except for the minimal change in the color produced. The chemical leading to fluorescence is pteridine. False-positive fluorescence can be shown by ointments, soap particles, scales, and fibers. Cloth particles can appear bright white.

Wood's lamp is practical in the mass screening and controlling epidemics in schools. The emergence of nonfluorescent hair on a Wood's lamp examination is the endpoint for treating tinea capitis.

Pityriasis Versicolor

Wood's lamp examination can diagnose the extent of infection and subclinical infection by *Malassezia furfur*. The infected areas emit yellowish-white or copper-orange fluorescence **(Fig. 6)**. The follicular disease causes bluish-white fluorescence, helping differentiate it from other types of folliculitis.

Infestations

Scabies

Wood's lamp examination or UV scab scanning can demonstrate burrows by applying fluorescent substances like tetracycline paste or fluorescein dye. It has been seen that naked-eye examination under UVA was much better than natural/artificial light. The body of the mite emits dot-like luminescence (white or green). Wood's lamp examination has the advantage of anogenital exploration because it is contactless.[7]

Porphyria (Table 3)

Wood's lamp examination can detect excess porphyrins in urine, feces, teeth, red blood cells, blister fluid, etc., in various porphyrias.

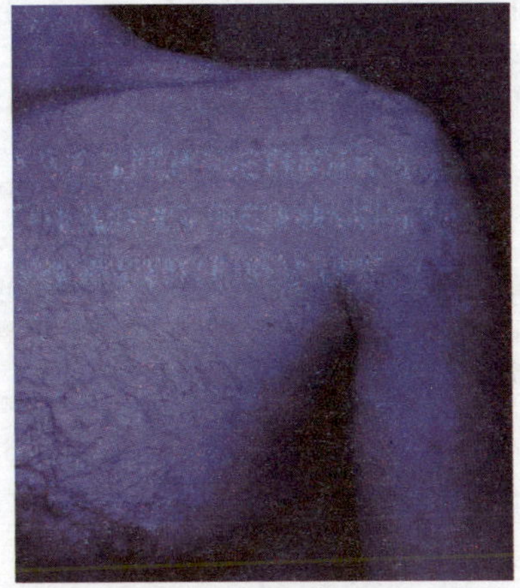

FIG. 6: Yellowish-white fluorescence of pityriasis versicolor under Wood's lamp.

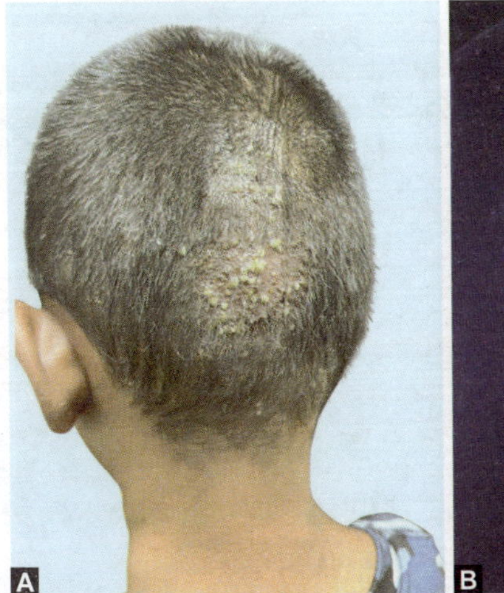

FIGS. 5A AND B: *Trichophyton schoenleinii* gives blue-green characteristic fluorescence.

Conversion of porphyrinogens to porphyrins can be achieved by adding hydrochloric acid to the sample, thereby intensifying the fluorescence. In porphyria cutanea tarda, liver biopsy samples show fluorescence due to accumulated porphyrins in liver. During acute crisis in variegate porphyria, urine shows fluorescence **(Fig. 7)**, while fluorescence from stool remains positive even during remission. Stool samples, when mixed with equal parts of amyl alcohol, glacial acetic acid, and ether, fetch better results. Gunther's disease or congenital porphyria shows fluorescence in bone marrow, teeth **(Fig. 8)**, and urine. There is transient fluoresce in red blood cells, while the urine does not in erythropoietic protoporphyria. Excess of protoporphyrin and coproporphyrin can emit an intense red fluorescence. Lead poisoning and anemic states show high levels of erythrocyte protoporphyrin. δ-aminolevulinic acid (δ-ALA) and porphobilinogen found in acute intermittent porphyria are not porphyrins; thus, fluorescence is not seen.[8]

Tumors

As early as 1943, Auler found that hematoporphyrin was retained in the tumor on injection. Under Wood's lamp examination, tumor borders were visible better. Necrosis of tumor cells is brought about by a combination of hematoporphyrin and UV light, forming the principle of photodynamic therapy. However, presently UV light is not being used to detect or differentiate tumors.[9]

TABLE 3: Wood's lamp application of porphyria and malignancy.

Diagnosis	Sample	Fluorescence
Porphyria cutanea tarda	Urine and feces	Red-pink
Erythropoietic protoporphyria	Red blood cells (RBCs), gallstones, and stool	Red-pink
Hepatoerythropoietic porphyria	RBCs, urine, and stool	Red-pink
Variegate porphyria	Urine and stool	Red-pink
Nonmelanoma skin cancers (squamous cell cancers and basal cell carcinoma)	5-aminolevulinate-induced protoporphyrin IX	Coral red

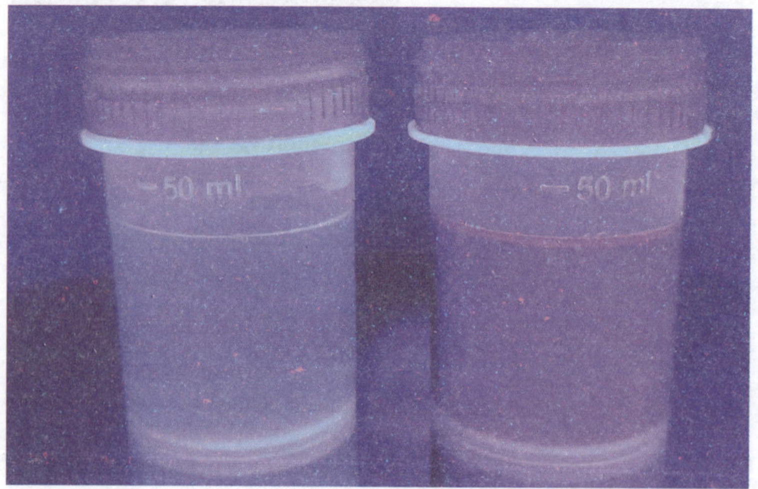

FIG. 7: Normal and congenital erythropoietic porphyria urine samples under Wood's lamp.

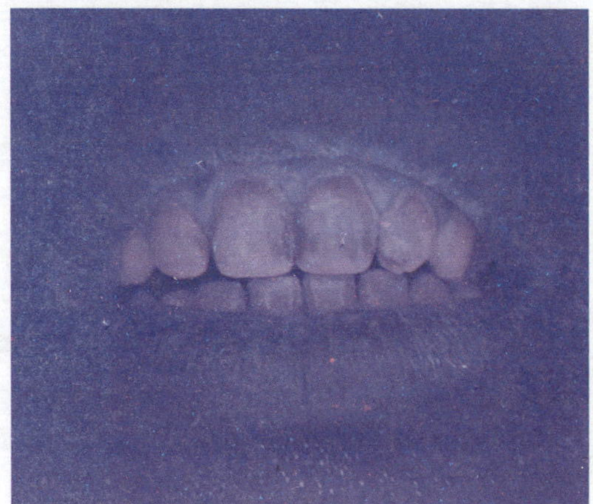

FIG. 8: Erythrodontia in congenital erythropoietic porphyria under Wood's lamp.

Surgical Applications

Wood's lamp can aid in the delineation of appropriate surgical margin. It helps in outlining the borders and complete excision of lesions in lentigo maligna by accentuation of hyperpigmentation in the epidermal layer. In a study, Wood's lamp was used to delineate margins before surgical removal of lentigo maligna which helps surgeons only to resect damaged tissue and rescue as much healthy skin as possible. Photodiagnosis is a preoperative technique that helps surgeons only to remove affected tissue and saving as much healthy tissue as possible by using methyl aminolevulinate (MAL) cream as a phosphor. After MAL application and Wood's lamp examination, the cancerous area of basal cell carcinoma (BCC) emits bright-red fluorescence; a fainter fluorescence termed "gray zone" is also seen. Photodiagnosis has helped surgeons in radical excision to save healthy tissue and better results.[10]

Miscellaneous Medical Applications

- Wood's lamp can help prevent overtreatment of any areas with chemical peeling. Adding salicylic acid and fluorescein sodium to chemical peels causes fluorescence; salicylic acid emits green fluorescence, and the fluorescein sodium is yellow-orange.[8]
- Wood's lamp can help assess adequate sunscreen application, especially in inaccessible areas like the back.[11]
- Adherence to tetracyclines can be confirmed by Wood's lamp examination of toenails for yellow fluorescence. Wood's lamp can help to differentiate tetracycline adverse reactions and other pathological causes of yellow nails which emit negative fluorescence on Wood's lamp examination.[12] Recently, patients under molnupiravir [an antiviral with action against severe acute respiratory syndrome coronavirus 2 (SARS-CoV-2)] have shown bright-blue fluorescent transverse bands over the lunula of nails under Wood's lamp, which persisted as late as 90 days after the last dose.[13] Favipiravir has also shown to emit fluorescence in nails.[14]
- Dihydroxyacetone (DHA) is a chemical used to artificially pigment lesions. Wood's lamp helps assess the extent of vitiligo in patients using DHA for camouflage, as DHA emits salmon color fluorescence while vitiligo lesions are bright blue-white.[15]
- Milia appear bright yellow under the Wood's lamp due to autofluorescence produced by keratin in the milia cavity.[16]
- Porokeratosis may show a diamond necklace-like or ring-like structure under Wood's light.[17]
- Early morphea lesions not apparent under visible light can be diagnosed with Wood's light. Wood's lamp helps demarcate new lesions well before the appearance of induration.[18]
- Detection of serum and blood in forensics.
- In cosmetic allergies, for the detection of allergens.
- Wood's lamp can be used for photopatch testing. The use of fluorescent markers requiring identification of the skin site

after 24 or 48 hours can be done by using Wood's lamp. It also aids in the diagnosis of photosensitizing disorders like solar urticaria.

- Gray hair (partial, complete, and even colored stands out compared to normally pigmented hair in Wood's light. It helps evaluate premature graying of hair and helps assess regrowing hair in alopecia areata (new hair is lighter in color). People with blonde hair, however, are an exception.[19]
- Circulation time can be calculated by injecting intravenous fluorescein.
- Fluorescent tags can determine cutaneous penetration and epidermal turnover.
- The sterilization effect of Wood's lamp can be used to sterilize culture media.

NONMEDICAL USES[20]

Besides medical applications, Wood's lamp has proved to be of use in other fields as well.

- Detection of hard water and fraudulent currency.
- In the food industry, it can be used to test contamination of food products. Wood's lamp can detect *Pseudomonas* infection of milk through infected water.
- Vitamin D is necessary for maintaining bone health and regulating the immune system. Sun exposure is required to produce vitamin D. Increasing the concentration of vitamin D2 in mushrooms by UV exposure using Wood's lamp is under research. It has been seen that mushrooms can retain this amount of vitamin D for up to 7 days after UV exposure, if refrigerated.
- Verification of signatures and detection of cracks in ceramics or metals.

LIMITATIONS[21,22]

- Wood's lamp examination helps to differentiate tinea capitis from other types of alopecia. However, most fungi do

BOX 1	**False-positive fluorescence under Wood's lamp examination.**

- Colored markers, like highlighters
- Soap particles and detergents with optical brighteners
- Thick scales
- Invisible ink
- Lemon juice
- Fiber/Cloth
- *Natural secretions*: Semen, serum, saliva, and milk
- Dyes and cosmetics
- Sunscreens and ointments
- Wet ear wax

not emit fluorescence; therefore, Wood's lamp cannot exclude the diagnosis of tinea capitis.
- Erythrasma fluorescence coral-red; however, fluorescence might not be observed if the affected area was washed just before Wood's lamp examination.
- Wrong interpretations
- False-positive or false-negative result **(Box 1)**
- Corneal issues if the device is used for a long time without protective goggles

CONCLUSION

Wood's lamp, a valuable diagnostic tool in dermatology, has demonstrated its versatility in various medical applications. Its ability to emit long-wave UV radiation, also known as black light, provides dermatologists with a noninvasive, quick, and accurate method for diagnosing a spectrum of skin conditions. From pigmentary disorders such as melasma and vitiligo to infections and infestations such as bacterial and fungal infections, Wood's lamp aids in revealing subtle changes not easily discernible under visible light. Moreover, its applications extend to surgical settings, assisting in delineating surgical margins and improving outcomes. Beyond the medical field, Wood's lamp finds utility in detecting hard water, counterfeit currency, and even in the food industry. Despite its widespread applications, it is crucial to acknowledge its limitations, including the potential for wrong interpretations and false results. As technology continues to advance, Wood's lamp remains a valuable and accessible tool in dermatology, contributing to enhanced diagnostic capabilities and improved patient care.

Key Messages

- Wood's lamp is a small, durable, portable, and easy-to-use office-based device for clinical diagnosis in dermatology.
- It majorly helps diagnose pigmentary disorders, infections, and porphyria.
- Advances in its use have helped in toxicological analysis and nonmedical fields.
- However, it has certain limitations like false-positive results in various cases.

REFERENCES

1. Margarot J, Deveze P. Aspect de quelques dermatoses lumiere ultraparaviolette. Note preliminaire. Bull Soc Sci Med Biol Montpellier. 1925;6:375-8.
2. Sanchez NP, Pathak MA, Sato S. Melasma: a clinical, light microscopic, ultrastructural, and immunofluorescence study. J Am Acad Dermatol. 1981;4:698-710.
3. Asawanonda P, Taylor CR. Wood's Light in Dermatology. Int J Dermatol. 1999;38:801-7.
4. Westerhof W, Relyveld GN, Kingswijk MM, de Man P, Menke HE. Propionibacterium acnes and the pathogenesis of progressive macular hypomelanosis. Arch Dermatol. 2004;140:210-4.
5. Amichai B, Finkelestein E, Halevy S. Early detection of pseudomonas infection using a Wood's lamp (letter). Clin Exp Dermatol. 1994;19:449.
6. Cornelius CE, Ludwig GD. Red fluorescence of comedones: production of porphyrins by Corynebacterium acnes. J Invest Dermatol. 1967;49:368-70.
7. Scanni G. Facilitations in the Clinical Diagnosis of Human Scabies through the Use of Ultraviolet Light (UV-Scab Scanning): A Case-Series Study. Trop Med Infect Dis. 2022;7(12):422.
8. Dyer JM, Foy VM. Revealing the Unseen: A Review of Wood's Lamp in Dermatology. J Clin Aesthet Dermatol. 2022;15(6):25-30.
9. Klatte JL, van der Beek N, Kemperman PM. 100 years of Wood's lamp revised. J Eur Acad Dermatol Venereol. 2015;29(5):842-7.
10. Borroni RG, Barruscotti S, Carugno A, Barbaccia V, Arbustini E, Brazzelli V. Usefulness of in vivo photodiagnosis for the identification of tumor margins in recurrent basal cell carcinoma of the face. Photodermatol Photoimmunol Photomed. 2015;31(4):195-201.
11. Light JG, Frantz T, McNamara K, Bashyam AM, Feldman SR. Efficacy of Applicator Devices for Self-Application of Topicals to the Back. J Cutan Med Surg. 2020;24(3):249-52.
12. Hendricks AA. Yellow lunulae with fluorescence after tetracycline therapy. Arch Dermatol. 1980;116(4):438-40.
13. Huang X, Asawanonda P, Oon HH. Molnupiravir-associated nail and hair fluorescence on Wood's lamp examination. Clin Exp Dermatol. 2023;48(4):381-2.
14. Demir B, Cicek D, Turkoglu S, Bozdemir NY, Sarikurt F, Banoglu E. Wood's lamp examination of hair and nails related to COVID-19 treatment. Dermatol Ther. 2021;34(6):e15174.
15. Jankowski M, Nowowiejska L, Czajkowski R. Wood's lamp fluorescence of dihydroxyacetone treated skin. J Eur Acad Dermatol Venereol. 2016;30(11):e12-e126.
16. Lee JH, Kwon HS, Jung HM, Kim GM, Bae JM. Wood's lamp-induced fluorescence of milia. J Am Acad Dermatol. 2018;78(5):e99-e100.
17. Sun R, Chen H, Zhu W, Lian S. Wood's lamp image of porokeratosis. Photodermatol Photoimmunol Photomed. 2017;33(2):114-6.
18. Curtiss P, Singh G, Lo Sicco K, Franks AG Jr. Wood's lamp as a tool in the evaluation of morphea. J Am Acad Dermatol. 2018;78(2):e33-e34.

19. Kaliyadan F, Jayasree P, Ashique KT. Looking for a grey needle in a 'hair' stack! Using a Wood's lamp for evaluating canities. Indian J Dermatol Venereol Leprol. 2023;89(4):636-7.

20. Cardillo H, Kohler J, Kriner E, Mehta K. Applications of Wood's Lamp technology to detect skin infections in resource-constrained settings. Silicon Valley, California: 4th IEEE Global Humanitarian Technology Conference; 2014. pp. 548-54.

21. Al Aboud DM, Gossman W. Wood's Light. Treasure Island (FL): StatPearls Publishing; 2023.

22. Silverberg JI, Silverberg NB. False "highlighting" with Wood's lamp. Paediatric Dermatol. 2014;31(1):109-10.

Diascopy

Pankaj Das, Silky Priya

INTRODUCTION

Diascopy is a test for blanchability of skin lesions that has been used for over a century by dermatologists and other clinicians. It is a simple, inexpensive, and noninvasive technique that can provide valuable information about the nature and etiology of various skin disorders. Diascopy can help distinguish between lesions that are due to blood within superficial vessels (inflammatory or vascular lesions) or due to hemorrhage (petechiae or purpura). It can also help identify some specific conditions that have characteristic color changes under pressure, such as sarcoidosis and erythrasma. Diascopy can also help define the extent and borders of pigmented lesions before excision. It is not a substitute for histopathological examination, but rather a complementary tool that can aid in the clinical diagnosis and management of skin diseases.[1,2]

HISTORY

The term diascopy was coined by the German dermatologist Paul Gerson Unna in 1886, from the Greek words dia (through) and skopein (to look). Unna was interested in the microscopic examination of skin lesions and devised a method of applying pressure with a glass slide to expel the blood from the tissue and observe the changes in color and structure. He used diascopy to study various skin conditions, such as lupus erythematosus, leprosy, syphilis, and tuberculosis. He also introduced the concept of the "apple jelly" color that is seen in sarcoid skin lesions under diascopy.[3,4]

Unna's technique was further developed and popularized by other dermatologists, such as L Goldman, H Plotnick, and I Balinkin, who published a comprehensive study on diascopy in 1957. They described the principles, methods, and applications of diascopy in detail and proposed a classification of skin lesions based on their blanchability. They also introduced the use of a black light (Wood light) to enhance the visibility of some lesions under diascopy, such as erythrasma and *Pseudomonas* infection.[5]

PRINCIPLES

Diascopy is based on the principle that the color of a skin lesion depends on the amount and distribution of blood in the superficial vessels and the optical properties of the skin and the lesion. When pressure is applied with a finger or a glass slide, the blood is displaced from the vessels and the color of the lesion changes accordingly. The degree and duration of the color change depend on the size, depth, and elasticity of the vessels, as well as the nature and thickness of the lesion.[6]

Diascopy can be performed in natural or artificial light, depending on the type and location of the lesion. A Wood light (black light) can enhance the visibility of some lesions that fluoresce under ultraviolet light, such as erythrasma, *Pseudomonas* infection, and some types of tinea capitis. Diascopy can also be combined with other techniques, such as dermoscopy, to improve the accuracy and specificity of the diagnosis.

METHODS

Diascopy is a simple and quick procedure that can be done in any clinical setting. The following steps are recommended for performing diascopy:

1. Select a suitable lesion that is not ulcerated, crusted, or infected.
2. Clean the lesion and the surrounding skin with alcohol or water.
3. Apply pressure with a finger or a glass slide on the lesion for a few seconds and observe the color change. If using a glass slide, hold it at an angle of 45° to avoid reflection and distortion of the image.
4. Release the pressure and observe the color return. Note the degree and duration of the blanching and the original color of the lesion.
5. Repeat the procedure on different parts of the lesion and on the normal skin for comparison.
6. Record the findings and interpret them according to the classification of skin lesions based on diascopy.[7,8]

CLASSIFICATION

Skin lesions can be classified into three main categories based on their blanchability under diascopy:

1. *Positive diascopy*: The lesion blanches completely or partially under pressure, indicating that the erythema is due to blood within superficial vessels. This category includes inflammatory and vascular lesions, such as acne, rosacea, psoriasis, eczema, urticaria, angioedema, hemangioma, and telangiectasia. Some of these lesions may have a characteristic color change under diascopy, such as the "apple jelly" color of sarcoidosis and the "salmon pink" color of pityriasis rosea.
2. *Negative diascopy*: The lesion does not blanch under pressure, indicating that the erythema is due to hemorrhage or nonvascular tissue. This category includes petechiae, purpura, and nevi. Some of these lesions may have a characteristic color change under diascopy, such as the "blue-gray" color of melanoma and the "brown-black" color of seborrheic keratosis.
3. *Variable diascopy*: The lesion blanches partially or inconsistently under pressure, indicating that the erythema is due to a combination of blood within superficial vessels and hemorrhage or nonvascular tissue. This category includes some pigmented lesions, such as lentigo, dysplastic nevus, and basal cell carcinoma.[9]

APPLICATIONS

Diascopy can be used for various purposes in the diagnosis and management of skin disorders, such as:

- To differentiate between vascular, non-vascular, and hemorrhagic lesions, which can have different causes, treatments, and prognoses[10]
- To identify some specific conditions that have characteristic color changes under diascopy, such as sarcoidosis, erythrasma, and *Pseudomonas* infection[11]
- To define the extent and borders of pigmented lesions before excision, which can help in planning the surgery and assessing the margins

- To monitor the response to treatment and the evolution of lesions, such as the fading of inflammatory lesions or the growth of tumors[12]

Besides the above, diascopy finds its utility in the evaluation of a wide spectrum of dermatological conditions, particularly those characterized by erythema or discoloration. Examples include the following:

- *Differentiation of erythema*: Diascopy helps distinguish erythema caused by vasodilation from that due to hemorrhage or pigmentation. Vasodilatory erythema, such as erythema solare or rosacea, blanches completely under diascopy, while nonblanching erythema suggests deeper causes, such as inflammation or pigmentation **(Figs. 1A and B)**.
- *Assessment of petechiae and purpura*: Diascopy is a crucial tool for differentiating petechiae, which are small, nonblanching, red spots caused by extravasation of erythrocytes into the skin, from purpura, larger nonblanching lesions due to deeper hemorrhage **(Figs. 2A and B)**.
- *Evaluation of granulomatous nodules*: Diascopy can aid in the diagnosis of granulomatous nodules, such as sarcoidosis, granuloma annulare, and lupus vulgaris. These lesions often exhibit a characteristic "apple jelly" appearance upon diascopy. This refers to a translucent or yellow-brown coloration seen when pressure is applied to the lesion. The mechanism behind this

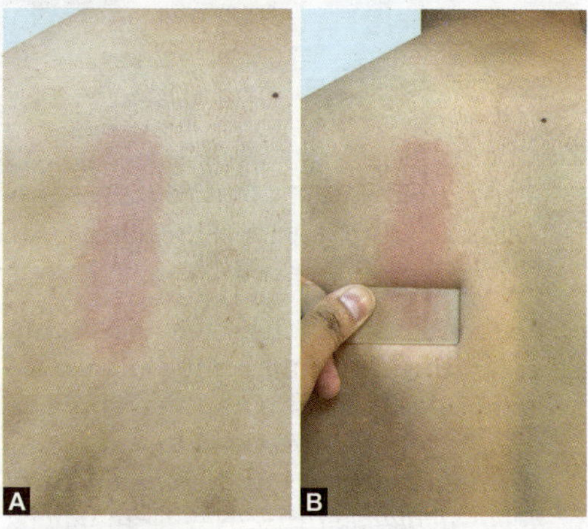

FIGS. 1A AND B: Dermographism in a patient of urticaria lesion blanches partially under pressure, indicating that the erythema is due to blood within superficial vessels.

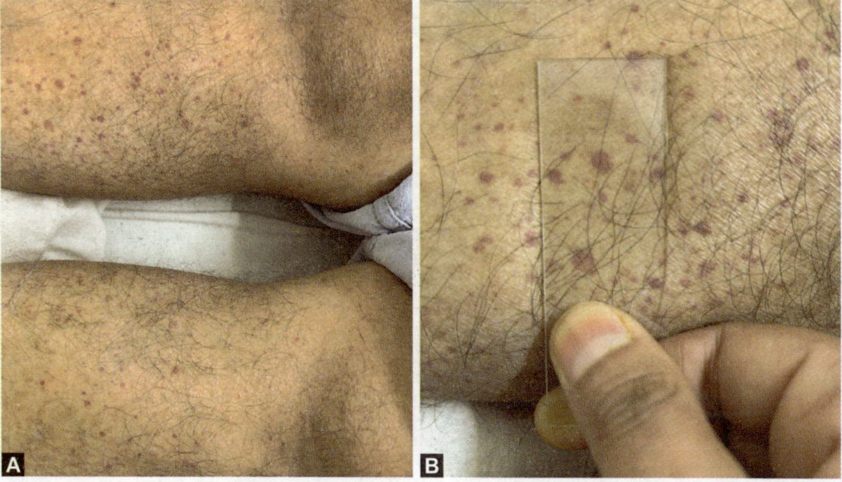

FIGS. 2A AND B: Petechiae or purpura does not blanch under pressure, indicating that the erythema is due to hemorrhage or nonvascular tissue.

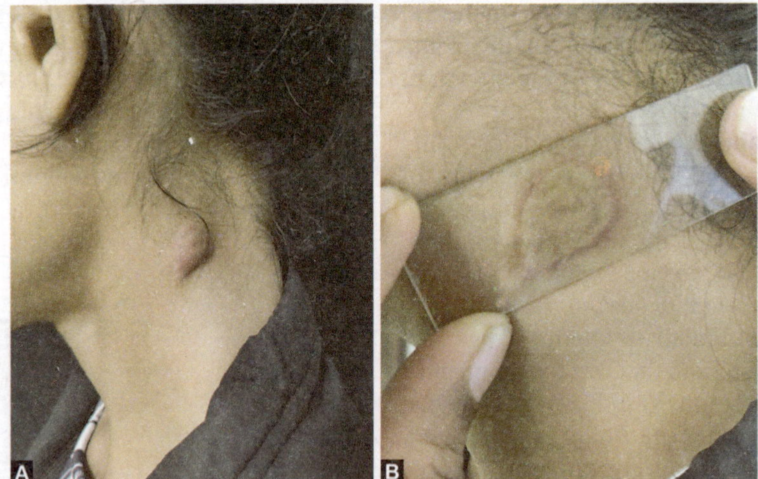

FIGS. 3A AND B: Lupus vulgaris exhibiting a characteristic "apple jelly" appearance upon diascopy.

phenomenon involves the disruption of erythrocytes and the release of hemosiderin, leading to the distinctive color change (**Figs. 3A and B**).

- *Distinguishing nevus anemicus from nevus depigmentosus*: Nevus anemicus typically exhibits a blanching or partial blanching response during diascopy due to vasoconstriction of blood vessels, resulting in reduced blood flow. This phenomenon leads to a paler appearance of the lesion when pressure is applied, with the color change being more noticeable under diascopic examination. In contrast, nevus depigmentosus does not undergo significant color changes under diascopy. The condition is characterized by the absence or reduction of melanin in the affected area, and since diascopy primarily assesses vascular changes rather than pigmentation, nevus depigmentosus is less likely to show alterations in color during diascopic evaluation (**Figs. 4A to D**).

- *Identification of telangiectasia*: Telangiectasia refers to the dilatation of small blood vessels near the surface of the skin, resulting in visible red or purple discolorations. When pressure is applied

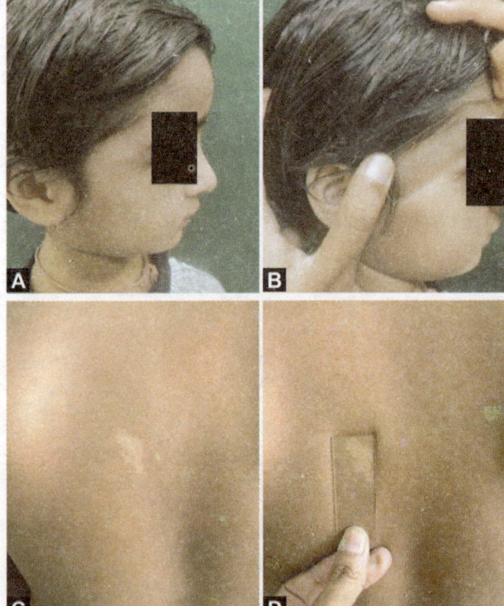

FIGS. 4A TO D: (A and B) Nevus anemicus typically exhibits a blanching or partial blanching response during diascopy while (C and D) nevus depigmentosus does not undergo significant color changes under diascopy.

during diascopy, the central "feeder" vessel of the telangiectasia may become more apparent. The vessel appears as a central channel or line within the lesion, and its visualization can provide important information about the morphology and distribution of the telangiectasia.

LIMITATIONS

Diascopy is not a definitive diagnostic test but rather a supportive tool that can provide useful clues and guide further investigations. Diascopy has some limitations, such as follows:

- It is not applicable to all skin lesions, especially those that are ulcerated, crusted, or infected, as they may interfere with the pressure and the color change.
- It is not specific to any condition, as some lesions may have similar or overlapping color changes under diascopy, such as the "apple jelly" color of sarcoidosis and tuberculosis.
- It is not sensitive to some conditions, as some lesions may not have any color change under diascopy, such as the "white" color of vitiligo and hypopigmented lesions.
- It is influenced by various factors, such as the amount and duration of pressure, the angle and type of light, the thickness and color of the skin and the lesion, and the subjective perception of the observer.[12]

CONCLUSION

Diascopy is a simple and useful diagnostic technique for skin disorders that has a long history and a wide range of applications. It can help differentiate between vascular, nonvascular, and hemorrhagic lesions, as well as identify some specific conditions that have characteristic color changes under diascopy. Diascopy can also help define the extent and borders of pigmented lesions before excision. It is not a substitute for histopathological examination but rather a complementary tool that can aid in the clinical diagnosis and management of skin diseases.

Key Messages

- Diascopy aids in diagnosing skin disorders by assessing blanchability of lesions.
- It is valuable for distinguishing between inflammatory, vascular, and hemorrhagic lesions.
- *Principles*: Lesion color changes with blood displacement under pressure, observed in natural or artificial light.
- It is a simple clinical procedure involving lesion selection, cleaning, pressure application, and color observation.
- Lesions are categorized into positive, negative, and variable diascopy, guiding diagnosis.
- Applications include differentiating lesion types, identifying conditions with characteristic color changes, and defining pigmented lesion borders.

REFERENCES

1. Sacchidanand S. IADVL Textbook of Dermatology, 5th edition. New Delhi: Bhalani Publishing House; 2022.
2. Griffiths C, Barker J, Bleiker T, Chalmers R, Creamer D (Eds). Rook's Textbook of Dermatology, 9th edition. Chichester: Wiley; 2016.
3. Lee H, Ramani LT, Parish LC, Lee JB. Tools of dermatology: A historical perspective. Clin Dermatol. 2021;39(4):555-62.
4. Campos-do-Carmo G, Ramos-e-Silva M. Dermoscopy: basic concepts. Int J Dermatol. 2008;47(7):712-9.

5. Goldman L, Plotnick H, Balinkin I. Investigative and clinical studies with diascopy in dermatology. AMA Arch Dermatol. 1957;75(5):699-705.

6. Torrelo A. Schachner and Hansen's Pediatric Dermatology, 5th edition. New Delhi: Jaypee Brothers Medical Publishers; 2022.

7. Rudd M, Eversole R, Carpenter W. Diascopy: a clinical technique for the diagnosis of vascular lesions. Gen Dent. 2001;49(2):206-9.

8. Nadeau C, Stoopler ET. The clinical value of diascopy. J Can Dent Assoc. 2013;79:d11.

9. Tanwar R, Sharma A, Suma G. (2017). Diascopy in oral lesions: An Old algorithm revisited. [online] Available from: https://www.semanticscholar.org/paper/Diascopy-in-Oral-Lesions%3A-An-Old-Algorithm-Tanwar-Sharma/1bca6043843ce99d9901d115bbc9aae82bc4ff12 [Last accessed February, 2024].

10. Sivakumar A, Thappa DM. Glass slide—an indispensable tool for the dermatologist. CosmoDerma. 2022;2:27.

11. Matos D, Coelho R. "Apple Jelly" sign: Diascopy in Cutaneous sarcoidosis. Acta Med Port. 2015;28(3):394.

12. Perez-Lopez D, Pena-Cristobal M, Otero-Rey E, Tomas I, Blanco-Carrion A. Clinical value of diascopy and other non-invasive techniques on differential diagnosis algorithms of oral pigmentations: A systematic review. J Clin Exp Dent. 2016;8(4):e448-58.

CHAPTER 13

Intradermal Tests

Sampoorna Choudhary, Shekhar Neema, Dilip Paudel

INTRODUCTION

Intradermal tests are minimally invasive tests and are widely employed to support the diagnosis of various dermatological and nondermatological diseases. Despite the evolution of medical diagnostics, in the hands of experienced dermatologists, they still hold important diagnostic and prognostic value. They are aimed at detecting both immediate and delayed type hypersensitivity reactions mounted against exogenous and endogenous antigens. They are inhibited by antihistamines, tricyclic antidepressants, and steroids (both topical and systemic), and therefore, short-acting antihistamines should be stopped for 72 hours prior to testing.[1,2]

The various diseases for which they are utilized are listed in **Table 1**. Various preprocedural requirements and important

TABLE 1: Classification of intradermal tests.[11]

Bacterial	Fungal	Protozoal test
Infectious disease:	• Candidin test	• Filarial skin test
• Anthraxin	• Coccidioidin test	• Leishmanin test
• Dick's test	• Histoplasmin test	• Onchocerciasis skin test
• Ito Reenstierna test	• Trichophytin test	
• Lepromin test		
• Foshay test		
• Frei's test		
• Schick test		
• Tuberculin test (Mantoux test)		
Noninfectious disease:		
• Autologous serum skin test		
• Autoerythrocyte sensitization test		
• Histamine test		
• Intradermal sensitivity test (IDST) for drug		
• Kveim–Siltzbach test		
• Pathergy test		
• Pilocarpine test		

procedural steps are listed in **Boxes 1 and 2**, respectively. Intradermal tests can elicit pain, which may be reduced by the use of a topical anesthetic cream such as the eutectic mixture of local anesthetics (EMLAs), which reduces the flare but not the wheal responses.[3] They can provoke a low rate of untoward, large local (immediate and late) and systemic reactions, with an incidence ranging from 0.02 to 1.4% of the tested patients.[4] Some fatalities have also been reported.[5] A waiting period of 20 minutes is recommended before the patient is released, and this period may be extended for high-risk patients, especially those on beta blockers. The tests that are commonly used and are historically important are covered in subsequent paragraphs.

INFECTIOUS DISEASE

Bacterial Infections

Anthraxin[6]

The anthraxin skin test measures cell-mediated immunity to anthrax antigens and has also been recommended by the World Health Organization for evaluation of the immunological memory against anthrax. Anthraxin, a cell-wall extract from the vegetative, noncapsulated Sterne strain of *Bacillus anthracis*, consists mainly of a complex of peptidoglycans and polysaccharides. Skin reactions are considered positive if an erythema of a minimum 8 mm in diameter with subsequent twofold thickening of the skin appeared 24 hours following inoculation. In a study conducted by Shlyakhov E et al., the test was found positive in 81.8% of cases in the first 3 days of the disease and in 97–99% of cases in the next two to three weeks. Thus, it is a valuable method for early diagnosis of acute anthrax as well as the only method available for retrospective diagnosis of human anthrax. Skin test screening can be applied successfully with antigens extracted from the anthrax bacillus cell wall, but not by using the protective antigen, which is the major antigen of the anthrax vaccine. Therefore, the anthraxin skin test can differentiate between exposed and unexposed individuals, even if they have been immunized. However, as

---

BOX 1 | Preprocedural preparation.

- Control—normal saline
- Antigenic suspension (test specific)
- Intradermal test recording sheet
- Pen
- 1.0 mL syringes or insulin syringe
- 27G needles
- Sterile gloves
- Sharps bin
- Sterile gauze
- Ruler
- Timer/Clock/Watch
- Anaphylactic tray

BOX 2 | Important steps while performing intradermal tests.

- Explain the procedure in detail
- Obtain informed consent
- Ensure the patient is in a comfortable sitting or lying (preferably) position
- Clean the test site (midvolar aspect of the forearm of a nondominant hand)
- Mark the test site with a pen and endorse the date and time at which the antigen is being injected
- Aspirate the antigen suspension into the insulin syringe (26G or 27G)
- Insert the needle into the skin at an angle of 10–15° and advance through the epidermis so that the needle tip bevel is just under the skin
- Inject the allergen suspension (~0.1 mL) slowly into the superficial dermis with the bevel end of the needle pointing upward in order to raise the bleb 4–6 mm in diameter on the skin surface
- Inject the control agent (preferably normal saline) into the contralateral side
- Read the result at the test-specific designated time

Note: Conventionally, the test is given on the left forearm to avoid errors in reading. However, the right arm may be used in case there is any contraindication to using the left arm.

it is a skin test, an individual may become sensitized following repeated testing, and a false-positive reaction may occur.

Dick's Test[7]

It was developed in 1924 by American physicians George Dick and Gladys Dick and helps in determining susceptibility to scarlet fever. The antigen injected is 0.1 mL of scarlet fever toxin on the test arm and neutralized toxin (control) on the other arm. The test is read after 24 hours, and erythema larger than 1 cm in diameter indicates a lack of immunity to the disease and makes an individual susceptible to scarlet fever. The incidence of scarlet fever has significantly reduced since the introduction of antibiotics.

Foshay's Test[8]

The test was developed by Dr Lee Foshay and involves the intradermal injection of a suspension of killed *Bartonella henselae*, the causative agent of cat-scratch disease. The antigen is prepared from the sterile lymph node material obtained from a patient with cat-scratch disease. The appearance of an area of erythema >5 mm in diameter after 48 hours at the injection site is considered a positive reaction. It can also be employed in tularemia patients, where the antigen used is a suspension of killed *Francisella tularensis*.

Frei's Test[9,10]

The *Frei's test* was developed in 1925 by a German dermatologist, *Wilhelm Siegmund Frei*, and aids in the diagnosis of lympho-granuloma venereum (LGV), a sexually transmitted infection caused by *Chlamydia trachomatis* serovars L1, L2, and L3. The antigen used is Frei's antigen, which is a heat-inactivated LGV grown in the yolk sac of an embryonated egg. The control usually employed is also prepared from a noninfected yolk sac. After 48–72 hours, an inflamed nodule >6 mm in diameter is considered significant.

Ito Reenstierna Test[11]

In 1913, Hayazo Ito, a Japanese surgeon, devised a specific intradermal test for chancroid using inactivated Ducrey-Krefting bacillus *(Haemophilus ducreyi)*, the diagnostic value of which was later confirmed by Reenstierna. Hence, it is known as the Ito-Reenstierna reaction. A positive reaction indicates delayed hypersensitivity against *H. ducreyi*, the causative organism of chancroid, and can occur in an ongoing or old infection.

Lepromin Test[11,12]

Kensuke Mitsuda developed the first immunological test for leprosy in 1919. It is a prognostic test and is utilized in determining the pole of a leprosy patient. Being an indirect marker of cell-mediated immunity, it measures the degree of *hypersensitivity* of the individual against *Mycobacterium leprae* antigens. The antigen most commonly used is lepromin (Hayashi-Mitsuda antigen), which is prepared by grinding 1 g of autoclaved bacteriologically positive tissue in 20 mL of normal saline in a concentration of 1:20. This being a crude and nonspecific antigen, two methods have been devised for separating bacilli from the tissue and making standardized suspensions. Fernandez and Olmos Castro separated them by centrifuging, first in strong saline to float them and then in alcohol to deposit them. A large proportion of the bacilli are lost during the process, and this method is little used. Dharmendra separated the bacilli by grinding the tissue material in chloroform, evaporating off the chloroform, taking up the residue in ether, and centrifuging the other suspension. The lepromin prepared from the bacilli so separated contains very little tissue element; it produces well-marked early reactions but weaker late reactions and no ulceration. The response after intradermal injection is typically biphasic, with an early Fernandez reaction and a late Mitsuda reaction. The interpretation of the test is listed in **Table 2**.

TABLE 2: Interpretation of lepromin test.

Response	Time	Reading	Interpretation
Fernandez reaction (early)	48–72 hours	Erythema or induration <5 mm	Negative
		Erythema and induration 5–10 mm	Weakly positive (+)
		Erythema and induration 10–15 mm	Moderately positive (++)
		Erythema and induration >15 mm	Strongly positive (+++)
Mitsuda reaction (late)	3–4 weeks	Nothing to see/feel	Negative
		Papule <3 mm	Doubtful
		Erythematous papule 4–7 mm	One plus positive (+)
		Erythematous papule 7–10 mm	Two plus positive (++)
		Erythematous papule >10 mm or of any size with ulceration	Three plus positive (+++)

Schick Test[13]

The Schick test was developed in 1913 by Dr *Béla Schick*, an Austrian pediatrician, and is a method for determining susceptibility to *diphtheria*. A small amount (0.1 mL) of diluted (1/50 minimal lethal dose) diphtheria toxin is injected intradermally into one arm of the person and a heat-inactivated toxin on the other as a control. A wheal >5 mm at the site of injection after 3 days indicates a positive reaction (absence of circulating antibody) or a pseudo-positive reaction (hypersensitivity to the toxin). A positive reaction can be distinguished by the use of a control injection of the same amount of heated toxin (toxoid) into the other forearm.

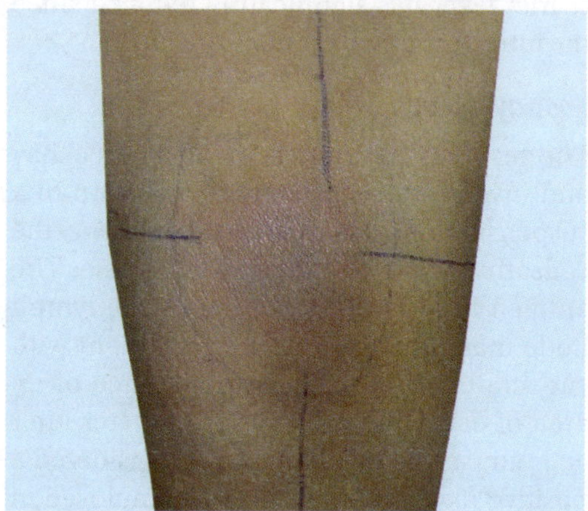

FIG. 1: A positive tuberculin test seen in a patient with cutaneous tuberculosis.

Tuberculin Test[11,14]

First developed in 1907 by Clemens von Pirquet and later modified by Charles Mantoux in 1908. It is an epidemiological tool and is utilized to detect tuberculous infections. The antigen used in India is one tuberculin unit (1TU) of purified protein derivative (PPD) RT23 with tween 80. Tween 80 is a stabilizing agent to protect the absorption of tuberculin on glass surfaces. PPD was developed by American biochemist Florence Seibert, while PPD RT23 with tween 80 was prepared by the Statens Serum Institute (SSI), Denmark from *Mycobacterium tuberculosis*. In India, it is reconstituted and supplied by BCG (Bacillus Calmette–Guérin) vaccine Laboratory, Guindy, Chennai, as an isotonic buffer solution. Other antigens include PPD-S (Siebert) and PPD-G. The test is read after 48–72 hours (Mantoux method) **(Figs. 1 and 2)**. The interpretation of the result is listed in **Table 3**. Tuberculins from atypical mycobacteria or environmental bacteria have also been prepared. They include PPD-B for Battey mycobacteria, PPD-Y for *Mycobacterium kansasii*, scrofulin for *Mycobacterium scrofulaceum*, and burulin for *Mycobacterium ulcerans*.

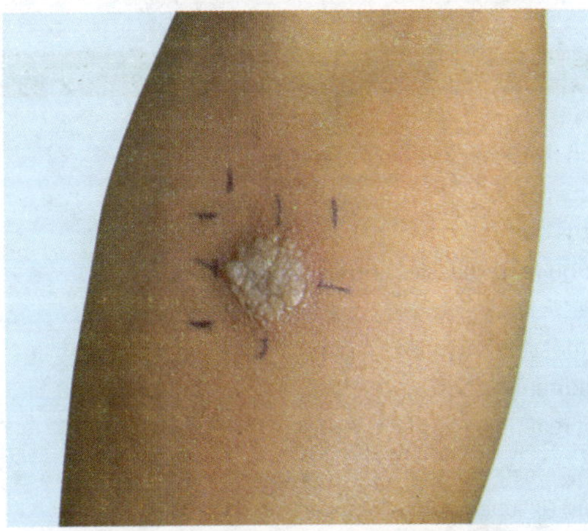

FIG. 2: Bullous Mantoux seen in a child with cutaneous tuberculosis.

Fungal Infections

Histoplasmin Test

Histoplasmin skin testing is useful in epidemiological studies but is not predictive of histoplasmosis. 0.1 mL of 1:100 diluted antigen containing the M and H precipitins is injected intradermally and is read after 48 hours. A test is considered positive when the induration measures 5 mm or more. It is seldom employed as a diagnostic tool as it cannot differentiate between active and past infections.

Trichophytin Test[15]

This test is performed to detect allergic hypersensitivity toward dermatophytes and

TABLE 3: Interpretation of Mantoux test.

Interpretation	Reading	Patient's group
Positive	>5 mm	• HIV-positive person • Recent contacts of active TB cases • Persons with nodular or fibrotic changes on chest X-ray consistent with old healed TB • Organ transplant recipients and other immunosuppressed patients who are on cytotoxic immunosuppressive agents such as cyclophosphamide or methotrexate • Patients on long-term systemic corticosteroid therapy (>6 weeks) and those on a dose of prednisone ≥ 15 mg/day or equivalent • End-stage renal disease
	>10 mm	• Recent arrivals (<5 years) from high-prevalence countries • Injectable drug users • Residents and employees of high-risk congregate settings (e.g., prisons, nursing homes, hospitals, homeless shelters, etc.) • Mycobacteriology laboratory personnel • Persons with clinical conditions that place them at high risk (e.g., diabetes, prolonged corticosteroid therapy, leukemia, end-stage renal disease, chronic malabsorption syndromes, low body weight, etc.) • Children <4 years of age, or children and adolescents exposed to adults in high-risk categories • Infants, children, and adolescents exposed to adults in high-risk categories
	>15 mm	• Persons with no known risk factors for TB. Reactions >15 mm are unlikely to be due to previous BCG vaccination or exposure to environmental mycobacteria
False positive		• Infection with nontuberculous mycobacteria • Previous BCG vaccination • Incorrect method of TST administration • Incorrect interpretation of reaction • Incorrect bottle of antigen used

Continued

Continued

Interpretation	Reading	Patient's group
False negative		• Cutaneous anergy • Recent TB infection (within 8–10 weeks of exposure) • Very old TB infection (many years) • Very young age (<6 months old) • Recent live-virus vaccination (e.g., measles and smallpox) • Overwhelming TB disease • Some viral illnesses (e.g., measles and chicken pox) • Incorrect method of TST administration • Incorrect interpretation of reaction, insufficient dose, and inadvertent subcutaneous injection

(BCG: bacillus Calmette–Guérin; HIV: human immunodeficiency virus; TB: tuberculosis; TST: tuberculin skin test)

act as an aid in diagnosing mycoses of the glabrous skin. The active principle of the pathogenic fungus in the skin was first isolated by Scholtz in 1918. Several trichophytins have been made by various authors from different fungi, but a standardized and universally recognized preparation is still lacking. The commonly used trichophytin antigen is a glycopeptide extracted (using the acetone-ethylene glycol extraction method) from the spores and mycelia of dermatophytes, mostly *Trichophyton mentagrophytes*. Other antigens employed include *Trichophyton* extract, which contains *Trichophyton gypsum* 40%, *Trichophyton cerebriforme* 20%, *Trichophyton microides* 20%, *Trichophyton rosaceum*, *Trichophyton violaceum*, and *Trichophyton crateriforme* in equal parts to 20% and is used in sterile distilled water in dilutions of 1:20 and 1:50. *Trichophyton* in a concentration of either 10 µg, 1 µg, or 0.1 µg in 0.1 mL of normal saline is injected intradermally into the flexor forearm. The test is read after 20 minutes for an immediate reaction and after 24 or 72 hours for a delayed response. Erythema, edema, and induration are generally seen, and a papulovesicular or ulcerative lesion can also occur. A wheal >10 mm in diameter at 20 minutes and induration >5 mm at 72 hours are considered positive responses. False-positive trichophytin tests may be obtained if the extract is contaminated with bacteria. Intradermal tests with trichophytin are an aid in diagnosing mycoses of the glabrous skin.

Protozoal Test

Filarial Intradermal Skin Test[16]

The intradermal test with the filariasis polypeptide antigen (FPT) purified from *Dirofilaria immitis* was developed in China as a surveillance tool to study the annual positive conversion rate of Filaria. The skin papule measuring >9 mm was considered a positive test. It can also be utilized to study filariasis transmission in an endemic zone.

Leishmanin Test (Montenegro Test)[17-19]

The *leishmanin skin test* (LST), also called the *Montenegro test*, is an immunological test that measures delayed-type hypersensitivity to *Leishmania* antigen. It was first described by Brazilian physician João Montenegro in 1926 and is performed via intradermal injection of *Leishmania* antigens (leishmanin). The cultured promastigotes are washed in 0.5% phenol saline, diluted to 1×10^6/mL, and 0.1 mL is injected intradermally. The injection site is examined 48 hours later, and induration of ≥5 mm is considered a positive test. The LST is generally positive when lesions of cutaneous and mucosal leishmaniasis are present but negative in active visceral leishmaniasis. The presence of a positive skin test seems to be under genetic control and is a marker for resistance to the development of symptomatic visceral leishmaniasis. The test should not be repeated in less than 6 months, because the antigens are immunogenic and capable of inducing a positive response. Occasional false-positive reactions have been noted in patients with glandular tuberculosis and systemic fungal infections. It is a useful and important tool for epidemiological, immunological, and diagnostic studies and is an essential component of vaccine trials.

NONINFECTIOUS DISEASES

Autoerythrocyte Sensitization Test[20,21]

First described by Gardner and Diamond in 1955, it is used to diagnose autoerythrocyte sensitization syndrome, also known as Gardner–Diamond syndrome (GDS) or psychogenic purpura, which is a rare autoimmune vasculopathy. Autoerythrocyte sensitization test (AEST) is performed to confirm the red blood cell (RBC) antigenicity by injecting intradermally 0.1 mL of washed RBC on the flexural aspect of the forearm.

Steps to prepare washed RBCs are depicted in **Flowchart 1**. The test readings are taken at 30 minutes and 24 hours. Tenderness or ecchymosis at the injection site is considered positive.

Autologous Serum Skin Test[22]

Autologous serum skin test (ASST) is a simple in vivo clinical test for the detection of basophil histamine-releasing activity and to diagnose chronic autoimmune urticaria (CAU) among chronic spontaneous urticaria (CSU) patients. The test involves the aspiration of 2 mL of venous blood and allowing it to clot at room temperature, followed by the separation of serum by centrifuging at 2,000 rpm for 10–25 minutes. 0.05–0.1 mL of serum is injected intradermally, and equal amounts of normal saline (negative control) and histamine (10 µg/mL) (positive control) are injected intradermally 3–5 cm apart in the volar aspect of the same forearm. The wheal and flare responses are measured at 30 minutes. A positive test is defined as a serum-induced wheal response with a diameter of >1.5 mm or more than that of the saline-induced response. Interestingly, positive tests (ASST)

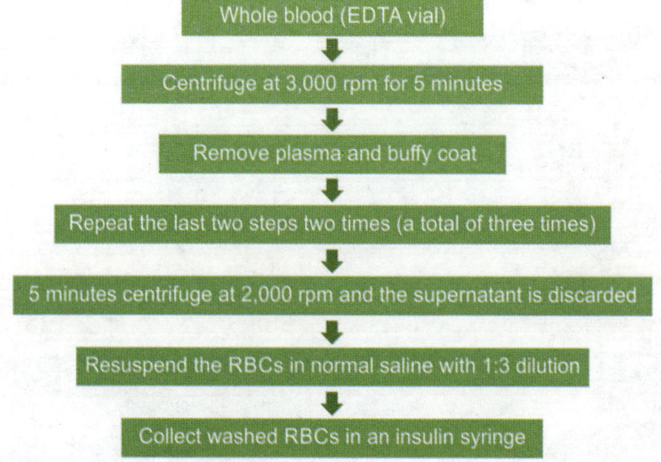

FLOWCHART 1: Steps to prepare washed RBCs in autoerythrocyte sensitization test.
(EDTA: ethylenediaminetetraacetic acid; RBCs: red blood cells)

have been reported to correlate strongly with disease severity, duration, the presence of *Helicobacter pylori* immunoglobulin G (IgG) antibodies, and multiple intolerances to nonsteroidal anti-inflammatory drugs **(Figs. 3 to 6)**.

Intradermal Sensitivity Test for Drug[23-25]

Intradermal testing is a rapid, convenient, and reproducible method of detecting immediate and delayed drug hypersensitivity (DH). It is also used to identify alternative drugs for patients with positive skin or provocation tests with suspected drugs. The guidelines discussed here are as per the European Academy of Allergy and Clinical Immunology (EAACI). First of all, prepare a stock solution by dissolving the parenteral powder in sterile isotonic saline, which should be used within 2 hours of reconstitution. 0.02–0.05 mL of drug is injected, and a bleb of 3 mm is raised. After 15–20 minutes, the site is examined, and if the diameter of the initial wheal is increased by 3 mm and associated with the surrounding flare, it is considered a positive test. For

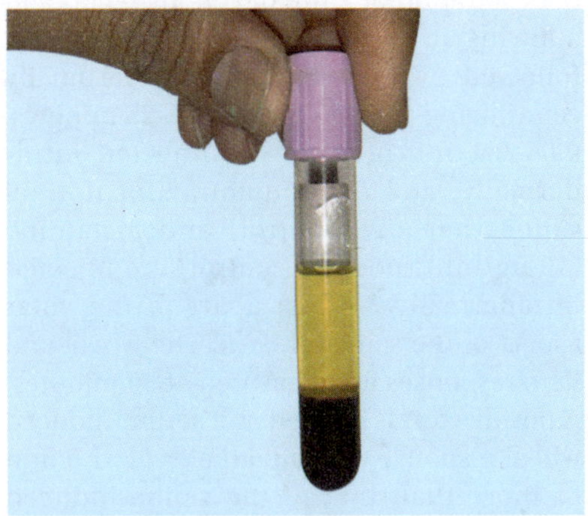

FIG. 3: Serum is separated by centrifugation (2,000 rpm for 10–25 minutes).

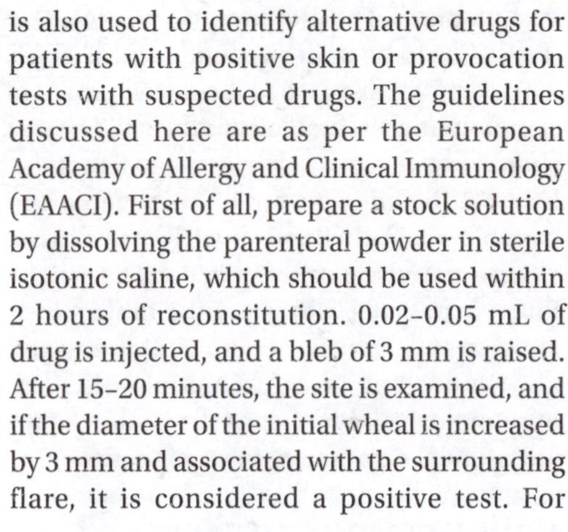

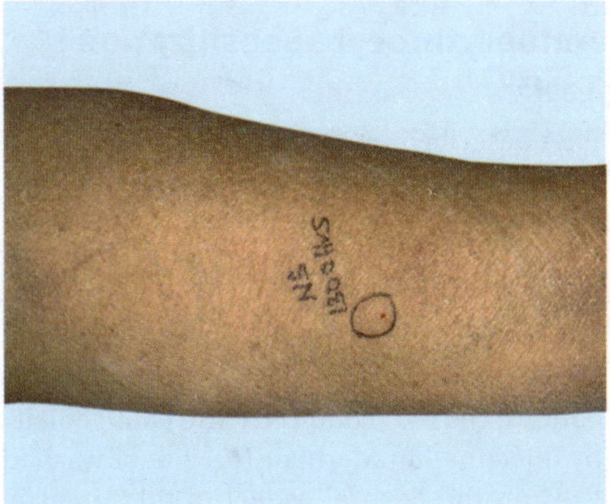

FIG. 5: Equal amount of normal saline is injected intra-dermally into same forearm 3–5 cm apart for control.

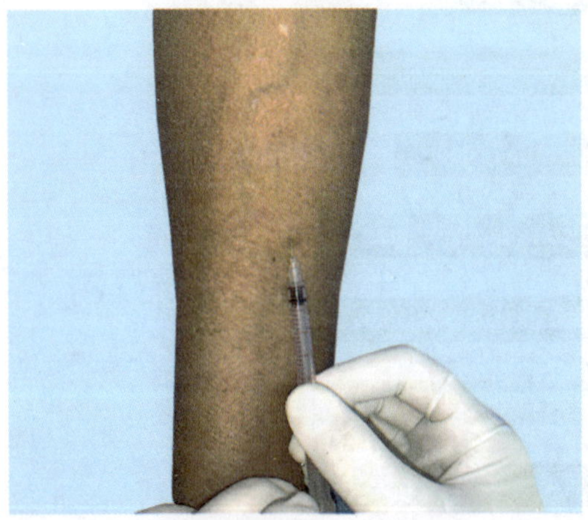

FIG. 4: 0.05 mL or serum being injected intradermally into the volar aspect of forearm.

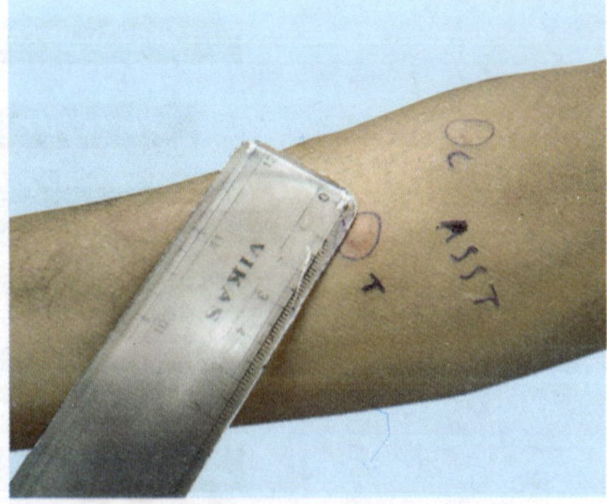

FIG. 6: A positive autologous serum skin test seen in chronic spontaneous urticaria.

delayed drug reactions, the site is reinspected after 24–72 hours and is considered positive if there is induration and erythema. Saline is used as a negative control on the contralateral side. The drugs for which this test is frequently warranted include penicillin, general and local anesthetic agents, tetanus toxoid, iodinated radiocontrast media, insulin, heterologous sera, and collagen chymopapain. Chances of anaphylaxis do persist, and therefore resuscitative measures and epinephrine injections should be kept ready. Intradermal sensitivity test (IDST) is contraindicated in severe cutaneous adverse drug reactions.

Kveim–Siltzbach Test[26]

The test was named after Norwegian pathologist Morten Ansgar Kveim, who first reported the test in 1941 using lymph node tissue from sarcoidosis patients. The test consists of injecting the Kveim reagent, a particulate suspension prepared from the granulomatous splenic tissue of a patient with sarcoidosis, into the skin of a person with suspected sarcoidosis. Approximately 50–80% of patients with sarcoidosis develop positive reaction and noncaseating granulomas in the injection site as seen on a skin biopsy 4–6 weeks later. The false-positive rate has been quoted at 1–5%. There is a concern that certain infections, such as bovine spongiform encephalopathy, could be transferred through a Kveim test.

Pathergy Test[27-29]

First described in 1937 by Blobner as a state of altered tissue reactivity in response to minor trauma, it is characterized by nonspecific pustules or papules, or the enlargement of preexisting wounds, developing on sites of minor trauma, including blunt trauma. It has been suggested that pathergy may be driven by either a nonspecific hyperinflammatory response to a traumatic insult, an exaggerated response to microbial antigens, or an interaction between genetic and environmental factors.

Sharp or blunted needles (20G needles) with 4–6 needle pricks are used, and response is evaluated after 24–48 hours. They are inserted either perpendicularly or obliquely through the skin. Needles can be blunted by hitting against a sterile plastic sheath cover. Once the needle is placed into the dermis, it can be twisted a couple of times to increase trauma. A total of 4–6 pricks are performed, with sensitivity varying from 28 to 33%. A test is evaluated by the naked eye, and an erythematous papule ≥2 mm or a pustule is regarded as a positive reaction. Sharp needles decreased both sensitivity and intensity of reaction.

Pathergy is characteristic of pyoderma gangrenosum (PG) and other neutrophilic skin conditions such as Behçet's disease (BD) and Sweet's syndrome. Other diseases where it can be seen include deficiency of interleukin 1 receptor antagonist (DIRA), Crohn's disease, atypical eosinophilic pustular folliculitis, neonates with Down syndrome, myeloproliferative disorders, non-Hodgkin lymphoma, and chronic myeloid leukemia treated with interferon-α. The development of a monocytic and neutrophilic cell infiltrate without true vasculitis can be seen on histopathology.

Pilocarpine and Histamine Tests

The pilocarpine and histamine tests are employed to assess the integrity of dermal nerves in patients with Hansen's disease. The tests read positive at the tuberculoid pole while showing a negative response at the lepromatous pole, as the nerve integrity is preserved until late.

The pilocarpine test verifies the integrity of the parasympathetic nervous system by stimulating the secretion of sweat. Iodine tincture is applied to a specific lesion (and normal skin as a control), followed by the injection of 0.2 mL of a 1 in 1,000 solution of pilocarpine. The areas are dusted with starch powder, which turns blue if there is sudoresis. In leprosy, sweat production is diminished or absent.

In the histamine test, the sympathetic nervous system is tested by placing a drop of histamine acid diphosphate 1 in 1,000 (1 mg/mL) on the lesion and on normal skin. Both areas are pricked with a needle, and after 10 minutes, a positive response manifests as erythema and the formation of a wheal. This test is especially valuable for hypopigmented leprosy lesions, in which there is no response to histamine.

CONCLUSION

In conclusion, intradermal tests remain integral in the diagnostic landscape of various dermatological and nondermatological diseases. Despite the continuous evolution of medical diagnostics, these tests, when administered by experienced dermatologists, continue to offer crucial diagnostic and prognostic insights. Their ability to detect both immediate and delayed hypersensitivity reactions against a range of antigens makes them versatile tools in clinical practice. Navigating through a spectrum of diseases, from anthrax to scarlet fever and cat-scratch disease to leprosy, each intradermal test plays a unique role in aiding diagnosis and providing valuable information about the patient's immune response. The historical significance of tests like Dick's, Foshay's, and Frei's underscores their enduring relevance in specific diagnostic contexts. However, it is crucial to acknowledge the potential challenges and risks associated with intradermal tests, including the possibility of pain and untoward reactions. The careful consideration of preprocedural requirements, procedural steps, and the management of adverse events is paramount to ensure the safety of patients undergoing these tests.

Key Messages

- Intradermal tests are minimally invasive yet powerful approach for diagnosing and assessing various diseases.
- The comprehensive coverage of intradermal tests, spanning bacterial, fungal, protozoa, and noninfectious diseases highlights their versatility and pivotal role in early and retrospective diagnosis.
- It is important to emphasize on procedural details, precautions, and awareness of potential risk-associated intradermal testing.

REFERENCES

1. Shah KM, Rank MA, Davé SA, Oslie CL, Butterfield JH. Predicting which medication classes interfere with allergy skin testing. Allergy Asthma Proc. 2010;31(6):477-82.

2. Gradman J, Wolthers OD. Suppressive effects of topical mometasone furoate and tacrolimus on skin prick testing in children. Pediatr Dermatol. 2008;25(2):269-70.

3. Sicherer SH, Eggleston PA. EMLA Cream for pain reduction in diagnostic allergy skin testing: effect on wheal and flare responses. Ann Allergy Asthma Immunol. 1997;78(1):64-8.

4. Calabria CW, Coop CA, Tankersley MS. The LOCAL Study: Local reactions do not predict local reactions in allergen immunotherapy. J Allergy Clin Immunol. 2009;124(4):739-44.

5. Lockey RF, Benedict LM, Turkeltaub PC, Bukantz SC. Fatalities from immunotherapy (IT) and skin testing (ST). J Allergy Clin Immunol. 1987;79(4):660-77.

6. Shlyakhov E, Rubinstein E. Anthraxin Skin Testing: an Alternative Method for Anthrax Vaccine and Post-Vaccinal Immunity Assessment. Zentralbl Veterinarmed B. 1996;43(8):483-8.

7. Britannica, The Editors of Encyclopaedia. (2022). "Dick test". Encyclopedia Britannica. [online] Available from https://www.britannica.com/science/Dick-test [Last accessed February, 2024].

8. Anderson B, Kelley C, Threlkel R, Edwards K. Detection of Rochalimaea henselae in cat scratch disease skin test antigens. J Infect Dis. 1993;168:1034-6.

9. Connor WH, Levin EA, Ecker EE. Flight test findings. J Infectious Dis. 1937;60(1):62-3.

10. Strauss MJ, Howard ME. Frei test for inguinal lymphogranuloma: experience with antigens made from mouse brain. J Am Med Assoc. 1936;106(7):517-20.

11. Nagar R, Pande S, Khopkar U. Intradermal tests in dermatology-I: Tests for infectious diseases. Indian J Dermatol Venereol Leprol. 2006;72: 461.

12. Hanks JH, Abe M, Nakayama T, Tuma M, Bechelli LM, Domínguez VM. Studies towards the standardization of lepromin: Progress and prospects. Bull World Health Organ. 1970;42(5):703 9.

13. Britannica, The Editors of Encyclopaedia. (2011). "Schick test". Encyclopedia Britannica. [online] Available from https://www.britannica.com/science/Schick-test [Last accessed February, 2024].

14. Nayak S, Acharjya B. Mantoux test and its interpretation. Indian Dermatol Online J. 2012;3(1):2-6.

15. Williams CM, Carpenter CC. Trichophytin in Diagnosis. Arch Dermatol Syphilol. 1932;25(5): 847-51.

16. Shi FT, Shi ZJ, Shi HH, Lin XM, Huang QA. Assessment of intradermal test in longitudinal surveillance of bancroftian filariasis. Chinese Medical J. 1990;103(1):29-33.

17. Cascio A, Iaria C. Appropriate Screening for Leishmaniasis before Immunosuppressive Treatments. Emerg Infect Dis. 2009;15(10):1706-7.

18. Sadeghian G, Ziaei H, Bidabadi LS, Nilforoushzadeh MA. Evaluation of Leishmanin Skin Test Reaction in Different Variants of Cutaneous Leishmaniasis. Indian J Dermatol. 2013;58(3):239.

19. Manzur A, Bari AU. Sensitivity of leishmanin skin test in patients of acute cutaneous leishmaniasis. Dermatol Online J. 2006;12(4):2.

20. Gardner FH, Diamond LK. Autoerythrocyte sensitization a form of purpura producing painful bruising following autosensitization to red blood cells in certain women. Blood. 1955;10(7):675-90.

21. Kumar P, Singh A, Prabha N, Ganguly S, Dudhe M. Role of Autoerythrocyte Sensitization Test in the Diagnosis of Recurrent Spontaneous Bruising. Indian Dermatol Online J. 2023;14(3):375.

22. Vikramkumar AG, Kuruvila S, Ganguly S. Autologous serum skin test as an indicator of chronic autoimmune urticaria in a tertiary care hospital in South India. Indian Dermatol Online J. 2014;5(Suppl 2):S87.

23. Barbaud A, Weinborn M, Garvey LH, Testi S, Kvedariene V, Bavbek S, et al. Intradermal tests with drugs: an approach to standardization. Front Med. 2020;7:156.

24. Brockow K, Romano A, Blanca M, Ring J, Pichler W, Demoly P. General considerations for skin test procedures in the diagnosis of drug hypersensitivity. Allergy. 2002;57:45-51.

25. Mertes PM, Malinovsky JM, Jouffroy L, Aberer W, Terreehorst I, Brockow K, et al.; Working Group of the SFAR and SFA. Reducing the risk of anaphylaxis during anesthesia: 2011 updated guidelines for clinical practice. J Investig Allergol Clin Immunol. 2011;21:442-53.

26. Kveim A. En ny og spesifikk kutan-reaksjon ved Boecks sarcoid. Nord Med. 1941;9:169-72.

27. Ergun T. Pathergy phenomenon. Frontiers in medicine. 2021;8:639404.

28. Varol A, Seifert O, Anderson CD. The skin pathergy test: innately useful? Arch Dermatol Res. 2010;302:155-68.

29. Honigman A, Kern JS, Frew JW. Pathergy: A review of potential mechanisms and novel therapeutic targets. Wound Pract Res. 2022;30(1):55-61.

Patch Test and Other Allergen Tests

Abirami C, Chakravarti R Srinivas, Jamyang Choden

INTRODUCTION

Clemens von Pirquet in the year 1906 termed the exaggerated immunological, harmful response to harmless substances as "allergies" or hypersensitive reactions (HSR).[1] These harmless materials that elicit allergy are called allergens. The first documented allergy test dates back to 1869 when Dr Charles Blakely introduced a minute quantity of pollen on wounded skin. Dr Joseph Jadassohn, a German physician of the 19th century, introduced patch testing and used it for diagnostic purposes. He is hence known as the "Father of Patch testing".

IMMUNOLOGY OF ALLERGEN TESTS

Allergens usually have a small molecular weight of < 500 Daltons, enabling it to cross the skin barrier.[2] Thus, patients with defective skin barrier such as atopic individuals and elderly are more susceptible to imbibe the allergen.

According to Gell and Coombs classification of hypersensitivity reactions, four types of HSR have been documented.[3] Out of these, type 4 is elicited with the help of an allergy test in an attempt to narrow down the exogenous allergen causing allergic contact dermatitis (ACD).

Allergic contact dermatitis is an example of type 4 HSR mediated by T lymphocytes and macrophages. Urticaria, angioedema, and anaphylaxis are mediated by immunoglobulin E (IgE) and mast cells and are an example of type 1 HSR.

PATCH TESTING

Patch testing refers to the application of a suspected allergen over a patch of skin, in known formulation and concentration to test its ability to elicit a reaction.

When to perform patch testing?[4]

- Patients in whom contact dermatitis is suspected.
- To rule out contact dermatitis as an aggravating factor of other skin conditions that may be aggravated by contact dermatitis (atopic dermatitis, seborrheic dermatitis, stasis, nummular eczema, psoriasis, and dyshidrosis).
- Chronic eczema patients with an unestablished etiology
- Suspected cases of occupational contact dermatitis
- Patients on long-term low-dose corticosteroids (< 10 mg/day) and/or antihistamines can also be enrolled for patch testing.

The North American Contact Dermatitis Group (NACDG) has published that a patient on immunomodulators such as azathioprine, cyclosporine, and calcineurin inhibitors may elicit a positive patch test irrespective of the immunosuppression; however, false-negative tests should not be neglected.

Materials Required

Standardized patch testing kits are available, with allergens commonly encountered (70–80%) in a particular region, {e.g., International Standard Series, Indian Standard Battery [Contact and Occupational Dermatoses Forum of India (CODFI)], British Standard Series (BSCA), American Core Series, etc.}. Special series such as Hairdressing series and Bakery series can also be employed if the allergen is narrowed down.

Table 1 gives the Indian Standard series, which is the most commonly applied patch test series.

The test units for the traditional patch test techniques are aluminum or polyethylene chambers, which hold the allergen and are placed over hypoallergenic adhesive strips. The commercially available chambers are Finns, van der Bend, and IQ chambers **(Fig. 1)**.

Finn's chamber is the commonly used test unit, made of stiff aluminum, with a diameter

TABLE 1: Indian Standard series.

Allergen	Concentration	Vehicle
Petrolatum (control)	100	
Potassium dichromate	0.5%	
Neomycin sulfate	20.0%	
Cobalt chloride hexahydrate	1.0%	
Benzocaine	5.0%	
p-Phenylenediamine (PPD)	1.0%	
Paraben mix	16.0%	Petrolatum base
Nickel sulfate hexahydrate	5.0%	
Colophonium	20.0%	
Gentamicin sulfate	20.0%	
Mercapto mix	2.0%	
Epoxy resin, bisphenol A	1.0%	
Fragrance mix I	8.0%	
2-Mercaptobenzothiazole (MBT)	2.0%	
Nitrofurazone	1.0%	
Chlorocresol	1.0%	
Lanolin alcohol	30.0%	
Peru balsam	25.0%	
Thiuram mix	1.0% pet	
Clioquinol	5.0% pet	
Black rubber mix	0.6% pet	
Para-tertiary butylphenol (PTBP)	1.0% pet	
Formaldehyde	1.0	Aqueous
Polyethylene glycol 400 (PEG 400)	100	Aqueous
Parthenolide	0.1	

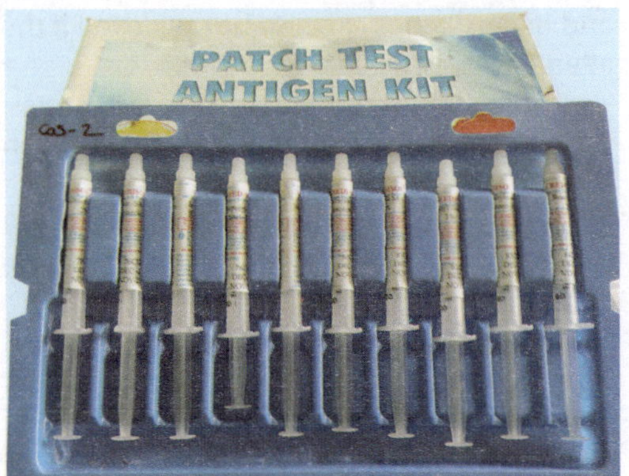

FIG. 1: A commercial patch testing kit with prefilled syringes.

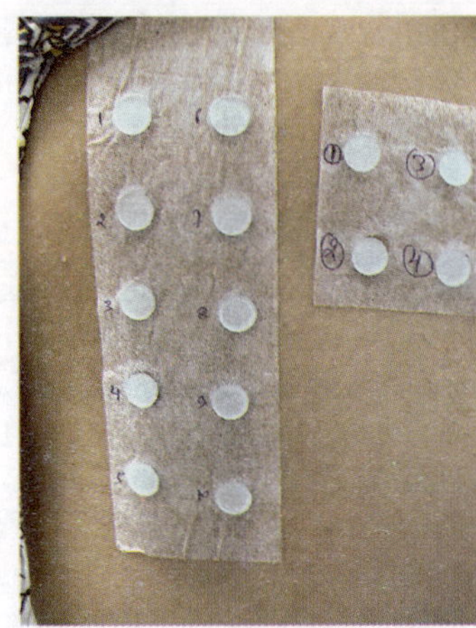

FIG. 2: Application of allergens on the upper back.

of 8 mm and depth of 0.5 mm, which houses the allergen suspended in a vehicle, the most common being white petroleum jelly. Other vehicles are water, ethanol, acetone, olive oil, etc. There is no single ideal vehicle, and it has to be selected based on the allergen. The allergen is kept in a prefilled syringe.

Commercially available thin-layer rapid-use epicutaneous (TRUE) test uses allergens, which are prefilled in the polyester chamber in a hydrophilic vehicle, such as SOFTSAN.[5]

Methodology

Site: Upper back (either side of the spine) > Upper extensor part of the arm > Upper thigh. The preferred site should be nonhairy to allow proper occlusion. If such a site is unavailable, shaving of hairs along the direction of hair growth may be done with a razor blade to prevent folliculitis.

Cleanse and degrease the area with alcohol. Apply the prepared panel and document the time of application along with allergens. Photographic documentation allows comparison while following up **(Fig. 2)**.

The patient is instructed not to wet the area and avoid activities that induce sweating such as exercise, and occlusive clothing.

Readings are to be taken at 24 hours if irritant contact dermatitis is suspected. If

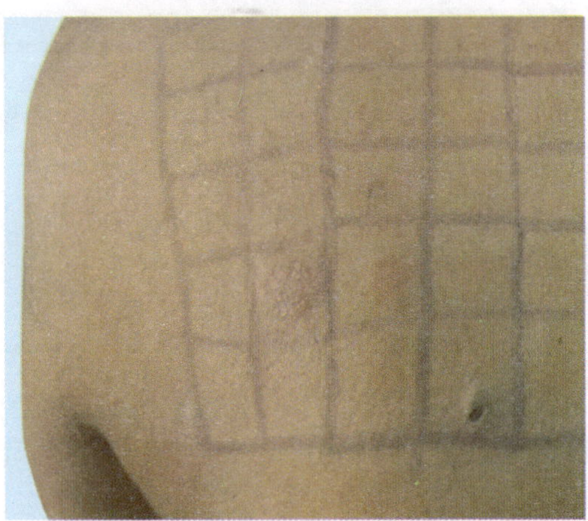

FIG. 3: Patch test reading noted at 48 hours.

the test is being done to elicit ACD, readings are to be taken at 48 hours and re-read at 72–96 hours. The second reading is to confirm the positive or negative reading taken at the end of the second day. Once the panel is removed, a window of 15–20 minutes is recommended to allow erythema and edema, which may appear due to local vasodilation to settle **(Figs. 3 and 4)**.

Interpretation (Table 2)

False-positive test could be due to a reaction to the vehicle or adhesive, improper suspension of the allergen in the vehicle, presence of

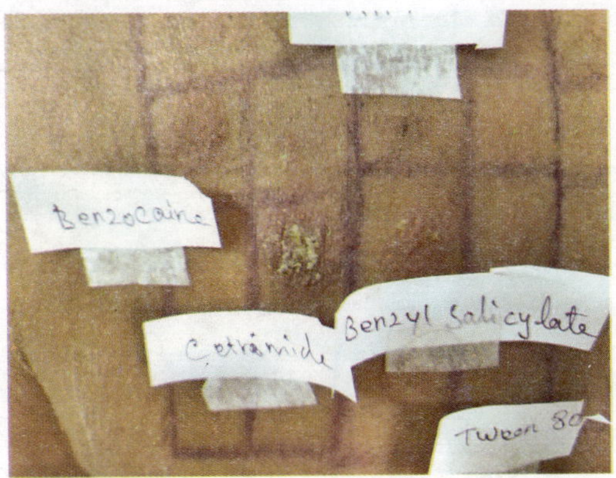

FIG. 4: Patch test reading noted at 72 hours.

TABLE 2: Interpretation of patch testing as per International Contact Dermatitis Research Group (ICDRG).

?+	Doubtful
+	Mild reaction, possible erythema, infiltration, and papules
++	Strong reaction, erythema, infiltration, papules, and vesicles
+++	Very strong reaction, intense erythema, infiltration, and coalescing vesicles
IR	Irritant reaction of various types
NT	Not tested

impurities in the test material, or in a patient with excited skin syndrome.[6] In all the above cases, consistent results are nonreproducible on repetition **(Fig. 5)**

False-negative tests could be due to inappropriate site selection, improper attachment of the panel, inadequate test material, wet panel, or premature or late reading. Delayed response is noted in patients on oral corticosteroids.

Complications[4]

- Severe local reactions
- Pigmentary changes (de/hyperpigmentation)
- Keloid/Scar formation
- Flare of preexisting eczema

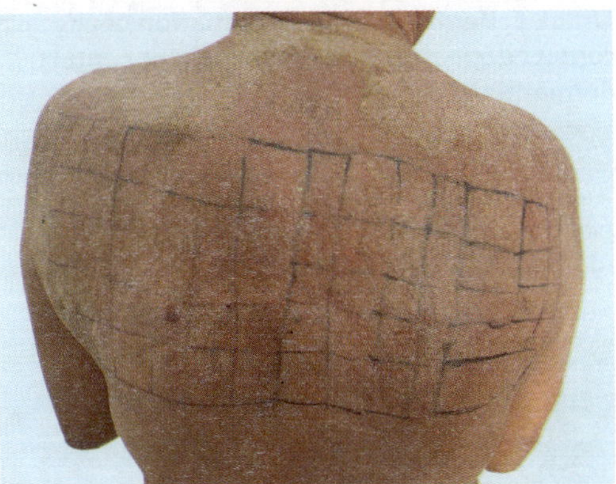

FIG. 5: Excited skin syndrome—when a panel of allergens are applied over the test skin leading to generalized erythema interpreted as positive patch test. The positive results are not reproducible on repetition.

- Persistent reaction which may last up to a few months
- Anaphylaxis (rare—reported in formaldehyde allergen)

Special Conditions/Innovations in Patch Testing

- *Unavailability of standardized kit*: Suspected allergen can be suspended in white petroleum jelly if lipophilic or water if hydrophilic and applied directly over the skin surface.
- The plastic cap over glass vials which are commonly disposed of can be used as an alternative to occlude the test material.
- Patch testing is not performed on a patient with active allergy to prevent the chances of id eruption and exacerbation of lesions.
- Patch test is generally avoided in pregnant patients—immunological changes might alter the results.
- In the pediatric population, the test is to be performed only after thorough history taking as the surface area to apply the panel is less.
- Defer patch test in those with oral corticosteroid intake > 10 mg/day, injectable steroids, and cyclosporine > 2 mg/kg/day,

TABLE 3: Dermoscopic differentiation of allergic contact dermatitis (ACD) from irritant contact dermatitis (ICD).[7]

ACD	ICD
Homogenous erythema, vesicles, and crusts with dotted vessels	Poral pattern or pore reaction pattern with perifollicular pattern

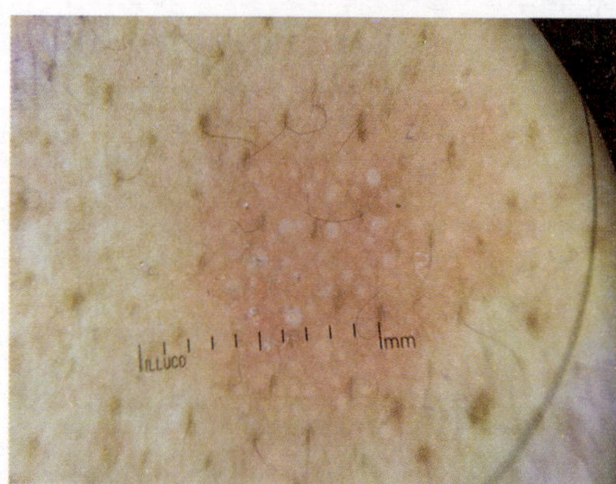

FIG. 7: Dermoscopy of allergic contact dermatitis (ACD) showing homogenous erythema, and vesicles. Poral pattern commonly seen in irritant contact dermatitis (ICD) is not appreciated here.

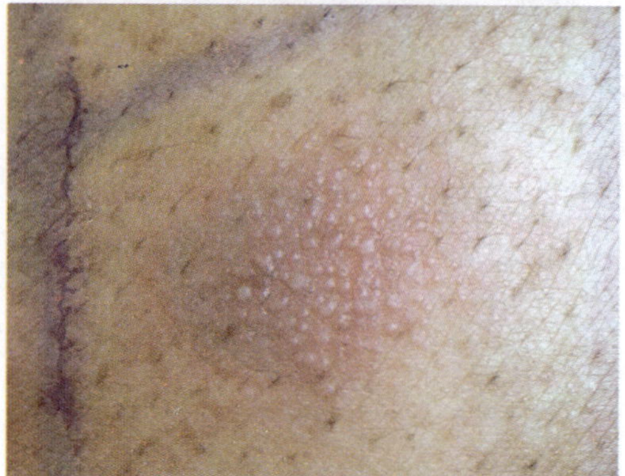

FIG. 6: Allergic contact dermatitis—gross appearance showing erythema, papules, and vesicles.

on phototherapy or severe recent sunlight exposure.

- Dermoscopic examination facilitates detection of faint erythema, which is missed in gross examination. **Table 3** shows dermoscopic differentiation of ACD from ICD **(Figs. 6 and 7)**.[7]

Open Tests

This is utilized as an initial screen test to identify the possibility of sensitivity and to present a heightened hypersensitivity response to unknown antigens.

The allergen in its form or diluted in a vehicle is applied over a diameter of 1 cm and readings are taken at 48 hours and 72–96 hours. The response is rather subtle and a positive reaction may present as papules.

Semiopen Tests

A suspected product with its offending ingredients (emulsifiers or solvents) is applied over the skin. An adhesive tape is applied over the site after it dries and readings are taken at 48 and 96 hours.

Repeated Open Application Tests

This test is used to confirm and reproduce the results obtained by closed tests. The formulation containing the sensitizing substance is applied twice a day over the exposed part of nonhairy skin, such as the anterior aspect of the arm and back. The development of eczematous changes on the site of the application indicates a positive test.

Photopatch Test

An allergen panel is arranged wherein each test material is duplicated side by side. This panel is then applied over the skin. Minimal erythema dose (MED) is calculated from a different site. After 48 hours of contact, one set of the allergens is exposed to ultraviolet A (UVA) at 50% of the calculated MED while the other set is protected from the irradiation. Development of reaction only of photo-exposed test area denotes a positive photo patch test.

Specific photo patch series are available for testing **(Fig. 8)**.

Patch testing of everyday materials

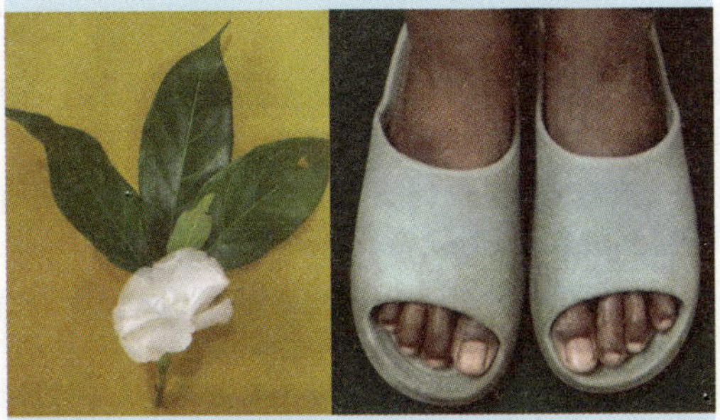

Crushed flower and leaf tested separately

Scrapings of footwear with normal saline as vehicle

FIG. 8: Examples of common items for which patch testing can be performed.

Prick Tests

It is used to demonstrate type 1 hypersensitivity reaction against the mounted allergen where IgE antibodies present in mast cells of the skin are activated. A wheal of > 3 mm and more than that of positive control (histamine) is read as a positive reaction. Negative control of saline is used.[8]

As chances of anaphylaxis prevail, these tests are to be performed in settings where resuscitation facilities are readily available.

- *Skin prick test*: After cleaning the surface of the skin, allergens are placed at intervals of 3–5 cm along with histamine-positive control. With the help of a 26G needle or lancet, a prick is made and the needle is gently lifted upward. A new needle is used for every prick and fresh allergen to prevent cross-contamination.
- *Intradermal test*: It is not performed routinely due to its practical downsides of sterility, invasiveness, and ethical considerations. A suspected allergen is injected intradermally with a 26G needle and response is read after 15–20 minutes.

Indications[9]

- Those food allergens which could not be identified by elimination or challenge, e.g., eggs and peanuts.
- Identification of allergens to improve quality of life in poorly controlled allergic conditions, such as bronchial asthma.
- Suspected allergy to medications of significant importance, e.g., penicillin wherein alternatives are limited.

Contraindications

- Strict—anaphylaxis episode up to 6 weeks before the date of testing.
- Avoid in children below the age of 2 years, elderly, and pregnant patients. Skin reactivity is dampened; hence, serum IgE level testing is preferred.
- Topical corticosteroids oral antihistamines and antidepressant usage have to be discontinued for 2–3 weeks and up to 10 days, respectively.

Serum Immunoglobulin E Testing[9]

A blood sample is taken and evaluated for circulating serum IgE antibody levels against a particular antigen. It is performed using enzyme-linked immunosorbent assay (ELISA) method or radioallergosorbent tests (RASTs) technique. The allergen to be tested can be single or series.

Indications

Exaggerated ongoing allergic response wherein sin prick test might yield a false-positive response.

- Children below the age of 2 years, elderly, pregnant patients, and those on antihistamines in whom skin prick is difficult to perform or less yielding.
- History of anaphylaxis
- Unavailability of suspected allergen in the prick test

Spot Test

These chemical tests are performed to identify the presence of an element in commonly utilized materials.

Nickel[10]

1% dimethylglyoxime (DMG) + nickel—a strawberry red coloration (in the presence of ammonia).

Dimethylglyoxime mixed in ethanol and 10% ammonia in water is added to a swab stick/earbud and rubbed on the metallic surface. The development of red color confirms the presence of Nickel in the material.

Cobalt

Cobalt commonly occurs as an impurity in alloys of Nickel. Thus, patients with sensitivity to Nickel have increased positivity to Cobalt as well. Thus, testing for Cobalt has to be performed before the DMG test to prevent false positivity.

Testing for cobalt may be done by Swab test with appropriate reagents or by allowing the suspected material to be immersed in a gel-containing the reagents. The presence of cobalt is identified by a change in yellow tinge to red.

Chromium

The test material is boiled or soaked in hot water and diluted sulfuric acid, water-soluble chromate mixed in ethanol is added to the boiled water. Lavender to Prussian blue tinge is noted in the presence of chromium.

CONCLUSION

Chronic urticaria is not an indication for allergen testing and has to be avoided. Both skin prick tests and serum IgE tests have low positive predictive value but high negative predictive value. Thus, those materials that did not elicit a reaction on testing can be routinely consumed/used by the patient, improving their quality of life and nutrition.

Key Messages

- Allergy is a common presentation to any clinic. It stands as a routine and recurrent reminder of one's immunity.
- Its management greatly depends upon the identification and avoidance of the allergen that might be hidden in plain sight.
- Successful management of allergy lies not only in the evasion of the suspect but also in empowering the patient with a better quality of life.
- Allergy tests aid in the detection of allergens, thereby preventing blanket avoidance.

REFERENCES

1. Von Pirquet C. Allergie. Münch Med Wochenschr. 1906;53:1457-8.
2. Murphy PB, Atwater AR, Mueller M. Allergic Contact Dermatitis. In: StatPearls [Internet]. Treasure Island (FL): StatPearls Publishing; 2023.
3. Uzzaman A, Cho SH. Classification of hypersensitivity reactions. Allergy Asthma Proc. 2012;33 Suppl 1:96-9.
4. Lazzarini R, Duarte I, Ferreira AL. Patch tests. An Bras Dermatol. 2013;88(6):879-88.
5. Jerajani HR, Melkote S. Thin-layer rapid-use epicutaneous test (TRUE test). Indian J Dermatol Venereol Leprol. 2007;73:292-5.
6. Duarte I, Almeida FA, Proença NG. Excited skin syndrome. Am J Contact Dermat. 1996;7(1):24-34.
7. Oppermann K, Cattani CAS, Bonamigo RR. Usefulness of dermoscopy in the evaluation of patch test reactions. An Bras Dermatol. 2021;96:706-11.

8. Heinzerling L, Mari A, Bergmann KC, Bresciani M, Burbach G, Darsow U, et al. The skin prick test - European standards. Clin Transl Allergy. 2013;3(1):3.

9. Muthupalaniappen L, Jamil A. Prick, patch or blood test? A simple guide to allergy testing. Malays Fam Physician. 2021;16(2):19-26.

10. Thyssen JP, Skare L, Lundgren L, Menné T, Johansen JD, Maibach HI, et al. Sensitivity and specificity of the nickel spot (dimethylglyoxime) test. Contact Dermatitis. 2010;62(5):279-88.

Calculation of Minimal Erythema Dose

Durga Madhab Tripathy, Senkadhir Vendhan, Jamyang Choden

INTRODUCTION

Phototherapy is a relatively safer and widely used mode of skin-directed therapy used in dermatology for the treatment of numerous skin diseases. Controlled use of the nonionizing ultraviolet (UV) part of the electromagnetic spectrum to induce physical, biochemical, and immunological alterations in the cutaneous biome forms the general pedagogy. Ultraviolet A (UVA) spectrum, UVA-1 spectrum, UVA spectrum with a psoralen sensitizer (PUVA), UVB spectrum, broadband UVB (BBUVB), and narrowband UVB (NBUVB) are the commonly employed light energies. The UVB spectrum is between 280 and 320 nm, which may be delivered as full-spectrum (broadband UVB 270–350 nm) or as small-spectrum (NBUVB 311–313 nm). UVB phototherapy has anti-inflammatory, immunosuppressive, and cytotoxic properties. It is hypothesized that the induction of Langerhans cell depletion, altered antigen presentation, amelioration of natural killer (NK) cell activity, and apoptosis of skin-homing T cells and keratinocytes are some of its therapeutic mechanisms.[1,2]

Posttreatment erythema, pruritus, and photosensitivity feature among the most common side effects of NBUVB. To combat these adverse effects, especially erythema, minimal erythema dose (MED) is calculated before administration of NBUVB. MED is defined as the dose (in mJ/cm^2) necessary to obtain minimum perceptible erythema that is measured usually 24 hours after irradiation. PUVA is a form of photochemotherapy where psoralen and UVA is concomitantly used. Minimal phototoxic dose (MPD) is the corresponding measurement used for the calculation of the initial dose in cases of administration of UVA. The skin phototype is a commonly used parameter to determine the dose of NBUVB before administration which is subjective and relatively vague. Moreover, the photosensitive effects significantly vary from individual to individual necessitating the use of an objective yardstick like MED.

INDICATIONS[2,3]

- *Psoriasis*: NBUVB is used as monotherapy in various forms of psoriasis except generalized pustular and erythrodermic psoriasis. It is considered safe in pregnancy and can be employed as an adjunct in impetigo herpetiformis.
- *Chronic eczema*: Eczemas such as prurigo nodularis, atopic dermatitis, and palmoplantar eczema are effectively managed with NBUVB.
- *Vitiligo*: NBUVB is used as a second-line therapy in vitiligo where topical therapy has been ineffective.
- *Mycosis fungoides (MF)*: NBUVB is effectively used for the patch stage of MF.

PUVA is reserved for the plaque stage. Increased inflammation and erythema are very common in the early stages which eventually settle.

- *Polymorphic light eruption (PLE)*: Both NBUVB and UVA are used for desensitization in cases of PLE. NBUVB is usually preferred because of its safer side effect profile. Post-treatment erythema can be combatted with topical steroids.
- *Cutaneous graft-versus-host disease (GVHD)*: NBUVB is sometimes used for a limited form of cutaneous GVHD. It can be used as an adjunct to immunomodulators.
- *Lichen planus*: In generalized lesions of lichen planus, NBUVB is effectively used as a third-line therapy or in combination with systemic steroids and retinoids.
- *Generalized pruritus*: The suppression of key inflammatory mediator interleukin-31 (IL-31) of the itch pathway, NBUVB has been beneficial in cases of cholestatic pruritus, chronic kidney disease-induced pruritus, and human immunodeficiency virus (HIV)-associated pruritus.
- *Pityriasis rubra pilaris (PRP)*: NBUVB along with acitretin is used for the management of PRP where phototherapy has an adjunctive role.
- *Miscellaneous*: Pityriasis lichenoides chronica, chronic urticaria, cutaneous mastocytosis, and generalized granuloma annulare are other dermatoses where NBUVB is used for management.

PROCEDURE[4-6]

The MED refers to the lowest amount of UV radiation exposure that results in erythema (reddening of the skin) after a specific period. Determining the MED is crucial in understanding an individual's sensitivity to UV radiation, particularly in the context of sun exposure or medical treatments involving UV radiation.

The standard methodology for calculating the MED involves a process known as the Fitzpatrick scale and utilizes a series of graded UV exposures on a small area of the skin, usually the back, under controlled conditions.

Fitzpatrick's Skin Types

- *Type I*: Always burns, never tans
- *Type II*: Always burns, sometimes tans
- *Type III*: Sometimes burns, always tans
- *Type IV*: Rarely burns, always tans
- *Type V*: Moderately pigmented skin (Asian)
- *Type VI*: Black skin (African)

STEP-BY-STEP METHODOLOGY FOR CALCULATING MED USING UVA AND NBUVB PHOTOTHERAPY

Step 1: Patient Selection and Preparatory Assessments

- *Patient selection*: Choose participants based on skin type, the condition being treated, and absence of contraindications for UVA or NBUVB therapy.
- *Informed consent*: Obtain informed consent from participants, detailing the procedure, potential risks, and benefits.

Step 2: Pretreatment Assessments

- *Skin typing*: Use standardized scales (e.g., Fitzpatrick scale) to categorize participants' skin types to understand baseline sensitivity.
- *Baseline evaluation*: Conduct a preliminary assessment to estimate initial skin response for setting starting points for UVA and NBUVB therapies.

Step 3: Test Site Preparation and Parameters

- *Test area selection*: Identify an unexposed skin area (e.g., back), ensuring it is free from recent sun exposure or skin conditions.

- *Grid marking*: Grids are created using an opaque material like a thick surgical gown, cardboard sheet, or at times an X-ray film is also used. Eight squares are cut on the surgical gown each of 4 cm × 4 cm which are subsequently irradiated incrementally **(Figs. 1A and B)**.

Step 4: Phototherapy Source Calibration and Dosimetry

- *Light source selection*: Utilize calibrated UVA and NBUVB phototherapy devices with known emission characteristics and spectral output.
- *Dosimetry calibration*: Calibrate devices using appropriate dosimeters for accurate and reproducible light dosing.

Step 5: Incremental Light Exposure for UVA

- *Dosing protocol for UVA*: Administer incremental doses of UVA therapy to grid sections, starting with lower doses and gradually increasing.

- *Example UVA dosing plan*: Begin with 0.1 J/cm² and increase by 0.05 J/cm² increments for subsequent exposures.

Step 6: Incremental Light Exposure for NBUVB

- *Dosing protocol for NBUVB*: Administer incremental doses of NBUVB therapy to grid sections, starting with lower doses and gradually increasing.
- *Example NBUVB dosing plan*: Start with 150 mJ/cm² and increase by 150 mJ/cm² increments for subsequent grid exposures.

Step 7: Skin Reaction Assessment

- *Erythema evaluation*: Document skin reactions postexposure, noting the presence and intensity of erythema in each grid section for both UVA and NBUVB. It is usually examined 48 hours in cases of UVB and 72 hours in UVA cases **(Fig. 2)**.
- *Data collection*: Record administered light doses, corresponding skin responses, and any observed adverse reactions.

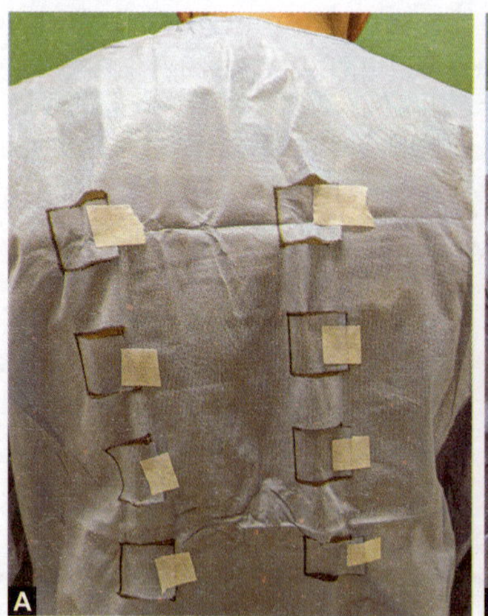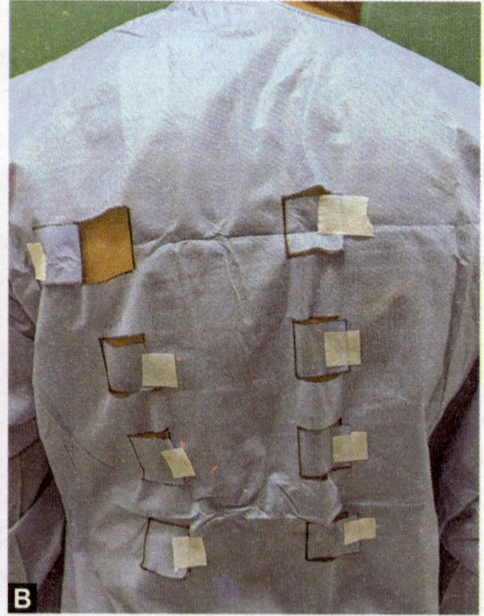

FIGS. 1A AND B: An unexposed surface in the form of the back is chosen as the site for the determination of minimal erythema dose (MED). A thick surgical gown is taken and eight 4 × 4 cm grids are cut out. One border of the square is left intact and a micropore tape strip is used to seal the grid when not irradiated.

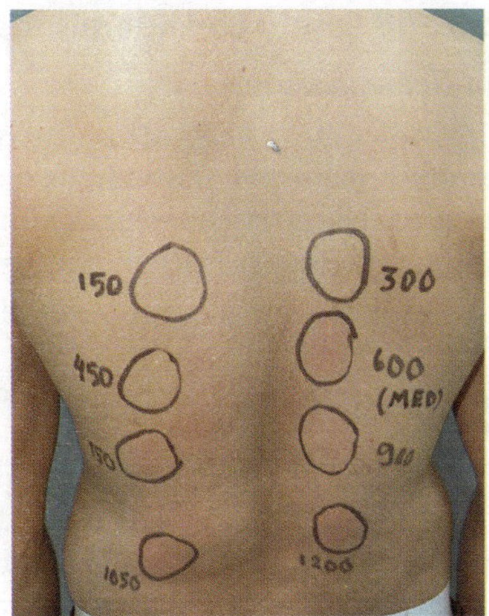

FIG. 2: Irradiation of incremental doses of ultraviolet B (UVB) with a starting dose of 150 mJ/cm^2 is performed and gradually subsequent grids are irradiated with an incremental dose of 150 mJ/cm^2, i.e., 150 mJ/cm^2 in the first grid, 300 mJ/cm^2 in the second, 450 mJ/cm^2 in the third, so on and so forth. The grids are examined for erythema after 48 hours and the grid which shows erythema at the minimal irradiation dose is designated as minimal erythema dose (MED) (600 mJ/cm^2 was determined as the MED in the index case).

Step 8: MED Determination and Validation

- *Dose-response analysis*: Analyze data separately for UVA and NBUVB to determine the MED, the lowest dose inducing the first perceptible erythema for each participant.
- *Repeatability and validation*: Repeat the procedure if necessary, adjusting parameters to validate and confirm the MED for both UVA and NBUVB.

Step 9: Data Analysis and Documentation

- *Data compilation*: Compile recorded data, including light doses, skin responses, patient demographics, and environmental conditions, separately for UVA and NBUVB.
- *Statistical analysis*: Perform separate statistical analyses (e.g., dose-response curve fitting) for UVA and NBUVB to validate MED calculations and assess relationships.
- *Documentation*: Prepare a comprehensive report following research or clinical guidelines, documenting methodology, observations, analyses, and conclusions for both UVA and NBUVB.

Step 10: Safety and Ethical Considerations

- *Safety protocols*: Strictly adhere to safety protocols to prevent overexposure and minimize risks to participants and researchers.
- *Ethical compliance*: Ensure adherence to ethical guidelines and regulations governing human research participation.

Step 11: Review and Future Implications

- *Peer review and collaboration*: Submit findings for peer review and collaborate to enhance methodological rigor and validity for UVA and NBUVB.
- *Continuous improvement*: Engage in ongoing research to refine methodologies, explore alternative dosing protocols, and validate findings across diverse patient populations.

HINDRANCES ENCOUNTERED[6]

The process of determining MED is not without its challenges and hindrances, which can affect accuracy and reliability.

Individual Variability

Skin Characteristics

The Fitzpatrick scale categorizes skin into types based on color, sun sensitivity, and tanning ability. However, even within these categories, individual skin responses can vary significantly, impacting the accuracy of MED determination.

Factors beyond Fitzpatrick Scale

Other skin attributes such as hydration levels, thickness, and preexisting conditions can affect how the skin reacts to UV radiation, making it challenging to standardize MED assessment across diverse individuals.

Equipment and Methodology

Calibration and Consistency

Variations in equipment calibration, such as UV lamps or solar simulators, can lead to inconsistencies in the administered UV doses. This can significantly impact the accuracy of MED determination.

Uniformity of Exposure

Ensuring even distribution of UV radiation across the skin surface during testing is crucial. Uneven exposure might result in misleading MED readings.

Environmental Factors

Ambient Conditions

Environmental factors such as humidity, temperature, and altitude can influence how the skin responds to UV radiation. These variables may not always be controlled during MED assessment, potentially affecting the results.

Natural Sunlight Variations

When using natural sunlight for MED testing, factors such as cloud cover, time of day, and geographic location can introduce variability in the intensity of UV radiation, complicating accurate measurements.

Subjective Interpretation

Observation and Assessment

Determining erythema can be subjective and reliant on individual interpretation. What one observer perceives as erythema might differ from another, leading to inconsistencies in MED determination.

Ethical and Safety Considerations

Risk of Overexposure

Testing to determine MED involves deliberately exposing individuals to UV radiation, which carries inherent risks of skin damage and increased susceptibility to skin cancer. Ensuring safety while conducting these tests is paramount.

Ethical Guidelines

Balancing the need for medical or research-related UV exposure with ethical considerations and informed consent from participants adds complexity to MED determination protocols.

Clinical Relevance

Translating to Real-world Scenarios

While MED determination provides valuable data, extrapolating these findings to real-life sun exposure scenarios can be challenging. Factors such as clothing, sunscreen use, and varying UV levels in different geographic regions affect actual sun protection needs beyond the determined MED.

Determining the MED is a complex process influenced by various intrinsic and extrinsic factors. Overcoming these hindrances requires standardized protocols, careful consideration of variables, and continual efforts to enhance accuracy while prioritizing participant safety.

Addressing these challenges is essential to refining MED determination methodologies, ensuring more precise evaluations of skin sensitivity to UV radiation, and providing personalized recommendations for sun safety and medical treatments.[4]

CONTRAINDICATIONS[6,7]

The MED assessment is a pivotal method to ascertain an individual's skin sensitivity to UV radiation.

Skin Health and Conditions

- *Active skin disorders*: Individuals with active skin conditions, such as eczema, psoriasis, or severe acne, exhibit compromised skin barriers. MED testing on affected areas may yield inaccurate results and potentially exacerbate these conditions.
- *History of skin cancer*: Patients with a history of skin malignancies or a predisposition to skin cancer should refrain from MED testing due to the heightened risk of further damage and cancer development associated with UV exposure.

Photosensitivity and Medications

- *Photosensitive disorders*: Subjects diagnosed with photosensitive disorders, like lupus erythematosus or certain porphyrias, are particularly susceptible to adverse reactions from UV exposure. MED testing can exacerbate these conditions, contraindicating their participation.
- *Medication-induced photosensitivity*: Certain medications, including antibiotics, diuretics, and nonsteroidal anti-inflammatory drugs (NSAIDs), can induce photosensitivity. Patients on these medications should avoid MED testing to prevent potential adverse reactions.

Age and Vulnerable Populations

Pediatric and elderly populations: Children, due to their more sensitive skin, and elderly individuals with age-related skin changes are at increased risk of UV damage. MED testing in these vulnerable populations requires careful consideration and might present contraindications due to heightened risks.

Pregnancy and Hormonal Factors

- *Pregnancy*: Due to potential risks to the developing fetus, MED testing during pregnancy is contraindicated. Hormonal changes during pregnancy can heighten skin sensitivity, increasing susceptibility to UV-related damage.
- *Hormonal fluctuations*: Hormonal variations during menstruation or hormone replacement therapy can impact skin sensitivity, affecting the reliability of MED testing results and warranting caution.

Ethical and Safety Considerations

- *Informed consent and safety protocols*: Ensuring participants comprehend associated risks and providing informed consent is imperative. Neglecting safety protocols, including adequate eye protection and controlled exposure, presents ethical contraindications for MED testing.

Acknowledging contraindications in MED testing is pivotal for ensuring participant safety, adhering to ethical guidelines, and maintaining the integrity of research protocols.

Healthcare providers and researchers must meticulously evaluate individual health statuses, considering potential risks before conducting MED assessments.

By respecting and integrating these contraindications into MED testing protocols, researchers and clinicians uphold ethical standards, safeguard vulnerable populations, and prevent adverse outcomes associated with UV exposure assessments.[5]

NEWER METHODS

Advancements in technology and research have led to the exploration of newer methods for calculating MED. Here are some of the newer approaches and technologies.

Optical Techniques[6,7]

- *Reflectance spectroscopy*: This method involves using reflectance spectroscopy to measure changes in skin reflectance before and after UV exposure. It allows for noninvasive monitoring of skin response, potentially providing insights into erythema development without causing actual skin damage.

- *Fluorescence imaging*: Utilizing fluorescence imaging techniques can detect subtle changes in skin autofluorescence induced by UV exposure. These changes can be indicative of skin damage and may aid in determining the MED.

Biophysical and Molecular Markers

- *Cytokine analysis*: Studying the levels of specific cytokines released by the skin after UV exposure can serve as markers for skin inflammation, providing a more detailed understanding of the skin's response and potentially aiding in MED determination.
- *Biomarkers of deoxyribonucleic acid (DNA) damage*: Assessing DNA damage markers in skin cells following UV exposure offers insights into the level of skin damage incurred, helping to determine an individual's MED.

Predictive Models and Algorithms

- *Mathematical models*: Developing mathematical models that incorporate various skin parameters, such as pigmentation, hydration, and genetic factors, to predict an individual's MED. These models aim to provide personalized predictions without the need for direct UV exposure.
- *Machine learning and artificial intelligence (AI)*: Using machine learning algorithms to analyze extensive datasets on skin responses to UV exposure, leading to more accurate predictions of MED based on a wide range of parameters.

Smart Sensors and Wearable Technology

- *UV dosimeters*: Advanced wearable UV dosimeters equipped with sensors can monitor UV exposure in real time. Integration of these devices with data analytics can aid in determining personalized MED by tracking individual UV exposure over time.
- *Smartphone applications*: Mobile apps utilizing smartphone sensors and algorithms to assess UV exposure and its impact on the skin. These apps may provide a convenient way to estimate an individual's MED.

In Vitro Testing

- *3D skin models*: In vitro testing using engineered 3D skin models provides an alternative to in vivo testing. These models mimic human skin and allow for controlled UV exposure to study erythema development and determine MED without subjecting individuals to direct radiation.

Integration of Imaging Technologies[8]

- *Multimodal imaging*: Combining different imaging modalities, such as optical coherence tomography (OCT) or confocal microscopy, to visualize skin changes at various depths and levels of resolution following UV exposure. This integrated approach offers a comprehensive view of skin response.

These newer methodologies and technologies offer promising avenues for refining the determination of MED. They strive to provide more precise, noninvasive, and personalized approaches to assess skin sensitivity to UV radiation, potentially improving both research methodologies and clinical applications related to sun safety and medical treatments involving UV exposure.[6,9]

CONCLUSION

In conclusion, the determination of the MED remains a pivotal aspect in understanding individual skin sensitivity to UV radiation. This chapter has highlighted the significance of accurately calculating the MED, a fundamental parameter in dermatology and photobiology research. By employing meticulous methodologies such as the use of phototesting protocols, standardized dosimetry, and precise measurement techniques, researchers can ascertain the MED with greater accuracy and reliability.

The MED serves as a critical benchmark in various fields, including determining safe sun exposure limits, assessing phototherapy effectiveness, and evaluating sunscreen efficacy. Its calculation aids in tailoring personalized recommendations for sun protection, minimizing the risk of sun-induced skin damage, and understanding skin phototypes.

However, challenges persist in achieving universal methodologies for MED determination due to factors such as individual variations, environmental influences, and evolving technology. Continuous advancements in instrumentation, data analysis, and understanding of biological responses to UV radiation are necessary to refine MED calculation techniques further.

As researchers delve deeper into understanding the complexities of skin response to UV exposure, collaborations across disciplines and concerted efforts are imperative to standardize protocols and enhance the accuracy and reproducibility of MED assessments. This ongoing pursuit will undoubtedly contribute to a more comprehensive comprehension of skin photobiology, ultimately promoting better public health strategies and personalized care in managing sun-related skin conditions.

Key Messages

- Phototherapy (UVA and NBUVB) is been extensively used for the management of a wide array of dermatoses.
- MED is a useful objective parameter to gauge the effects of phototherapy before administration for a prolonged period and to curtail untoward effects of phototherapy.
- MED is defined as the dose (in mJ/cm^2) necessary to obtain minimum perceptible erythema that is measured usually 24 hours after irradiation.
- Calculation of MED is a simple outpatient procedure requiring minimal skills to perform and interpret.
- Reflectance spectroscopy and fluorescent imaging have been used in determining MED recently making the procedure more robust.

REFERENCES

1. Ly K, Chang AY, Kiprono SK, Jose M, Smith MP, Beck K, et al. Implementation of an Ultraviolet Phototherapy Service at a National Referral Hospital in Western Kenya: Reflections on Challenges and Lessons Learned. Dermatol Ther (Heidelb). 2020;10(1):107-17.

2. Rathod DG, Muneer H, Masood S. Phototherapy. Treasure Island (FL): StatPearls Publishing; 2023.

3. Horio T. Indications and action mechanisms of phototherapy. J Dermatol Sci. 2000;23 Suppl 1:S17-21.

4. Dornelles S, Goldim J, Cestari T. Determination of the minimal erythema dose and colorimetric measurements as indicators of skin sensitivity to UV-B radiation. Photochem Photobiol. 2004;79(6):540-4.

5. Fors M, González P, Viada C, Falcon K, Palacios S. Validity of the Fitzpatrick Skin Phototype Classification in Ecuador. Adv Skin Wound Care. 2020;33(12):1-5.

6. Kim MA, Jung YC, Suh BF, Lee HN, Kim E. Skin biophysical properties including impaired skin

barrier function determine ultraviolet sensitivity. J Cosmet Dermatol. 2022;21(10):5066-72.

7. Heckman CJ, Chandler R, Kloss JD, Benson A, Rooney D, Munshi T, et al. Minimal Erythema Dose (MED) testing. J Vis Exp. 2013;(75):e50175.

8. Tejasvi T, Sharma VK, Kaur J. Determination of minimal erythemal dose for narrow band-ultraviolet B radiation in north Indian patients: comparison of visual and Dermaspectrometer readings. Indian J Dermatol Venereol Leprol. 2007;73(2):97-9.

9. Tan Y, Wang F, Fan G, Zheng Y, Li B, Li N, et al. Identification of factors associated with minimal erythema dose variations in a large-scale population study of 22146 subjects. J Eur Acad Dermatol Venereol. 2020;34(7):1595-600.

Pathergy Test

Rahul Thombre, Smriti Sharma, Pankaj Das

INTRODUCTION

The pathergy phenomenon is a nonspecific cutaneous hypersensitivity reaction in response to minor trauma. It has been well-known to dermatologists since it was first described in 1937 by Blobner and further investigated by Katzenellenbogen in 1960. The phenomenon can be elicited by a simple bedside pathergy test (PT) manifested clinically by erythematous induration at the site of sterile needle pricks, which may remain as papules or progress to sterile pustules. While pathergy has been reported in numerous diseases, pathergy testing is primarily used to diagnose Behçet's disease (BD).[1,2] It is used for diagnosis, indicates an active disease, and also serves as a model for clinical and histopathological research.[3]

EPIDEMIOLOGY

There is great variation between different geographic regions with a higher positivity in areas with higher prevalence of BD and vice-versa. The positivity is higher around the Silk Route, which extends from the Far East to the Mediterranean Basin, including the Gulf area. The reactivity of the "pathergy test" is suggested to be correlated with human leukocyte antigen (HLA)-B51 in Mediterranean countries.[4] In a landmark study conducted in Turkey, Tuzun et al. reported an 84% positivity rate in pathergy.

Positivity rates in other high-prevalence countries are 77% in Morocco; 71% in Iraq; 62% in China, Iran, and Egypt; and 44% in Japan. On the other hand, the positivity in low-prevalence countries such as Denmark and Sweden is low, i.e., 7.7 and 8.3% respectively. Although there may be procedural differences amongst the studies, the heterogeneity of disease phenotypes in different populations may be the reason behind the significant differences between the positivity rates.

Davatchi et al. reported positive lower skin pathergy reaction (SPR) (41%) in patients whose disease onset was after 1998 as compared to those who had disease onset before 1977 (61.5%). This change may be attributable to the revolutionary use of disposable needles after the discovery of HIV which are less traumatic than the earlier nondisposable ones.[3]

PATHOGENESIS

The underlying pathogenesis for the pathergy phenomenon is not fully understood. Cutaneous needle prick apparently incites an exaggerated inflammatory response due to an increased or aberrant release of cytokines by the keratinocytes or other cutaneous cells resulting in a perivascular inflammatory infiltrate seen on histopathology.[4]

The innate immunity of the human skin is capable of rapidly responding to any tissue damage and microbial invasion. Injured cells of the epidermis and dermis secrete various cytokines, chemokines, antimicrobial peptides, and growth factors leading to an inflammatory response. Sjögren et al. have suggested that even the minutest of trauma caused through insertion of sterile microcatheters in a healthy individual's normal skin produce proinflammatory cytokines, such as interleukin I beta (IL-1β), interleukin 6 (IL-6), and interleukin 8 (IL-8). These inflammatory mediators reach peak skin levels at 3–8 hours which is followed by a decline, but existing in small quantity at 24 hours. This sequence overlaps with histopathology where inflammatory infiltrate is evident by 4 hours, reaching a crescendo at 24 hours, followed by a decline. These data underline the role of trauma-induced activation of cutaneous innate immune response, which is already exaggerated due to underlying genetic factors in a subset of BD patients. A higher response rate with blunt and/or large needles and twisting motion while testing favors the possibility of reaction to mechanically damaged epidermal and dermal components. This is further supported by the fact that sterile areas such as eyes, joints, and blood vessels also develop hyperinflammatory responses due to trauma. Koebner phenomenon, which is the appearance of disease-specific skin lesions in an uninvolved area of the skin as a consequence of trauma, is a well-known aspect of some skin diseases, such as vitiligo, psoriasis, and lichen planus.

The putative role of microbial antigens as triggers is supported by the fact that the positivity of pathergy reduces when the skin is cleaned by surgical spirit or povidone iodide increased positivity of SPR after application of saliva to the test site before the test and higher sensitivity to pneumococcal vaccine also supports the hypothesis of microbial elements potential inducers of SPR.

PROCEDURE

There is no standardized consensus among clinicians as to the optimal method for performing the test.[5] Although intradermal, subcutaneous, intraoral, and intravenous testing have all been described, intradermal needle prick is the most commonly used method. Many investigators have also used intradermal injection of normal saline, monosodium urate crystals, or streptococcal antigens to perform the test.[2]

The two commonly used methods to elicit a pathergy response are (1) the skin and (2) oral pathergy tests **(Figs. 1A to D)**.

Skin Pathergy Test

Site

The glabrous skin over the forearm, legs, abdomen, and back can be used. The percentage of positive pathergy reaction (PR) has been reported as 64.2%, 46.4%, 44.6%, and 26.7% in the forearms, legs, back, and abdomen respectively.[6]

Routes of Needle Prick

Intradermal, intravenous, and subcutaneous routes for inducing tissue trauma have been studied. The intradermal route has been found to have higher sensitivity in BD patients both during active and remission phases.[4]

Procedure

Glabrous skin of the forearm is cleansed with an antiseptic, commonly alcohol, and 20G needles are inserted at an angle of 45° through the skin till a depth of 3–5 mm (level of the dermis) with the bevel edge facing up. Sharp or blunt needles can be used and four to six needle pricks are usually made. Prior to inserting, the needles can be made blunt by hitting them against a sterile plastic sheath cover. Once the needle is introduced into the dermis, it may be twisted to induce more trauma. Although results can be read at

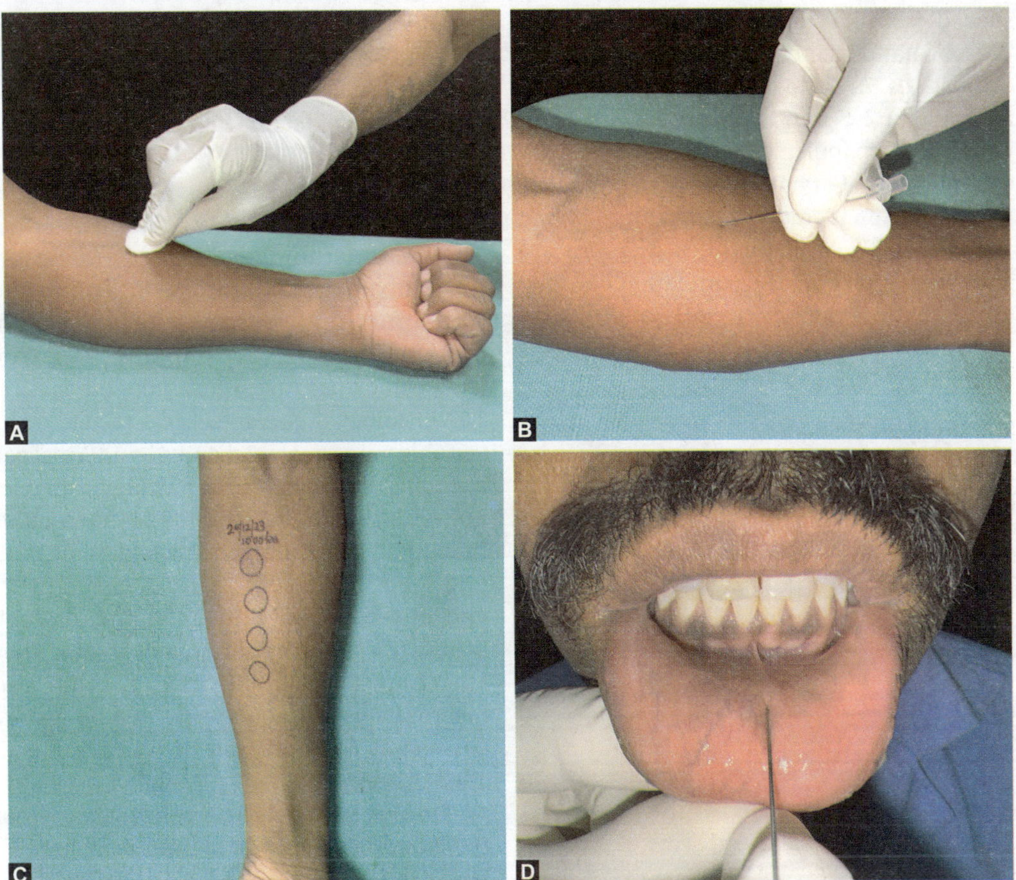

FIGS. 1A TO D: Procedure for skin and oral pathergy tests. (A) Clean the test site with normal saline; (B) Using a blunt-tipped 20G needle, three to four needle pricks are made on the volar aspect of the forearm, at an angle of 45°, to a depth of 3–5 mm, with the bevel edge facing upward; (C) The prick sites are marked and evaluated at 24–48 hours for the appearance of an erythematous papule or pustule; and (D) The oral pathergy test involves a sterile blunt 20G needle prick on the lower lip mucosa up till the level of submucosa.

either 24 or 48 hours, the latter have higher specificity. An erythematous papule $\geq$ 2 mm or a pustule is regarded as a positive reaction.[3]

Assessment of Response

Clinical Evaluation

Readings are taken after 48 hours of the needle prick. A $\geq$2 mm papule that is usually felt by palpation surrounded by an erythematous halo is formed on the skin. The papule may transform into a 1–5 mm pustule. The pustule becomes prominent in 24 hours, becomes maximum in size in 48 hours, and disappears in 45 days. Erythema without induration is interpreted as a negative result.[4]

Dilsen's method of assessing and grading pathergy tests is preferred by clinicians and is based on the readings at 48 hours after needle prick. Since the sharpness of the needle has a significant influence on the skin pathergy test (SPT), the criteria for assessment of blunt and sharp needle pathergy differs. The SPT is considered negative if there is only erythema. When a blunt needle is used, a papule < 2 mm is considered neither positive nor negative, but rather "suspect." Positive reactions are scored from 1+ to 4+ depending on the presence and size of erythematous papules or pustules. A grade of 1+ is assigned when a papule of 2–3 mm is observed with blunt needles, or a papule ≤ 3 mm is observed with sharp needles. For both types of needles, any papule > 3 mm is graded 2+, pustules 1–2 mm are graded 3+, and pustules > 2 mm are graded 4+. However, the correlation between the strength of the positive SPT and disease severity or disease activity in BD remains uncertain **(Fig. 2 and Table 1)**.[2]

Photographic Evaluation

This method was found a have a high variability and low sensitivity.

Dermoscopic Evaluation

Dermatoscopy is strongly recommended for the investigation of suspected BD patients since it can reveal evidence of inflammation, especially for small lesions (<2 mm). Dermatoscopy shows erythematous papule/pustule or ulcero-crusted lesions surrounded by erythema or edema in positive SPR.[7]

Histopathology and Immunohistochemistry

The histopathological spectrum points to a mixed inflammatory infiltrate and intraepidermal pustules on one end, and findings of vasculopathy and true leukocytoclastic vasculitis on the other end.[3] The histology of pathergy is characterized by variable epidermal thickening, epidermal cell vacuolization, subcorneal pustule formation, upregulation of cell adhesion molecules (including intercellular adhesion molecule 1, endoglin, E-selectin, and P-selectin 1) and mixed perivascular inflammatory cell infiltrates [neutrophils, clusters of differentiation 4 (CD4) positive T cells, and macrophages], which appear at 4 hours, are densest at 24 hours and begin to diminish after 48 hours.[8]

However, there is also controversy about the histopathology of pathergy response. Some authors claim mixed infiltration, while others report neutrophilic infiltration with leukocytoclastic vasculitis. A possible explanation for this discrepancy may be the different methods used to induce lesions (needle prick, histamine injection, etc.), variations in biopsy time, ethnic origin of patient, disease activity, and medication use.[9]

The histopathologic result of the pathergy test depends on the time of biopsy. In the first 6 hours, polymorphonuclear leukocytes are the dominant inflammatory cells. After 24 hours, mononuclear cell infiltration in dermal vessels, edema in vessel endothelium, edema, and leukocytoclasia in reticular dermis are seen.[10]

In the study by Ozluk et al., lobular panniculitis with or without vasculitis apart from mixed type inflammatory cell infiltration, neutrophil-rich infiltration, and

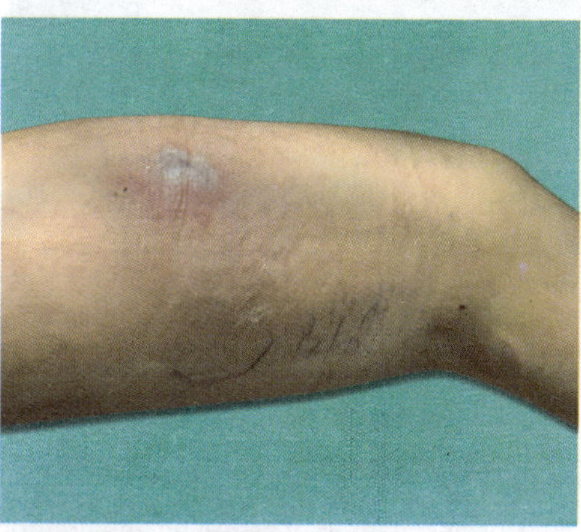

FIG. 2: Positive pathergy response.
Courtesy: Dr Somesh Gupta.

TABLE 1: Dilsen method of grading skin pathergy reaction (SPR).[2]

Grade	Clinical response
1+	2–3 mm papule
2+	>3 mm papule
3+	1–2 mm pustule
4+	>2 mm pustule

lymphocyte-rich infiltration were found to be the subcutaneous histopathologic findings of positive pathergy test in BD. In literature; panniculitis, lobular or mixed septal, and lobular in pattern were shown in erythema nodosum-like lesions of BD. Vasculitis was noted in most erythema nodosum-like lesions in BD.

Uveitis was found to be statistically significant in patients in whom vasculitis was observed. In light of this finding, a lookout should be kept in patients with findings of vasculitis against the development of uveitis.[11-14]

Immunohistochemical findings were HLA-DR expression by keratinocytes and inflammatory cells, predominant CD3(+), CD4(+), CD45Ro(+) cells, and small collections of neutrophil elastase positive cells in needle insertion sites, and E-selectin, P-selectin, intercellular adhesion molecule (ICAM), and CD105 expressions by endothelial cells. Ben Ahmed et al. reported significant increases in the messenger ribonucleic acid (RNA) expression of monocyte chemoattractant protein 1, interleukin-8, interferon-γ, interleukin-10 (IL-10), and interleukin-12 (IL-12) in BD lesions compared with normal skin thus signaling to a strong Th1 polarization with IL-10 probably having a role in preventing a more severe inflammatory response. In a comprehensive study, Melikoglu et al. investigated cellular and molecular elements of the inflammatory response to needle prick in BD and healthy control subjects at 0, 8, and 48 hours. Unlike controls, BD patients had increased influxes of mature dendritic cells, monocytes, and lymphocytes including T regulatory cells by 48 hours. Similarly, increases in cytokines IL-12 p40, IFN-γ, IL-10, IL-15, and IFN-γ-induced genes and transcription factors were found. Chemokines, IP-10, MIP3-α, Mig, and iTac leading to recruitment of dendritic cells, mononuclear cells as well as adhesion molecules [ICAM-1 and vascular cell

TABLE 2: Dermal histopathological findings of positive pathergy response reported by Ozluk E et al.[15]

Histopathological findings	Number of patients	Percentage
Erythrocyte extravasation	6	26
Endothelial swelling and thickening	4	17.3
Leukocytoclastic vasculitis	5	21.7
Lymphocytic vasculitis	3	13
Pustule formation in epidermis	6	26
Lymphocytic vascular reaction	2	8.6
Perivascular cell infiltration	3	13
Mixed-type inflammatory cell infiltration	10	43.4

adhesion molecule 1 (VCAM-1)] were noted. These results also support an exaggerated lymphoid Th1-type response in SPR. Alpsoy et al. investigated the androgen receptor index of SPR site as compared to nonlesional skin and found higher expression among males, concluding that androgens may have a possible role in reaction **(Tables 2 and 3)**.[3]

The clinical use of the pathergy test is very important in the diagnosis of BD. On the other hand, misinterpretation of tests might cause false-positive or false-negative results. For that reason, immunopathologic and histopathologic tests are recommended with the pathergy test.[11,12]

Oral Pathergy Test

The lower lip mucosa is pricked with a 20G disposable needle till the level of the submucosa and reading for a response is done at 48 hours. Although the sensitivity of the oral pathergy test is reported to be lower

TABLE 3: Subcutaneous histopathological findings of positive pathergy response reported by Ozluk E et al.[15]

Histopathological findings	Number of patients	Percentage
Mixed-type inflammatory cell infiltrate	9	39.1%
Neutrophil rich infiltration	2	8.6%
Lymphocyte rich infiltration	5	21.7%
Lobular panniculitis without vasculitis	2	8.6%
Normal fat tissue	5	21.7%

BOX 1 | **Conditions with a positive pathergy phenomenon.**

Behçet's disease:
- Pyoderma gangrenosum (PG): The pathergy test positivity at a rate of 25% has been reported in the literature in PG patients. Aggressive surgical debridement or skin grafting is discouraged in these patients because of the risk of a pathergic response.

Interferon alpha-treated chronic myeloid leukemia patients:
- Sweet syndrome
- Deficiency of interleukin 1 receptor antagonist (DIRA)[3]
- Eosinophilic pustular folliculitis
- Inflammatory bowel disease (8%)[16]
- Myeloproliferative disorders, non-Hodgkin lymphoma
- Healthy individuals
- Rarely in spondyloarthropathies
- Neonates with Down's syndrome
- Erythema elevatum diutinum[17]
- Blind loop syndrome[17]

than that of the SPT, it is easier to assess as the appearance of an ulcer or pustule of any size at the site of the prick is considered a positive response, and there is no need to measure the size of the lesions.[2] The oral pathergy test is reported as less painful than the SPT by many patients **(Box 1)**.

Factors determining sensitivity and specificity of the SPR: Pathergy positivity is influenced by various factors, such as a number of pricks, the size and sharpness of the needle, the method of disinfection, disease-related factors, concomitant treatment, and ethnic/geographic background.

- In a study conducted by Dilşen et al. 20 and 26G blunt needles were used for pathergy in 92 BD patients, 128 diseased, and 64 healthy controls. Significantly higher responses were obtained with 20G needles.
- Karadag et al. have compared blunt and sharp needles and found a significantly higher rate of positive tests in areas where blunt needles were used (85% vs. 32.5%). It is proposed that in the past the reusable needles that were reused after sterilization in boiling water became rough due to the deposition of calcium on the bent parts of the needles making them more traumatic than disposable ones, contributing to the higher pathergy positivity in the past.
- Positive PR rates are maximized by using four needle pricks but there is little advantage gained by more than four insertions. Increasing the number of pricks increases sensitivity to 19, 28, and 33% for two, four, and six pricks, respectively.
- Twisting motion while pricking the skin increases the traumatic insult and is found to have higher positivity rates.
- It was shown that surgical cleaning of the skin surface before the application of the needle reduced the test positivity. Some substances, bacteria, or skin products, eliminated by surgical cleaning, might play a role in the development of SPR.
- Pricking the skin with the needle bevel up was found to be associated with a higher pathergy positive response.[6]

- Another method of increasing the rate of positivity consists of resting the needle in the dermis for 90 seconds before taking it out.
- The positivity rate of the pathergy test in BD was found to vary from country to country. It is most prevalent around the Silk Route, which extends from the Far East to the Mediterranean Basin, including the Gulf area in comparison to its Western counterparts, especially in Europe and the USA.[4]
- Injection of polysaccharide 23-valent pneumococcal vaccine by 20G needles revealed higher sensitivity and specificity of 64.3 and 100% respectively. An increased IL-1β and IL-1Ra production in response to the 23-valent pneumococcal polysaccharide vaccine (PS-23) vaccine was observed in the group with active BD.[18]
- Pathergy response has been reported to be higher during the active stages of BD.
- Other than histamine and saline, injection of microbial or chemical compounds such as monosodium urate (MSU) crystals have been used to induce SPR and revealed a greater sensitivity compared to the classical pathergy test. However, unlike classical pathergy response with papular or pustular lesions, the reaction to MSU was characterized by erythema alone.[19]
- *Three-step pathergy test*: In the three-step pathergy test, the intravenous puncture was applied to the antecubital vein and 1 mL saline was injected intramuscularly to the upper external quadrant of the gluteus maximus on three consecutive days. The puncture sites were evaluated at 24 and 48 hours and the pathergy test was considered as positive in the presence of a positive reaction in at least one of the intravenous or intramuscular pathergy sites. The application and evaluation period of the three-step pathergy test was therefore longer and took 5 days.

The sensitivity and specificity of the three-step pathergy test were 43 and 96%, respectively whereas the intradermal pathergy test has a sensitivity of 30% and a specificity of 98%. The sensitivity of the three-step pathergy test was reported significantly higher than that of the intradermal pathergy test ($p < 0.05$). In the three-step pathergy test, a higher frequency of positivity was associated primarily with the intramuscular method, and the intravenous method did not contribute to the positivity of the test. Drawbacks of the three-step test were the need for multiple visits for the procedure and the longer assessment time.[19]

- Skin prick with self-saliva in which oral bacteria including streptococci are ordinarily contained was studied in comparison to pricks using sterilized saliva. The results revealed > 90% of BD patients showed erythematous reaction by prick with self-saliva and that a tiny spot or no reaction was seen by the prick with microfilter-sterilized saliva and control saline. The results also suggest that oral streptococci play an important role in the pathogenesis of recurrent aphthous stomatitis in BD patients and that the salivary prick is able to make a differentiation of BD from non-BD disorders.[20]
- There is a site-related variation in sensitivity with the highest sensitivity reported for forearms and the lowest for the abdominal skin pricks.

SKIN PATHERGY REACTION AND BEHÇET'S DISEASE

Behçet's disease was first described by Hulusi Behçet's in 1937 as an inflammatory process of unknown etiology, characterized by recurrent aphthous ulcers, genital ulcers with scarring, uveitis, and cutaneous lesions. It is also associated with other less frequent systemic manifestations, such as gastrointestinal, central nervous system, vascular, and joint infections.

In 1990, the International Study Group for Behçet's Disease established the existence of recurrent mouth ulcerations and at least two additional clinical manifestations, which may consist of recurrent genital ulcers, ocular lesions, arthritis, thrombophlebitis, neurological abnormalities, and cutaneous lesions or positive pathergy test, which occurs in 40–80% of the cases as key points for diagnosing BD. On the other hand, in the Japanese BD diagnostic criteria "pathergy test" is excluded, as the positivity is low among Japanese and is instead considered as one of the diagnostic references.[16,20-22] Recently, an international expert group analyzing clinical manifestations of 219 pediatric BD patients, proposed consensus classification criteria for pediatric Behçet's disease (PEDBD), which excluded SPR. These proposed criteria had a sensitivity and specificity of 91.7 and 42.9%, respectively and the addition of the SPR failed to improve the performance. The impact of the positive pathergy test on the performance of 16 available classification/diagnosis criteria sets for BD was analyzed. Accordingly, without SPR, 15 out of 16 criteria

set lost sensitivity, gained specificity, and lost accuracy, highlighting the diagnostic value of this test **(Figs. 3 and 4)**.[3]

In vitro, there is an increased chemotactic activity of polymorphonuclear leukocytes (PMNL) in BD patients compared to healthy subjects. The proportion of PMNL initially comes up to 100% in the skin window preparations, with a very rapid fall in patients with BD as compared to a distinctly slower drop in the controls. Conversely to the number of PMNL, the skin window cellular pattern was built up by monophagocytic cells replacing the PMNL. The phenomenon of "rapid depletion of PMNL," from the skin window can be considered an additional hint on the functional disturbance of the PMNL involved in the pathogenesis of BD.[23]

However, the positivity of the pathergy test in BD patients seems to be chronologically lower to <40% of BD patients seen in the 2007s, though >70% of the patients exhibited a positive to the pathergy test in the 1970s. Without PPT as a criterion for the diagnosis of BD, the sensitivity and accuracy of the sets of classification/diagnosis criteria decrease, while the specificity improves **(Box 2)**.[24]

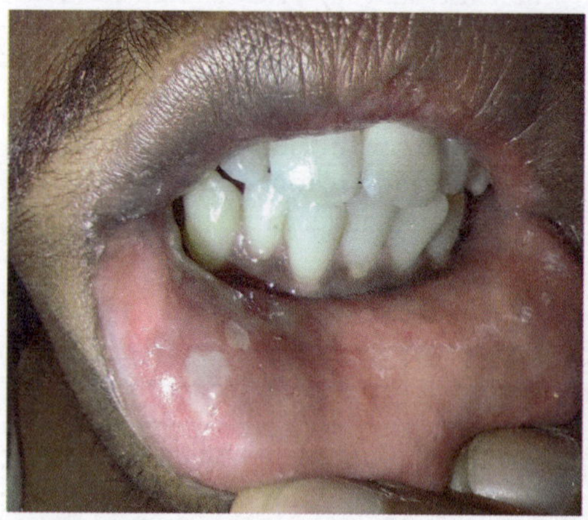

FIG. 3: Recurrent aphthous ulcers in a patient with Behçet's disease.

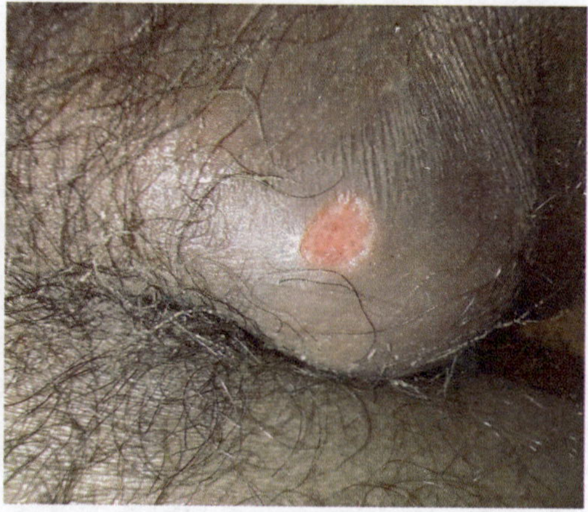

FIG. 4: Scarring genital ulcers in a patient with Behçet's disease.

<table>
<tr><td>BOX 2</td><td>Classification/criteria of Behçet's disease (BD).</td></tr>
</table>

- *Japanese BD diagnostic criteria*:
  - Major symptoms:
    - Recurrent oral aphthoid ulcer
    - Skin lesions
    - Ocular symptoms
    - Genital ulcer
  - Minor symptoms:
    - Arthritis without deformity and ankylosis
    - Epididymitis
    - Gastrointestinal lesions such as ileocecal ulcers
    - Vascular lesions
    - Central nervous system lesion
  - Complete type: Four major symptoms during the course.
  - Incomplete type: Three major symptoms, two major + two minor symptoms, typical ocular symptoms + one major symptom, or two minor symptoms
- *International Study Group*:
  - Major criteria
  - Recurrent oral ulceration
  - Minor criteria:
    - Recurrent genital ulceration
    - Eye lesions
    - Skin lesions
    - Pathergy test

Major + two minor criteria indicate BD

- *International criteria for BD*:

Ocular lesions	2 points
Oral aphthosis	2 points
Genital aphthosis	2 points
Skin lesions	1 point
Central nervous system involvement	1 point
Vascular manifestations	1 point
Positive pathergy test	1 point

Note: Scores ≥ 4 indicate BD.

PATHERGY PHENOMENON IN ORGANS OTHER THAN SKIN

Pathergy is not limited to skin in BD patients and a similar hyperreactivity can be seen in any surgical or mechanical trauma in various tissues and organs. BD patients can experience exacerbation of uveitis following eye surgery or intraocular injections and synovitis following arthrocentesis.[26] Vascular interventions such as angiography and vascular surgery may lead to arterial thrombus or aneurysm; venipuncture may induce superficial thrombophlebitis, and segmental bowel resection may trigger intestinal ulcers. Other examples of pathergy phenomenon are pustular lesions after laser hair removal, the appearance of oral ulcers after dental interventions, and the placement of orthodontic braces. These findings support the notion that hyperinflammatory response triggered by trauma is a feature of the disease itself, rather than being an organ-specific phenomenon.[3]

COMPLICATIONS OF PATHERGY TEST

There are no serious adverse effects of the pathergy test itself. However, the pathergy phenomenon could lead to numerous serious complications in patients with BD due to an exaggerated inflammatory response to a mechanical or surgical intervention in organs other than the skin as stated in the aforementioned section.

Complications due to pathergy in PG patients have also been well reported. Surgical debridement of PG ulcers has resulted in a rapid increase in the size of the ulcers. Procedures such as venipuncture and intravenous line placement too have been reported to induce new PG lesions; hence, it is important to be aware of the complications due to pathergy in patients so that clinicians can minimize interventions that may worsen their disease.[2]

DRAWBACKS OF THE PATHERGY TEST

- Decreasing prevalence of disorders with a pathergy phenomenon
- Low yield of positive pathergy
- Lack of standardization in performance and evaluation
- Low reproducibility
- Decrease in sensitivity over decades
- Ethnic variation in positivity rates[4]

FUTURE SCOPE OF THE PATHERGY TEST

In spite of impressive advances in this field, much remains unknown about the immunopathogenesis of BD and SPR may serve as an in vivo model for investigating the cellular and molecular elements of the immune response. Using novel non/minimally invasive research techniques such as skin dialysis or microneedle patches for sampling cellular and molecular mediators of inflammation may cast some light on the inflammatory pathways and lead to a detailed knowledge of skin homeostasis to minimal trauma in both health and disease.

Future research should focus on methods of improving the sensitivity of SPR, identifying possible triggers, T-cell repertoire, the effector dendritic cell subtypes, and also mechanisms of dysregulated intrinsic tolerogenic mechanisms. Such advancements may enable the development of targeted therapies in this era of biologics and small molecules.[3]

Some studies have suggested positive pathergy tests to be an independent risk factor for postoperative complications in patients with BD. Surgical intervention may be required at times for BD when, for example, patients manifest ischemia from thromboembolism or have an impending aneurysm rupture. In such situations, a positive pathergy test can help identify the subset of patients at higher risk of postoperative complications and guide the initiation of immunosuppressive treatments in such patients.[2]

It will be of great interest to systematically perform and study pathergy tests in patients with diseases other than described earlier since it may provide invaluable insight into their pathophysiology and possibly guide their management.

CONCLUSION

Due to its broad clinical spectrum, multidisciplinary treatment is important to make an early and efficient diagnosis of BD, so as to prevent aggravation and to provide adequate treatment, in order to offer the patient an improved quality of life. Emphasis is laid on the importance of the dentist's knowledge about the BD, its characteristics, and its forms of oral and general manifestations, as in view of the seriousness of this pathology and its similarity to other diseases, it is difficult to diagnose and treat.

Though the likelihood of positive findings has decreased over time, a positive pathergy test has demonstrated specificity as high as 98.4% for BD. Therefore, this test remains a powerful tool in resolving various diagnostic dilemmas for diseases that may have a similar initial presentation.[9,25] Despite its limitations, the pathergy test is an easy and inexpensive test to perform and its positivity beyond aiding diagnosis also indicates an active disease and hence is still performed widely.[3]

Key Messages

- Pathergy test is a simple bedside test to elicit the pathergy phenomenon, wherein cutaneous trauma-induced nonspecific hypersensitivity leads to the appearance of a papule, pustule or ulcer at the site of trauma.
- It has classically been described in relation to BD. Other conditions where the phenomenon is seen are pyoderma gangrenosum, Sweet syndrome, inflammatory bowel disease, myeloproliferative disorders, and deficiency of interleukin-1 receptor antagonists.
- There are two types of pathergy tests, i.e., (1) oral and (2) SPTs.
- Pathogenesis is marked by a cascade of inflammatory events at the test site, initiated by trauma-induced keratinocyte damage and/or insertion of yet undefined microbial antigen into the skin, expression of Toll-like and NOD-like receptors, activation of intracellular signaling pathways, release of IL-6, tumor necrosis factor alpha (TNF-α), and IL-1β. These cytokines activate dermal dendritic cells, which in turn lead to Th1 responses through releasing IL-12, IL-23, and INFs, release chemokines CXCL8-11 which attract neutrophils, mature dendritic cells, and activated T-lymphocytes to the dermis eventually causing collections of polymorphonuclear cells, dermal mixed inflammatory infiltrate as seen on histopathological examination.
- The reactivity of the test depends of multiple factors such as the sharpness and size of the needle, number of pricks, procedural variations, disease-related factors, sterility of the test site, medications being used, and ethnicity/geographic regions.
- Although the positivity of the pathergy phenomenon has declined over the decades, it still holds an important place in the diagnosis of BD and research model for the various conditions with a positive pathergy phenomenon.

REFERENCES

1. Camargo CMDS, Brotas AM, Ramos-e-Silva M, Carneiro S. Isomorphic phenomenon of Koebner: Facts and controversies. Clin Dermatol. 2013;31(6):741-9.

2. Rahman S, Daveluy S. Pathergy Test. In: StatPearls. Treasure Island (FL): StatPearls Publishing; 2024.

3. Ergun T. Pathergy phenomenon. Front Med (Lausanne). 2021;8:639404.

4. Sequeira FF, Daryani D. The oral and skin pathergy test. Indian J Dermatol Venereol Leprol. 2011;77(4):526-30.

6. Ozden MG, Bek Y, Aydin F, Senturk N, Canturk T, Turanli AY. Different application techniques of pathergy testing among dermatologists. J Eur Acad Dermatol Venereol JEADV. 2010;24(10):1240-2.

7. Ozdemir M, Balevi S, Deniz F, Mevlitoğlu I. Pathergy reaction in different body areas in Behçet's disease. Clin Exp Dermatol. 2007;32(1):85-7.

8. Scherrer MAR, de Castro LPF, Rocha VB, Pacheco L. [The dermatoscopy in the skin pathergy testing: case series in patients with suspected Behçet's Disease]. Rev Bras Reumatol. 2014;54(6):494-8.

9. Gül A, Esin S, Dilsen N, Koniçe M, Wigzell H, Biberfeld P. Immunohistology of skin pathergy reaction in Behçet's disease. Br J Dermatol. 1995;132(6):901-7.

10. KARADAĞ A, AKBAY G, AYDIN M, ASTARCI H, EKŞİOĞLU M. Comparison of Clinical and Histopathologic Findings of Pathergy Test with Disposable/Sharp and Nondisposable/Blunt Needles in Behcet´s Disease. Turk J Med Sci. 2009;39(1):47-51.

11. Haim S, Sobel JD, Friedman-Birnbaum R, Lichtig C. Histohogical and direct immunofluorescence study of cutaneous hyperreactivity in Behçet's disease. Br J Dermatol. 1976;95(6):631-6.

12. Jorizzo JL, Solomon AR, Cavallo T. Behçet's syndrome. Immunopathologic and histopathologic assessment of pathergy lesions is useful in diagnosis and follow-up. Arch Pathol Lab Med. 1985;109(8):747-51.

13. Ergun T, Gürbüz O, Harvell J, Jorizzo J, White W. The histopathology of pathergy: a chronologic study of skin hyperreactivity in Behçet's disease. Int J Dermatol. 1998;37(12):929-33.

14. Chun SI, Su WP, Lee S. Histopathologic study of cutaneous lesions in Behçet's syndrome. J Dermatol. 1990;17(6):333-41.

15. Kim B, LeBoit PE. Histopathologic features of erythema nodosum--like lesions in Behçet disease: a comparison with erythema nodosum focusing on the role of vasculitis. Am J Dermatopathol. 2000;22(5):379-90.

16. Ozluk E, Balta I, Akoguz O, Kalkan G, Astarci M, Akbay G, et al. Histopathologic Study of Pathergy Test in Behçet's Disease. Indian J Dermatol. 2014;59(6):630.

17. Hatemi I, Hatemi G, Celik AF, Melikoglu M, Arzuhal N, Mat C, et al. Frequency of pathergy phenomenon and other features of Behçet's syndrome among patients with inflammatory bowel disease. Clin Exp Rheumatol. 2008;26 (4 Suppl 50):S91-5.

18. Davatchi F, Chams-Davatchi C, Ghodsi Z, Shahram F, Nadji A, Shams H, et al. Diagnostic value of pathergy test in Behcet's disease according to the change of incidence over the time. Clin Rheumatol. 2011;30(9):1151-5.

19. Deniz R, Emrence Z, Yalçınkaya Y, Artım Esen B, İnanç M, Öcal ML, et al. Improved sensitivity of the skin pathergy test with polysaccharide pneumococcal vaccine antigens in the diagnosis of Behçet disease. Rheumatology (Oxford). 2023;62(5):1903-9.

20. Lacin A, Uzun CA, Gunendi Z, Gogus F; Physical Medicine and Rehabilitation; Division of Rheumatology; et al. Comparison Of Different Methods Of Skin Pathergy Test In Patients With Behçet's Syndrome. [online] Available from https://acrabstracts.org/abstract/comparison-of-different-methods-of-skin-pathergy-test-in-patients-with-behcets-syndrome/ [Last accessed February, 2024]

21. Kaneko F, Togashi A, Nomura E, Nakamura K. A New Diagnostic Way for Behcet's Disease: Skin Prick with Self-Saliva. Genet Res Int. 2014;2014: 581468.

22. Davatchi F. Diagnosis/Classification Criteria for Behcet's Disease. Pathol Res Int. 2012;2012:607921.

23. Diaz G. Behcet's Syndrome – Diagnosis. [online] Available from https://grepmed.com/images/12917/behcets-diagnosis-syndrome-rheumatology-disease [Last accessed February, 2024].

24. Djawari D, Hornstein OP, Luckner L. Skin Window Examination According to Rebuck and Cutaneous Pathergy Tests in Patients with Behçet's Disease. Dermatologica. 1985;70(6):265-70.

25. Davatchi F, Abdollahi BS, Chams-Davatchi C, Shahram F, Ghodsi Z, Nadji A, et al. Impact of the positive pathergy test on the performance of classification/diagnosis criteria for Behcet's disease. Mod Rheumatol. 2013;23(1):125-32.

26. Helm TN, Camisa C, Allen C, Lowder C. Clinical features of Behçet's disease: Report of four cases. Oral Surg Oral Med Oral Pathol. 1991;72(1): 30-4.

Bedside Tests in Psoriasis

K Lekshmipriya, Sushmita Mishra

INTRODUCTION

The use of bedside clinical tests is necessary even for an experienced dermatologist for confirmation of diagnosis, especially for similar-looking lesions. These are being replaced by evolving technology and advancements in investigative procedures. However, these simple tests remain the main method of diagnostic confirmation in routine dermatological practice, especially in resource-poor settings.[1]

LIST OF BEDSIDE TESTS DONE IN PSORIASIS (BOX 1)

Psoriasis is a common, relapsing chronic inflammatory condition affecting about 1.5–3% of the world's population, causing significant morbidity. The presence of a well-defined margin and a silvery white scale, over a glossy homogenous membrane, is clinically diagnostic of psoriasis.[2]

Psoriasis is a genetically determined, inflammatory, and proliferative disease of the skin characterized by dull red, sharply demarcated scaly plaques. The two clinical signs, the Auspitz sign, and the Grattage test have been described as pathognomonic of psoriasis by Hellgren et al.[2]

GRATTAGE TEST

When the scaling is not evident, it can be induced by light tangential scratching with the edge of the glass slide (Grattage).[2]

AUSPITZ SIGN

The successive removal of the psoriatic scales usually reveals an underlying smooth, glossy red membrane with multiple bleeding points where thin suprapapillary epithelium is torn off.[2]

It is usually elicited using the Grattage test where the superficial scales are scraped off with the help of a glass slide which reveals a shiny glistening membrane referred to as the Bulkeley's membrane corresponding to the thinning of suprapapillary plate. On further scraping, there is the appearance of punctate bleeding spots due to the presence of dilated dermal capillaries.[3]

BOX 1	List of bedside tests done in psoriasis.

- Grattage test
- Auspitz sign
- PASI score
- Koebner phenomenon
- Dermoscopy
- Tender and swollen joint count for psoriatic arthritis

METHOD

Grattage Test

Gentle scratching and rubbing alter the visibility of scaling. Scratching scale in psoriasis makes the scale appear more silvery in color by introducing air-keratin interfaces **(Figs. 1A and B)**.

On Grattage, the characteristic coherence of the scales can be seen as if one scratches a wax candle—*signe de la tache de bougie* **(Figs. 1C and D)**.

In nonscaly lesions, indentation by a fingernail leaves an opaque mark resembling that made by scratching a tallow wax candle.[4]

Auspitz Sign

Named after Heinrich Auspitz this was first described by Daniel Turner in the 19th century.[4] When the scales are completely scraped off, the stratum mucosum (basement membrane) is exposed and is seen as a moist red surface (membrane of Bulkeley) **(Figs. 2A and B)** through which dilated capillaries at the tip of elongated dermal papillae are torn, leading to multiple bleeding points **(Figs. 2C and D)**. This is a characteristic feature of psoriasis and is known as the *Auspitz sign*.[4]

It is attributed to parakeratosis, suprapapillary thinning of the stratum malpighii, elongation of dermal papillae and dilatation, and tortuosity of the papillary capillaries.[3]

If the surface of psoriatic plaque is scraped with a blunt scalpel, squamae falls off as layers of white lamellae that exhibit coherence after removal, much like candle wax. This desquamation is sometimes referred to as the "wax spot phenomenon." It is a sign of parakeratotic hyperkeratosis. If

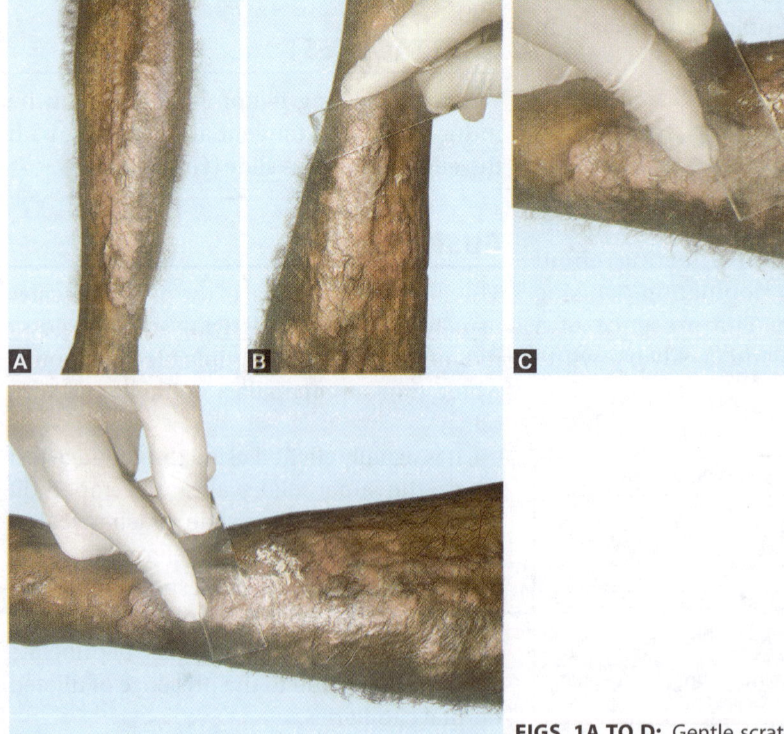

FIGS. 1A TO D: Gentle scratching and rubbing done in Grattage test showing *signe de la tache de bougie*.

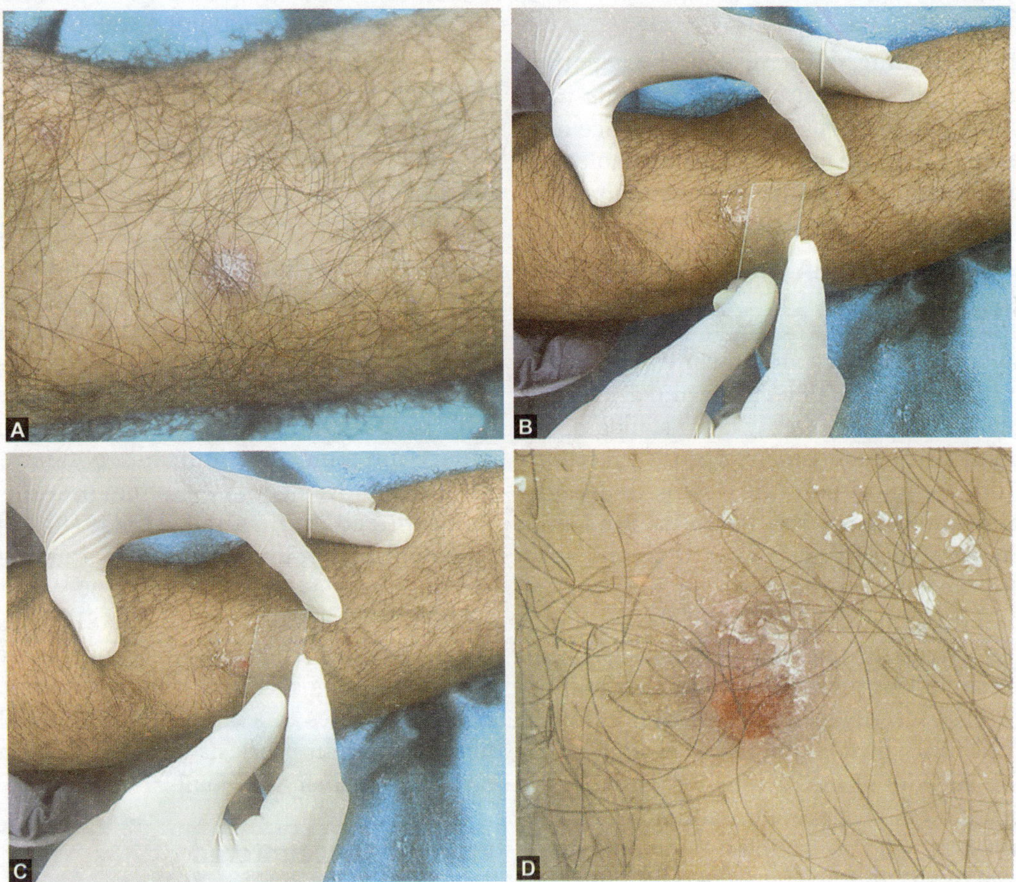

FIGS. 2A TO D: Bulkeley membrane and multiple bleeding points seen in Auspitz sign.

psoriatic plaque is scraped further, a wet layer adhered to the lesion can be revealed.[5] This is the last layer of the dermal papillae of the epidermis, and it is a pathognomonic sign of psoriasis, known as the "last membrane phenomenon."[6]

Significance

Clinically psoriasis vulgaris can be diagnosed (>80%) by the presence of micaceous scales, along with the Grattage test and Auspitz's sign.[3]

Problems Encountered

- Not sensitive
- Not seen in inverse psoriasis; pustular, erythrodermic psoriasis; guttate psoriasis, rupioid variant, and also in case of treated cases.[1]
- Psoriasis has many different clinical variants and can resemble other skin diseases, such as secondary syphilis, dyshidrotic eczema, seborrheic dermatitis, pityriasis rosea, psoriasiform drug rash, and parapsoriasis.
- Besides, the same patient can present at different times with a different clinical presentation or variant.[4]
- However, their absence warrants a detailed histological examination in a clinical setting suggestive of psoriasis.
- Not specific because it is also seen in nonpsoriatic scaling disorders, including Darier's disease and actinic keratosis.[7]

Summary

These findings are considered as "pathognomonic" clinical signs in patients with suspected psoriasis and their presence may even obviate the need for a histopathological examination in resource-limited settings.[2]

PSORIASIS AREA AND SEVERITY INDEX SCORE

In clinical practice and in clinical research, it is important to objectively and accurately measure disease severity using standardized methods. The assessment of psoriasis severity from a clinical point of view is frequently performed using the Psoriasis Area and Severity Index (PASI).[8]

The clinical diagnosis of psoriasis is based on the assessment of the patient's history and the presence of skin lesions with characteristic morphology and distribution. Disease severity is usually assessed through the PASI, which combines an evaluation of the severity of the lesions with erythema, infiltration, and peeling, scored on a scale of 0–4 (0 = none, 1 = mild, 2 = moderate, 3 = marked, and 4 = very marked) and the percentage of skin involved on the head, trunk, upper limbs, and lower limbs. Moderate or severe disease can be defined by a PASI score of 5–10 or a PASI score of >10, respectively.[9]

Method

Psoriasis Area and Severity Index is determined by assessing severity in four anatomical regions (head/neck, upper extremities, trunk, and lower extremities). Each of the three primary clinical signs of psoriasis—(1) erythema, (2) induration, and (3) desquamation—is ranked as an average severity across each region using a scale of 0 (none) to 4 (maximum) and added together generating an overall severity score for each body region. Next, the area of involvement in the body region is determined and assigned area scores based upon the proportion of the anatomical region involved with psoriasis. Area scores are multiplied by severity scores for a region-proportionate score.[10]

Significance

The PASI is a scoring system to evaluate baseline and response of therapy in psoriasis. The British Association of Dermatologists (BAD) recommends PASI 75 for measuring the primary response of psoriasis in patients with psoriatic arthritis (PsA). PASI 75 is a binary outcome that indicates a 75% or greater improvement in PASI from baseline. Randomized controlled trials (RCTs) commonly report this and other measures of response, such as PASI 50 and PASI 90.[11]

A 75% reduction in the PASI score (PASI 75) is the current benchmark of primary endpoints for most clinical trials of psoriasis. PASI 50 equates to a clinically meaningful improvement in psoriasis and represents a discerning primary endpoint.[12]

Problems Encountered

Despite some limitations, exemplified by different measures provided by the same rater or different measures provided by distinct raters when assessing the same patient, the PASI has been widely accepted as a very useful tool.[13]

Simple sensitivity analyses will assume different values of the thresholds for the change in PASI, such as using the upper end of the range and the midpoint.[11]

The PASI is not a precise measure of severity with less precision when the regional area of involvement is <10% of the body surface area (BSA) of a specific anatomical region.[10]

It has substantial limitations, such as low response distribution, no consensus on interpretability, and low responsiveness in mild disease.[14]

It involves estimating the percentage of BSA involvement, for which there is high interobserver variability particularly, in patients with limited psoriasis. As a result, the PASI is poor in detecting changes in mild or moderate psoriasis (the most prevalent type of psoriasis). Patients with very different clinical manifestations of psoriasis could have the same PASI score (e.g., if one has widespread but minimal psoriasis and another has localized but severe psoriasis). Because plaque elevation, scaling, and erythema are rated equally, treatments that temporarily affect scaling or erythema will affect the PASI score more than equally effective treatments that do not.[15]

Summary

The gold standard for assessing the severity of psoriasis is the PASI, which combines the assessment of the severity of lesions and the extent of the affected area in a single index score. We have previously observed that the PASI score was a more important factor than the Dermatology Life Quality Index (DLQI) in the decision to initiate biological treatment.[16]

Psoriasis Area and Severity Index has been criticized for being resource intensive, complex, lacking sensitivity, low in accuracy, and having a nonlinear scale. Nevertheless, the PASI is often used as the standard measurement in the validation of new measures and correlated well in most cases with other physician-based assessments.[14]

THE KOEBNER PHENOMENON

The Koebner phenomenon (KP), is the appearance of new skin lesions on previously unaffected skin secondary to trauma. This phenomenon is also termed the isomorphic (from Greek, "equal shape") response, given the fact that the new lesions that appear.[17]

Koebner phenomenon lesions are typically linear in shape as they follow the route of cutaneous injury.

In other words, a patient with psoriasis who exhibits koebnerization (and is said to be "Koebner-positive") will develop new psoriasiform lesions along sites of skin injury, even if trivial **(Figs. 3A and B)**. Koebner phenomenon can develop in any anatomic site, including in classic areas of psoriatic involvement and in regions that are usually spared, such as the face. The phenomenon shows dynamic behavior. Patients may be "Koebner-negative" at one point in life but may later become "Koebner-positive.[17]"

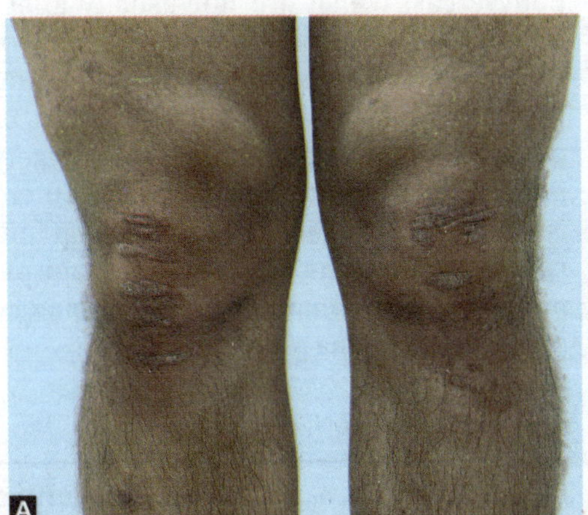
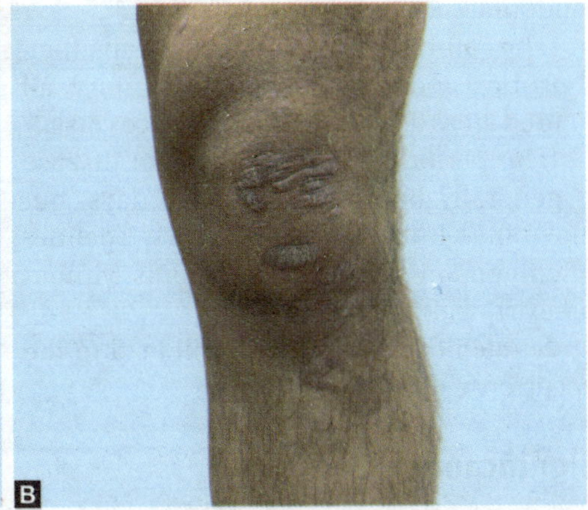

FIGS. 3A AND B: New psoriasiform lesions along sites of skin injury demonstrating the Koebner phenomenon.

Method

Different types of cutaneous injury may trigger this phenomenon, a number of agents/triggers have been reported to induce the development of new psoriatic lesions in healthy skin areas and these include, tattooing skin, radiations, skin incision, viral infections, and striae. The other factors/agents that are reported to exacerbate psoriasis as *Koebner reaction* include megavoltage irradiations, radiotherapy for carcinoma of the breast, exposure to purified protein derivative (PPD)/Mantoux test, surgical incision during breast reconstruction, needle acupuncture, prosthesis after amputation of the leg, secondary syphilis, cupping therapy, a traditional Chinese medicine, striae distensae, and striae gravidarum, electrocardiogram (ECG), itching (one of the core features of psoriasis)-induced skin injury and viral infection-induced hand-foot-and-mouth disease. The occurrence of psoriatic lesions at unusual areas of the body regions, such as on the penis, around the eyes, and on keloid suggests that the Koebner phenomenon may be responsible for these psoriatic lesions. Moreover, the development of dactylitis (inflammation of an entire digit, finger, or toe) in PsA has been linked with the deep Koebner phenomenon of the flexor tendon-associated accessory pulleys.[18]

The "all-or-none principle" means that, if psoriasis occurs in one area of injury, all injured areas develop psoriasis or vice versa.[19]

The period from injury to skin disease is generally between 10 and 20 days, but may range from 3 days to 2 years. Koebner phenomenon can occur in patients without preexisting dermatosis.[20]

Scratching over the skin will lead to the occurrence of new lesions.[2]

Significance

Koebnerization may significantly impact patients with psoriasis, as any insult to their skin, including tattoos and injections, can cause their disease to flare.

Koebner phenomenon is also instrumental in the occurrence, progression, persistence, and relapse of the primary disease. Koebnerization might function as a clinical indicator of disease activity, as well as serve as a predictor of treatment response.[17] The presence of the Koebner phenomenon appears to be associated with rapid disease progression and a lower response to treatment. Therefore, we need to evaluate the disease stage, select the appropriate treatment for the Koebner phenomenon, and control the development of lesions at the earliest.[21]

Problems Encountered

This isomorphic phenomenon is now known to involve numerous diseases, among them vitiligo, lichen planus, and Darier disease, and thus not specific for psoriasis. The pathogenesis of the Koebner phenomenon is still obscure but may involve cytokines, stress proteins, adhesion molecules, and autoantigens.[22]

Summary

The presence of psoriatic lesions in those body areas, which are not usually affected by psoriasis suggest the key role of the Koebner phenomenon in spreading psoriasis. It is essential that any sort of persistent inflammations/injurious triggers are effectively controlled; otherwise, there is a tendency to transform and develop into cancers. Understanding the key mechanisms may help in combating the inflammatory processes including psoriatic lesions.[18]

DERMOSCOPY

Dermoscopy is a noninvasive in-office method, which enables the diagnosis of many dermatoses and reduces the need for performing biopsies. There is an accumulating body of evidence that dermoscopy (both handheld and videodermoscopy) is a useful tool in differential diagnosis in doubtful cases of psoriasis of the skin, scalp, nails, palms, soles, and genital region.[23]

Method

Dermoscopic examination of a psoriasis plaque should be done in three categories (1) background, (2) vessels, and (3) scales. The examination should be done with minimal pressure to visualize vessels better and with immersion oil if possible.[24]

The regular arrangement of red-dotted vessels is the most common vascular feature of psoriasis vulgaris, as seen using dermoscopy **(Figs. 4A to C)**.[24] The background color was described as reddish or pinkish with white or yellowish scales. The most frequent dermoscopic (trichoscopic) feature of scalp psoriasis was the presence of red dots/globules and twisted red loops. Typical dermoscopic (onychoscopic) signs of nail psoriasis were onycholysis, salmon patches, and splinter hemorrhages.[23]

White scale is one of the characteristic manifestations of psoriasis and its corresponding histopathological features are orthokeratosis and/or parakeratosis. Light red is the most common background color for psoriasis and in children and adolescents, some researchers have described the background color as milky pink.[25]

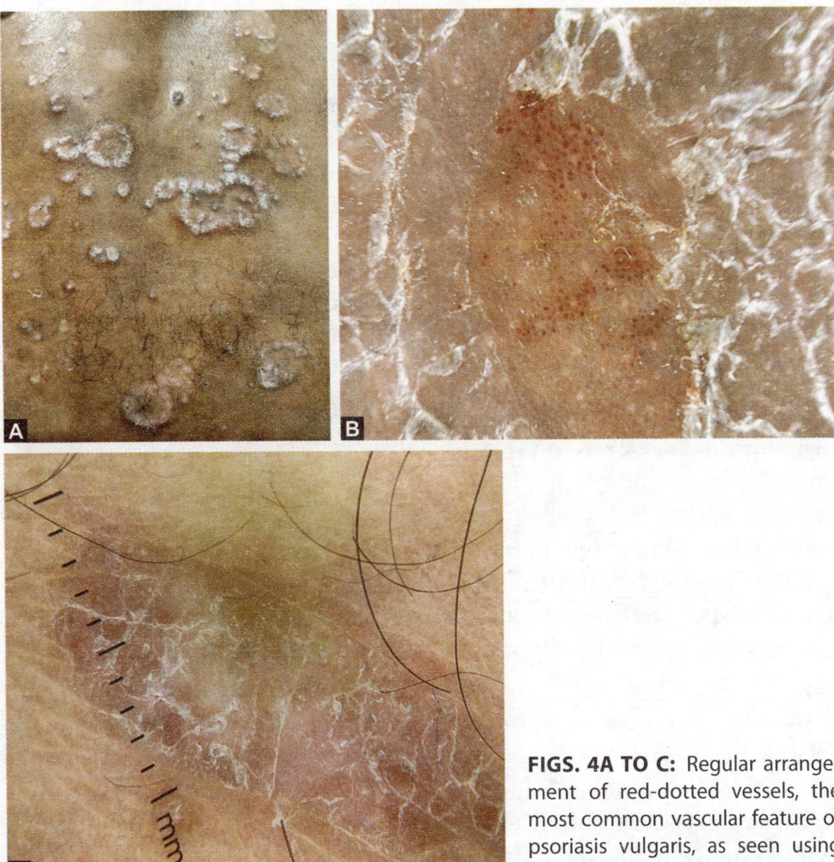

FIGS. 4A TO C: Regular arrangement of red-dotted vessels, the most common vascular feature of psoriasis vulgaris, as seen using dermoscopy.

Nail matrix involvement has been shown to manifest as deep pitting, red spots in the lunula, and leukonychia. Nail bed involvement manifested as salmon patch/oil drop sign, onycholysis, and splinter hemorrhage.[25]

Significance

In a study by Lallas et al., if all three features were present, psoriasis vulgaris was highly predicted, with a diagnostic specificity of 88.0% and a sensitivity of 84.9%.

Although the shape, size, and distance of the vessels in these diseases are nonhomogeneous, the specificity of the regular distribution of vessels in the diagnosis of psoriasis has been found to be 100%.[25]

Problems Encountered

Dermoscopic findings of psoriasis such as dotted vessels may be similar to skin diseases, which are characterized by erythematous plaques with scales, such as dermatitis, tinea corporis, pityriasis rosea, pityriasis rubra pilaris, lichen planus, and nonpigmented squamous cell carcinoma in situ.[24]

Based on the locations of the lesion and skin phototypes, there are some differences in the vascular patterns. In the palmar and plantar areas, the frequency of dotted vessels has been found to be the lowest and in the intertriginous areas (axilla, submammary, and groin), dotted vessels with regular distribution were more common; whereas, the vessels in the back were usually patchy. Patients with darker skin types (V or VI) were observed to be similar to those patients with lighter skin types (I–III); however, the frequency of specific vascular patterns was lower.[25]

Summary

- The most common dermoscopic findings of psoriasis vulgaris are dotted vessels in a regular arrangement over a light red background and white scales in a diffuse arrangement.[24]
- Dermoscopy is a tool of great clinical value in the diagnosis of psoriasis vulgaris.
- Dermoscopy is highly accurate in the diagnosis of nail psoriasis.[25]
- Dermoscopy, as an economical, noninvasive, and rapid examination technique, has good clinical value in the diagnosis and differential diagnosis of psoriasis and shows great promise for severity assessment and efficacy prediction monitoring. However, due to the short development time, dermoscopy is still in the exploratory stage for the diagnosis and treatment of psoriasis, and further large-scale research is needed to establish the diagnostic criteria and explore the corresponding mechanism.[25]

PSORIATIC ARTHRITIS

Psoriatic arthritis is a common condition that significantly impacts affected patients. The introduction of novel therapeutic agents for PsA has generated considerable interest in both clinical trials and clinical care. Thus, there is a great need for standardized outcome measures to assess the activity of disease and the response to therapy. Because psoriasis is a heterogeneous and multifaceted condition, defining outcome measures has been a challenge. To date, such measures have largely been adapted from related diseases, as described in this essay. Further research is needed to further develop outcome measures for PsA to facilitate optimal treatment of patients with PsA.[26]

Assessment of articular involvement uses a count of swollen and tender joints. Psoriatic arthritis, unlike rheumatoid arthritis (RA), usually presents with oligoarticular, asymmetric involvement. Psoriatic arthritis, however, may also cause polyarticular involvement that includes the distal interphalangeal (DIP) joints.[27]

Unlike RA, the pattern of joint involvement in PsA is usually asymmetric and frequently involves the DIP joints. Peripheral joints are assessed for tenderness and swelling. There is no validated measure to assess peripheral joints in PsA. The measure used is the American College of Rheumatology (ACR) joint count initially developed in 1949 for the assessment of patients with RA.[3] The ACR joint count ranges from 28, 44, 68, and 78 for tenderness; 28, 44, 66, and 76 for swelling (excluding hips from assessment of swelling).[28]

Method

The SJC66/TJC68 joint count **(Table 1)**. The 66 swollen and 68 tender joints are assessed (the hips are not assessed for swelling). The joint count is scored as a sum of the tender joints and a sum of the swollen joints **(Fig. 5)**.[29] This scoring (ACR joint count) was developed in 1949 for the evaluation of RA and is now also used for measuring disease activity in PsA.[30]

Significance

The 68/66 Joint Count is the most thorough clinimetric.[27] Tender counts joint counts

TABLE 1: Swollen and tender joint count.

Joints	Swollen joints	Tender joints
Temporomandibular joint	(0–2)	(0–2)
Sternoclavicular joints	(0–2)	(0–2)
Acromioclavicular joints	(0–2)	(0–2)
Glenohumeral(s)	(0–2)	(0–2)
Elbow(s)	(0–2)	(0–2)
Wrists(s)	(0–2)	(0–2)
Metacarpal phalangeal joints	(0–10)	(0–10)
Finger proximal interphalangeal joints	(0–10)	(0–10)
Finger direct interphalangeal joints	(0–8)	(0–8)
Hip(s)	NA	(0–2)
Knee(s)	(0–2)	(0–2)
Ankle(s)	(0–2)	(0–2)
Tarsus/midfoot (feet)	(0–2)	(0–2)
Metatarsal phalangeal joints	(0–10)	(0–10)
Toe proximal interphalangeal joints	(0–10)	(0–10)
Total joint counts	(0–66)	(0–66)

(TJC) and swollen joint counts (SJC) are items of disease activity scores in RA and PsA. In PsA, the role of tenderness and swelling of joints for reflecting active inflammation has not been well studied so far. SJC are more closely linked with ultrasound (US) signs of inflammation as compared to TJC in PsA. While swelling of a joint predicts US inflammation after a year, the information on whether the joint is additionally tender or not gives no additional predictive information.[31]

Problems Encountered

A study by the Group for Research and Assessment of Psoriasis and Psoriatic Arthritis (GRAPPA) showed that reduced joint counts do not properly assess active PsA.[7] Reduced counts of 28 or 44 swollen joints are not suitable for this condition.[27]

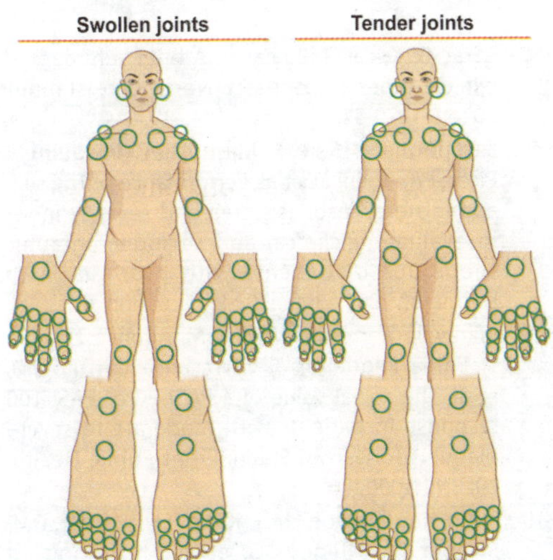

FIG. 5: Diagram representing the 68/66 joint count.

Summary

Although developed for RA, it has been shown to have good interobserver and intraobserver reliability in PsA. The ACR joint count has become a standard measure, both in RA and in PsA, in part because of its inclusion in key composite criteria.[26]

CONCLUSION

The clinical signs of psoriasis include micaceous scales, the Grattage test, and Auspitz's sign, all considered pathognomic for diagnosing psoriasis. The PASI score has been crucial for objectively measuring disease severity, combining evaluations of erythema, induration, and scaling. The Koebner phenomenon, the appearance of new lesions on injured skin, is discussed as a significant marker of disease activity. Dermoscopy has come up as an important tool for the diagnosis of psoriasis with findings of dotted vessels and white scales. The 68/66 joint count, adapted from RA assessment, is introduced as a thorough clinimetric for evaluating tender and swollen joints in PsA.

Key Messages

- Clinical signs such as micaceous scales, the Grattage test, and the Auspitz sign are considered pathognomic for diagnosis of psoriasis.
- The gold standard for assessing psoriasis severity is the PASI score despite its limitations and remains crucial in clinical trials and treatment decisions.
- The Koebner phenomenon may serve as a clinical indicator of disease activity and a predictor of treatment response.
- Dermoscopy, a noninvasive, shows promise in diagnosing and differentially diagnosing psoriasis.

REFERENCES

1. Sivakumar A, Thappa DM. Glass slide—An indispensable tool for the dermatologist. CosmoDerma. 2022;2:27.
2. Mehta S, Singal A, Singh N, Bhattacharya SN. A study of clinicohistopathological correlation in patients of psoriasis and psoriasiform dermatitis. Indian Journal of Dermatol Venereol Leprol. 2009;75(1):100.
3. Kangle S, Amladi S, Sawant S. Scaly signs in dermatology. Indian Journal of Dermatol Venereol Leprol. 2006;72(2):161-4.
4. Venna AB, Chittla S, Malkud S. A Clinico-Pathological Study of Psoriasis and Psoriasiform Dermatitis. J Evid Based Med Healthc. 2020;51(7):2349-562.
5. Madke B, Nayak C. Eponymous signs in dermatology. Indian Dermatology Online J. 2012;3(3):159-65.
6. Teledermatology for PG entrance. Psoriasis. [online]. Available from: http://drsaurabhjindal. blogspot.com/2015/01/psoriasis.html [Last accessed February, 2024].
7. Sarac G, Koca TT, Baglan T. A brief summary of clinical types of psoriasis. North Clin Istanbul. 2016;3(1):79-82.
8. Sampogna F, Sera F, Mazzotti E, Pasquini P, Picardi A, Abeni D, et al. Performance of the self-administered psoriasis area and severity index in evaluating clinical and sociodemographic subgroups of patients with psoriasis. Arch Dermatol. 2003;139(3):353-8;discussion 357.
9. Maravilla-Herrera P, Merino M, Alfonso Zamora S, Balea Filgueiras J, Carrascosa Carrillo JM, et al. The social value of a PASI 90 or PASI 100 response in patients with moderate-to-severe plaque psoriasis in Spain. Front Public Health. 2023;11:1000776.
10. Papp KA, Lebwohl MG, Kircik LH, Pariser DM, Strober B, Krueger GG, et al. The proposed PASI-HD provides more precise assessment of

plaque psoriasis severity in anatomical regions with a low area score. Dermatol Ther (Heidelb). 2021;11(4):1079-83.

11. Rodgers M, Epstein D, Bojke L, Yang H, Craig D, Fonseca T, et al. Etanercept, infliximab and adalimumab for the treatment of psoriatic arthritis: a systematic review and economic evaluation. Southampton (UK): NIHR Journals Library; 2011.

12. Carlin CS, Feldman SR, Krueger JG, Menter A, Krueger GG. A 50% reduction in the Psoriasis Area and Severity Index (PASI 50) is a clinically significant endpoint in the assessment of psoriasis. J Am Acad Dermatol. 2004;50(6):859-66.

13. Silva MF, Fortes MR, Miot LD, Marques SA. Psoriasis: correlation between severity index (PASI) and quality of life index (DLQI) in patients assessed before and after systemic treatment. An Bras Dermatol. 2013;88(5):760-3.

14. Spuls PI, Lecluse LL, Poulsen ML, Bos JD, Stern RS, Nijsten T. How good are clinical severity and outcome measures for psoriasis?: quantitative evaluation in a systematic review. J Invest Dermatol. 2010;130(4):933-43.

15. Lew-Kaya D, Lue J, Sefton J, Walker P. Evaluating psoriasis severity: limitations of the PASI and advantages of the overall lesional assessment. J Am Acad Dermatol. 2004;50(3):P153.

16. Hägg D, Sundström A, Eriksson M, Schmitt-Egenolf M. Severity of psoriasis differs between men and women: a study of the clinical outcome measure psoriasis area and severity index (PASI) in 5438 Swedish register patients. Am J Clin Dermatol. 2017;18(4):583-90.

17. Sanchez DP, Sonthalia S. Koebner phenomenon. In: StatPearls [Internet]. Treasure Island (FL): StatPearls Publishing; 2024.

18. Ji YZ, Liu SR. Koebner phenomenon leading to the formation of new psoriatic lesions: evidences and mechanisms. Bioscience Rep. 2019;39(12):BSR20193266.

19. Kalayciyan A, Aydemir EH, Kotogyan A. Experimental Koebner phenomenon in patients with psoriasis. Dermatology. 2007;215(2):114-7

20. Arias-Santiago S, Espiñeira-Carmona MJ, Aneiros-Fernández J. The Koebner phenomenon: psoriasis in tattoos. CMAJ. 2013;185(7):585.

21. Zhang X, Lei L, Jiang L, Fu C, Huang J, Hu Y, et al. Characteristics and pathogenesis of Koebner phenomenon. Exp Dermatol. 2023;32(4):310-23.

22. Sagi L, Trau H. The koebner phenomenon. Clinics in dermatology. 2011;29(2):231-6.

23. Golińska J, Sar-Pomian M, Rudnicka L. Dermoscopic features of psoriasis of the skin, scalp and nails - a systematic review. J Eur Acad Dermatol Venereol. 2019;33(4):648-60.

24. Gokyayla E, Cetinarslan T, Ermertcan AT. Dermoscopic Differential Diagnosis of Psoriasis. In: Aghaei S (Ed). Psoriasis-New Research. London: IntechOpen; 2022.

25. Wu Y, Sun L. Clinical value of dermoscopy in psoriasis. J Cosmet Dermatol. 2024;23(2):370-81.

26. Kavanaugh A, Cassell AK. The assessment of disease activity and outcomes in psoriatic arthritis. Clin Exp Rheumatol. 2005;23(5 Suppl 39):S142-7.

27. Sandoval DC, Fernández-Ávila DG. Assessment tools in psoriatic arthritis: A review. Revista Colombiana de Reumatología. 2023;30(Suppl 1):S75-86.

28. Wong PC, Leung YY, Li EK, Tam LS. Measuring disease activity in psoriatic arthritis. Int J Rheumatol. 2012;2012:839425.

29. Duarte-García A, Leung YY, Coates LC, Beaton D, Christensen R, Craig ET, et al. Endorsement of the 66/68 joint count for the measurement of musculoskeletal disease activity: OMERACT 2018 psoriatic arthritis workshop report. J Rheumatol. 2019;46(8):996-1005.

30. Mease PJ, Antoni CE, Gladman DD, Taylor WJ. Psoriatic arthritis assessment tools in clinical trials. Ann Rheum Dis. 2005;64(Suppl 2):ii49-54.

31. Bosch P, Lackner A, Dreo B, Husic R, Anja F, Gretler J, et al. The role of tender and swollen joints for the assessment of inflammation in PsA using ultrasound. Rheumatology (Oxford). 2022;61(SI):SI92-6.

Bedside Tests in Autoimmune Bullous Disorders

Sidharth Bhat, K Lekshmipriya, Binu Kunwar

INTRODUCTION

Autoimmune bullous disorders (AIBDs) encompass a diverse group of dermatological conditions characterized by the development of blisters and erosions on both the skin and mucous membranes. These conditions arise from immune-mediated attacks on the structural components of the skin, resulting in the loss of cellular adhesion, a phenomenon referred to as acantholysis. The clinical presentation of AIBDs varies considerably, spanning a spectrum from relatively mild to potentially life-threatening. This chapter focuses on the crucial role played by bedside tests in the diagnosis of AIBD.

The identification and knowledge of specific clinical signs and test holds paramount importance in the bedside diagnosis of AIBD. These tests not only assist in distinguishing AIBD from other skin conditions but also provide valuable insights into the underlying disease mechanisms, aiding in the differentiation of various AIBD subtypes. Given the broad range of clinical presentations and the potential for significant health impacts, a comprehensive understanding of these signs and test is indispensable for healthcare practitioners in managing autoimmune bullous skin disorders.

Within this chapter, we will delve into several clinical signs and tests associated with AIBD, which include the well-recognized Nikolsky's sign and its variations, the bulla spread sign, Lutz sign, and the Tzanck smear test. Each of these will be explored in depth, highlighting their diagnostic significance, techniques for elicitation, and the conditions with which they are associated. Through this exploration, the chapter aims to equip dermatologists with the necessary knowledge to effectively identify and assess these disorders.

CLASSIFICATION OF AUTOIMMUNE BULLOUS DISORDER AND RELEVANT BEDSIDE TESTS

The classification of AIBD plays a pivotal role in comprehending their diverse presentations and guiding appropriate management approaches. These disorders are typically categorized into two primary groups based on the location of blister formation within the skin: intraepidermal and subepidermal blistering diseases. **Table 1** provides an enumeration of various intraepidermal and subepidermal blistering disorders.

Intraepidermal Blistering Diseases

These conditions are distinguished by the formation of blisters within the epidermal layer of the skin. Among the most prevalent diseases in this category are various forms

TABLE 1: Classification of intraepidermal and subepidermal bullous dermatoses.

Intraepidermal bullous disorders	Pemphigus vulgaris
	Pemphigus foliaceus
	Pemphigus erythematosus
	Paraneoplastic pemphigus
Subepidermal bullous disorders	Bullous pemphigoid
	Mucous membrane pemphigoid
	Linear immunoglobulin A (IgA) disease
	Dermatitis herpetiformis
	Epidermolysis bullosa acquisita
	Pemphigoid gestationis

of pemphigus, such as pemphigus vulgaris (PV) and pemphigus foliaceus. These disorders are characterized by the presence of autoantibodies that target desmosomal proteins (specifically, desmoglein 1 and 3), resulting in acantholysis or the loss of cohesion among keratinocytes. Bedside tests, such as the Nikolsky's sign, play a critical role in diagnosing these diseases, as they reveal the compromised integrity of the epidermis.

Subepidermal Blistering Diseases

In these conditions, blisters develop at the junction between the epidermis and the dermis. This category encompasses diseases such as bullous pemphigoid (BP), epidermolysis bullosa acquisita, and dermatitis herpetiformis. These disorders are frequently associated with antibodies that target components of the basement membrane zone, leading to separation at the dermoepidermal junction. The bulla spread sign (also known as the Lutz sign) serves as a valuable clinical test in these cases, as it can illustrate the extension of subepidermal blisters.

HISTORY

The Nikolsky's sign, an important clinical assessment tool in the field of dermatology, was originally documented by the Russian dermatologist Pyotr Vasilyevich Nikolsky during the late 19th century. Pyotr Vasilyevich Nikolsky (1858–1940) was born in Usman, a town located in Lipetsk Oblast, Russia. He pursued his medical education at St Vladimir Emperor University in Kiev, which is now recognized as Taras Shevchenko National University of Kyiv.[1] Between 1884 and 1897, he worked as an assistant to Mikhail Stukovenkov, a pioneering dermatologist and venereologist at the Kiev Clinic for Skin and Venereal Disease. Stukovenkov was the first to propose the use of mercury for treating syphilis. Nikolsky assumed the role of the Head of the Department of Dermatology at Warsaw University from 1898 to 1915. Subsequently, he relocated to the University School of Medicine in Rostov-on-Don, Russia, where he continued to serve as the Head of the Department until 1930.[2]

Nikolsky authored a book titled "L'etat de la dermatologie et de la syphiligraphie en Russie jusqu'à 1884" (The State of Dermatology and Syphiligraphy in Russia up until 1884). In 1884, he publicly introduced his eponymous observation. In 1896, he published his doctoral thesis, in which he reported that when patients with pemphigus foliaceus had their skin rubbed; it resulted in epidermal denudation, revealing a glistening surface underneath. He observed that this reduced cohesion between epidermal layers was not limited to the affected lesions but also affected the normal-appearing skin, which he labeled as "keratolysis universalis". This observation went beyond being merely a clinical curiosity; it provided a deeper insight into the pathological processes underlying conditions like pemphigus.

The Nikolsky's sign brought about a significant transformation in the diagnostic approach to blistering skin disorders. It highlighted a compromised connection and contact between the layers of the epidermis, particularly the corneal and granular layers. Nikolsky's groundbreaking work, later corroborated by other dermatologists such as Alan Lyell, extended the applicability of the sign to various dermatological conditions, including toxic epidermal necrolysis (TEN).

Another notable scientist who made significant contributions to the field of dermatology was Dr Nikolay Dmitriyevich Sheklakov (1918–1989), a medical mycologist and dermatologist. Dr Sheklakov was not only a distinguished professional but also a remarkable humanist who played a vital role in saving thousands of lives in the Sachsenhausen and Bergen–Belsen German death camps, where he was affectionately known as "Doctor Nicolaus". In addition to his contributions to the study of immunobullous disorders, he was a trailblazer in Soviet dermatology for developing a clinical classification system for mycoses.[3]

Dr Sheklakov is credited with describing the sign of perifocal subepidermal separation, often referred to as the "false Nikolsky's sign", which is now known as the "Sheklakov's sign". In contrast to the authentic Nikolsky's sign, the Sheklakov's sign involves the induction of perifocal subepidermal separation at the periphery of blisters. This is achieved by gently pulling the peripheral remaining blister roof, leading to the extension of erosions into adjacent normal skin. These erosions remain limited in size, do not spontaneously expand, and tend to heal relatively quickly.

Furthermore, Sheklakov made modifications to the classic description of the Nikolsky's sign and introduced the term "marginal Nikolsky's sign". This sign entails the application of lateral pressure to a preexisting bullous lesion using items such as a cotton-tipped swab, tongue depressor, or pencil eraser, resulting in the lateral extension of the bulla.

Additionally, Dr Sheklakov demonstrated the ability to elicit the Nikolsky's sign in the oral mucosa of patients afflicted with PV. His pioneering work in dermatology and immunobullous disorders significantly enriched our understanding of these conditions and their diagnostic indicators.

NIKOLSKY'S SIGN

Definition

It refers to the formation of an erosion on applying a lateral/tangential pressure on a perceivably normal skin (direct Nikolsky) or perilesional skin (marginal Nikolsky). It helps in differentiating intraepidermal from subepidermal blister, thus helping to distinguish pemphigus from BP.[4]

Procedure

The sign is elicited by applying lateral pressure with thumb or finger pad on skin over a bony prominence. This results in a shearing force that dislodges the upper layer of epidermis from the lower layer of the epidermis.

The Nikolsky's sign, in its classic form, is not a singular phenomenon but presents in various subtypes, each with specific diagnostic relevance:

- *Direct Nikolsky's sign*: Direct Nikolsky's sign involves inducing erosion on normal skin far from lesions. Its presence suggests a widespread weakening of epidermal cohesion, typical in severe cases of pemphigus and other intraepidermal disorders. This sign can be indicative of more extensive epidermal involvement, seen in various intraepidermal blistering diseases **(Fig. 1)**.
- *Marginal Nikolsky sign*: This subtype involves the extension of erosion to the surrounding normal skin, elicited by

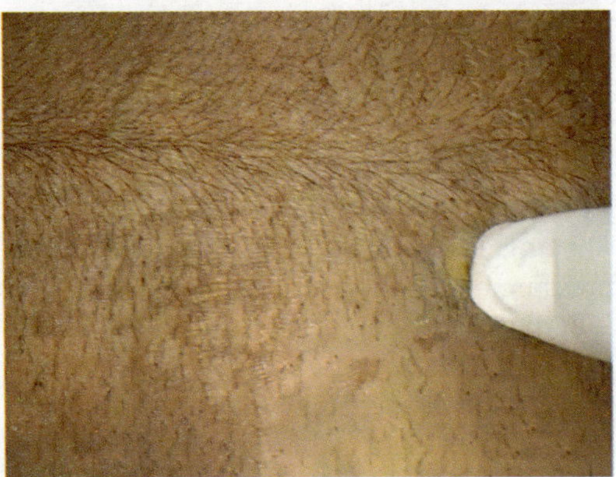

FIG. 1: Direct Nikolsky's sign.

rubbing the skin around preexisting lesions.

- *Wet Nikolsky's sign*: When pressure is applied, and the base of the blister appears moist and glistening, it is referred to as the "wet Nikolsky's sign". This subtype is particularly seen in conditions with intraepidermal blistering, such as PV. The moist base is indicative of a more active disease process, with ongoing epidermal disruption and inflammation.
- *Dry Nikolsky's sign*: Contrasting the wet subtype, the dry Nikolsky's sign features a dry base upon pressure application. The dry aspect of the eroded skin suggests a lessened inflammatory process and re-epithelialization beneath a PV blister and so can suggest a less active disease. It can also possibly indicate a subcorneal blistering disorder like Pemphigus foliaceous.[5]
- *Modified Nikolsky's sign*: This is peripheral extension of the blister on applying pressure on their surface. This is helpful in those patients in whom a new bulla is not available for biopsy. The advantage here is that artificially extended blister does not show epithelial regeneration which may sometimes be seen on the floor of older subepidermal blisters making them appear as intraepidermal.

- *Nikolsky phenomenon*: This is a term used when superficial layer of epidermis is felt to move on the deeper layer of the epidermis. In this region unlike in case of Nikolsky where an erosion is formed, a blister develops after sometime.[6]
- *False Nikolsky's sign (Sheklakov's sign)*: Also known as the Sheklakov's sign, the false Nikolsky's sign is elicited in subepidermal blistering disorders, such as BP. It is observed by pulling the peripheral remnant roof of a ruptured blister, extending the erosion on the surrounding normal skin. This subtype suggests a subepidermal cleavage, which is limited in size and tends to heal rapidly.[6]
- *Pseudo-Nikolsky's sign/epidermal peeling sign*: This is elicited just like the normal Nikolsky's sign in an erythematous skin of the patients of Stevens–Johnson syndrome (SJS)/TEN, burns, and bullous ichthyosiform erythroderma. Here the underlying mechanism is necrosis of the epidermal cells and not true acantholysis.
- *Microscopic Nikolsky's sign*: In conditions like PV or pemphigus foliaceus, sometimes the lateral pressure does not cause visible epidermal separation but induces microscopic changes. This subtype requires histological confirmation. This is especially important for inducing blisters prior to biopsy in patients where there are no visible blisters but pemphigus is suspected. In such cases, similar methodology can employ prior to biopsying the lesion. Hameed and Khan's study revealed a positive microscopic Nikolsky's sign in 73.9% of pemphigus patients who underwent biopsies following lateral pressure application. In contrast, there were no observable changes in the biopsies of healthy control subjects.[7]

Uzun and Durdu conducted a study involving 123 pemphigus cases to assess the usefulness of Nikolsky's sign as a diagnostic tool. They discovered that Nikolsky's sign had moderate sensitivity but high specificity in diagnosing pemphigus. Specifically, the marginal Nikolsky's sign demonstrated higher sensitivity at 69%, while the direct Nikolsky's sign exhibited greater specificity at 100% for the diagnosis of pemphigus.[8]

BULLA SPREAD SIGN

The bulla spread sign, also known as the Asboe-Hansen's sign, is a sign named after Gustav Asboe-Hansen, a Danish physician who significantly contributed to the understanding of dermatological conditions. The bulla spread sign is primarily used to assess the spreadability of blisters in skin disorders and plays a vital role in differentiating between different types of blistering diseases.

Procedure

The margin of the bulla is marked using a pen. Slow careful unidirectional pressure is applied by a finger causing peripheral extension of the bulla beyond the marked margin. The pressure can be applied over the center (Asboe-Hansen's sign) **(Fig. 2)** or the periphery (Lutz sign) **(Fig. 3)** of the bulla. In conditions like PV, the blister extends toward the periphery under the pressure, indicating the presence of intraepidermal blisters.

Relevance of Angle in Bulla Spread Sign

The angle at which the blister extends upon pressure application in the bulla spread sign is of diagnostic importance. In PV, the blister extension often has a sharp angle, indicative of intraepidermal blister formation. In contrast, BP, a subepidermal blistering disorder, shows a rounded border upon extension **(Fig. 4)**.

TZANCK SMEAR IN AUTOIMMUNE BULLOUS DISEASES

The Tzanck smear, introduced by Arnault Tzanck in 1947, is a cornerstone diagnostic tool in dermatology. Diagnostic cytology, the study of individual cells and their characteristics, plays a crucial role in the analysis of cutaneous disorders particularly for identifying vesiculobullous disorders.

Procedure

After cleaning the vesicle with an alcohol swab, the blister roof is unroofed and the base is gently scraped with the back of a number 15

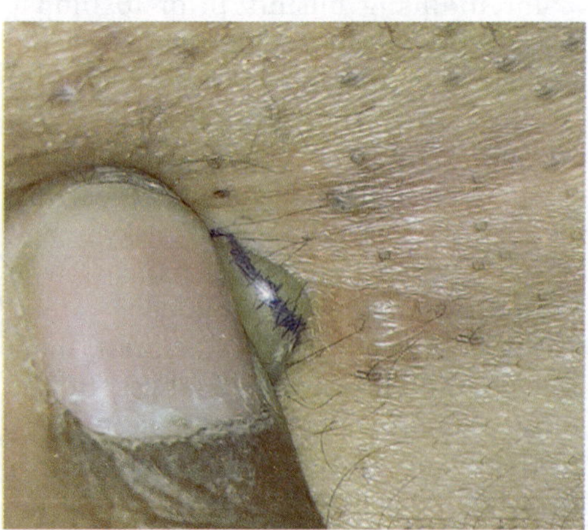

FIG. 2: Bulla spread sign (Asboe-Hansen's sign).

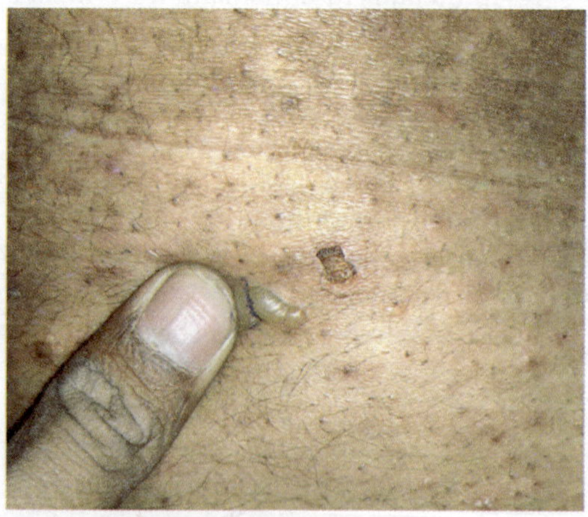

FIG. 3: Bulla spread sign (Lutz sign).

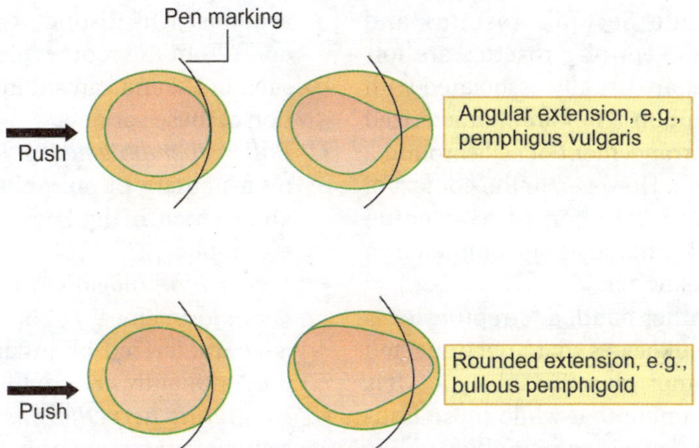

FIG. 4: Relevance of angle of extension in bulla spread sign.

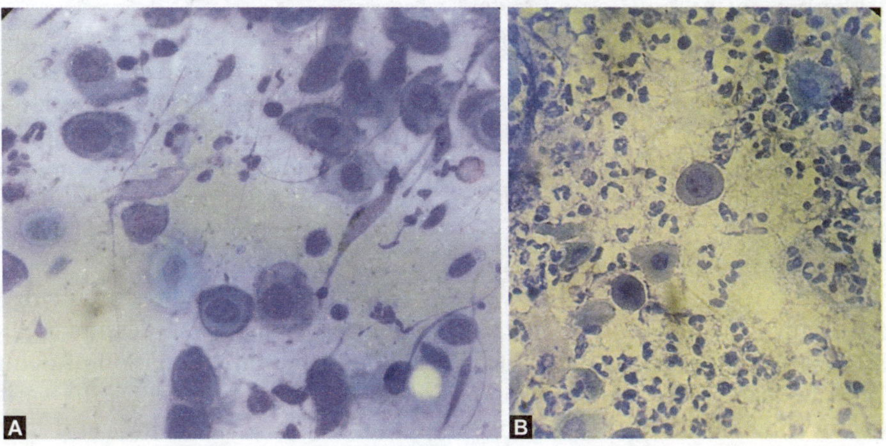

FIGS. 5A AND B: Tzanck cell (acantholytic cell).

scalpel or the edge of a spatula. The collected material is then transferred to a clean glass slide. It is then air or heat dried and stained for microscopic examination. Giemsa stain is commonly used, but other staining methods like Hemacolor, Diff-Quik, Wright's, methylene blue, Papanicolaou, and toluidine blue can also be employed.

Findings of Tzanck Smear in Various Autoimmune Bullous Diseases

- *Pemphigus vulgaris*: In PV, the Tzanck smear examination unveils the presence of multiple acantholytic cells, which are also referred to as Tzanck cells. These cells are characterized by their large size, rounded shape, hypertrophic nucleus, hazy or sometimes absent nucleoli, and an abundance of basophilic cytoplasm. Notably, they exhibit peripheral basophilic staining, giving rise to a distinctive "mourning edged" appearance under microscopic evaluation **(Figs. 5A and B)**.[9]

  In addition to the typical features seen in pemphigus, there are other findings that, while not pathognomonic for pemphigus, are frequently observed.

These include Sertoli's rosettes and "streptocytes." Sertoli's rosettes are formations that are usually associated with Sertoli cell tumors. They are characterized by a radial arrangement of cells around a central lumen. However, in the context of PV, Sertoli's rosettes consist of a central necrobiotic keratinocyte surrounded by a rosette of leukocytes.

On the other hand, a "streptocyte" is a chain of leukocytes that are connected by a filamentous, glue-like substance. It is important to note that while these findings are not specific to pemphigus, they can be observed in other conditions as well. Sertoli's rosettes are also associated with herpes zoster, and "streptocytes" may be seen in diseases within the pemphigoid group.[10]

The reported sensitivity of finding acantholytic cells in Tzanck smears for PV is 100%, indicating that this test is very effective at detecting acantholytic cells in individuals with PV.

However, the specificity is reported to be 43.4%, which suggests that while the presence of acantholytic cells in Tzanck smears is a strong indicator of PV, it may also be observed in some individuals without the condition, leading to a relatively higher rate of false-positive results.[11]

- *Pemphigus vegetans*: The cytologic characteristics closely resemble those of PV, with the notable addition of an increased number of inflammatory cells, notably eosinophils. The presence of these additional inflammatory cells can serve as a distinguishing feature when differentiating pemphigus vegetans from PV.
- *Pemphigus erythematosus and foliaceus*: In these conditions, acantholytic cells frequently exhibit a cytoplasm that has become hyalinized, which corresponds to the dyskeratosis observed in tissue

sections. This distinct feature sets them apart from the more typical presentation seen in PV and can aid in the differentiation of these variants.

- *Bullous pemphigoid*: BP is characterized by a paucity of epithelial cells and an abundance of leukocytes, particularly eosinophils.
- *Linear immunoglobulin A (IgA) bullous dermatosis*: Linear IgA bullous dermatosis is characterized by inflammatory cells, predominantly neutrophils.
- *Dermatitis herpetiformis*: Inflammatory cells, particularly neutrophils.

CONCLUSION

In conclusion, the Nikolsky's sign, bulla spread sign, and Tzanck smear are indispensable tools in the diagnosis of AIBDs. These bedside tests play a pivotal role in distinguishing between intraepidermal and subepidermal blistering, facilitating accurate disease classification and subsequent treatment decisions.

The Nikolsky's sign is inducing blister extension upon lateral pressure application, aiding in the differentiation of pemphigus from BP and other AIBDs. Its variations, including the wet, dry, and marginal Nikolsky's signs, offer nuanced insights into disease activity and extent.

The bulla spread sign provides an efficient means to assess blister spreadability, aiding in disease differentiation by revealing the angle of blister extension.

Meanwhile, the Tzanck smear offers a rapid and relatively cost-effective diagnostic approach for AIBDs by examining individual cells and their characteristics, providing early results that contribute to timely treatment initiation.

These tests, although rooted in the contributions of scientists like Pyotr Vasilyevich Nikolsky, Gustav Asboe-Hansen, and Arnault

Tzanck, continue to be invaluable in the modern diagnosis of AIBD. They not only complement clinical evaluation but also offer a cost-effective and timely means to confirm these complex dermatological conditions.

> ### Key Messages
>
> - Bedside tests play a crucial role in diagnosing ABD aiding in distinguishing them from other skin conditions.
> - Specific clinical signs and tests such as Nikolsky's sign, bulla spread sign, Lutz sign, and Tzanck smear test hold paramount importance in the bedside diagnosis of ABD.
> - These tests help differentiate between intraepidermal and subepidermal blistering disorders among others.
> - These tests provide a valuable insight into underlying disease mechanisms enriching the understanding of various subtypes of AIBD and aiding the healthcare practitioners in effective management.
> - A comprehensive understanding of these bedside tests is indispensable for dermatologists managing ABDs.

REFERENCES

1. Goodman H. Nikolsky sign: page from notable contributors to the knowledge of dermatology. AMA Arch Derm Syphilol. 1953;68(3):334-5.
2. Shakeri A. Pyotr Vasilyevich Nikolsky—The Man Behind the Sign. JAMA Dermatol. 2018;154(2):181.
3. Polemann G. Nicolai Sheklakov zum 60. Geburtstag [The 60th birthday of Nicolai Sheklakov]. Mykosen. 1978;21(7):199-200.
4. Channual J, Wu JJ. The Nikolskiy sign. Arch Dermatol. 2008;144:1140.
5. Urbano FL. Nikolsky's Sign in Autoimmune Skin Disorders. Hosp Physician. 2001;37:23-4.
6. Sachdev D. Sign of Nikolskiy and related signs. Indian J Dermatol Venereol Leprol. 2003;69: 243-4.
7. Hameed A, Khan AA. Microscopic Nikolsky's sign. Clin Exp Dermatol. 1999;24:312-4.
8. Uzun S, Durdu M. The specificity and sensitivity of Nikolskiy sign in the diagnosis of pemphigus. J Am Acad Dermatol. 2006;54:411-5.
9. Barr RJ. Cutaneous cytology. J Am Acad Dermatol. 1984;10:163-80.
10. Ruocco E, Brunetti G, Del Vecchio M, Ruocco V. The practical use of cytology for diagnosis in dermatology. J Eur Acad Dermatol Venereol. 2011;25:125-9.
11. Durdu M, Baba M, Seçkin D. The value of Tzanck smear test in diagnosis of erosive, vesicular, bullous, and pustular skin lesions. J Am Acad Dermatol. 2008;59:958-64.

Urticaria and Related Disorders

Karthi Kishore, Siva Chaitanya Senapathi, Sreechithra Menon

INTRODUCTION

Urticaria is defined as a skin disorder characterized by local transient skin or mucosal edema (wheal) and an area of redness (erythema) that typically accompanies itchy sensations and lesions diminish within a day.[1] It can be spontaneous or inducible. The characteristic skin lesion in urticaria is a *"wheal"* which is a well-demarcated superficial pale/pinkish swelling of the dermis, caused by the exudation of plasma in the skin that fades usually within hours without leaving any residual mark. Angioedema is a local and transient skin or mucosal edema that develops in deep tissues mostly without itching but may be accompanied by pain or burning sensations.[1] Bedside tests play a pivotal role in guiding clinicians through the intricate landscape of urticaria. They not only aid in confirming the diagnosis but also contribute to unraveling the underlying causes, thereby facilitating tailored treatment strategies. In this chapter we will navigate through the diverse array of bedside tests available, shedding light on their application, interpretation, and the valuable insights they provide for a comprehensive understanding of urticarial disorders.

BEDSIDE TESTS FOR INDUCIBLE URTICARIA

Dermographism (Skin Writing)

Dermographism refers to the phenomenon of exaggerated "Triple response" of skin. The "Triple response of Lewis" comprises of a cutaneous response to firm stroking of skin **(Fig. 1)**. The triple response consists of the following aspects:

- Red spot, caused by *capillary vasodilation* appears in 15 seconds.
- Flare, a redness in the surrounding area due to *arteriolar dilation mediated by axon reflex* takes about 45 seconds to form.
- Wheal, caused by *exudation of extracellular fluid* from capillaries and venules can take up to 3 minutes to form.

The various types of dermographism and the methods to elicit them are described further.

Symptomatic Dermographism

It is characterized by itching/burning skin sensations and the development of pruritic wheals and flare in areas exposed to shearing forces on the skin.[1]

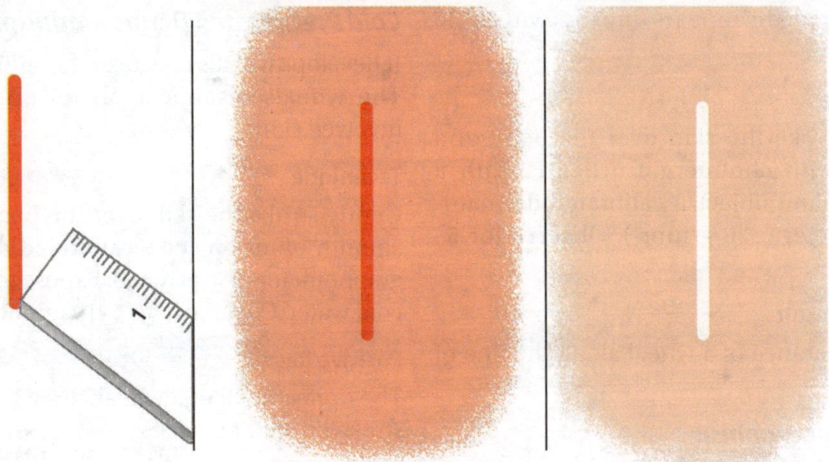

FIG. 1: Schematic diagram of the triple response of Lewis depicting the initial response of red dot, followed by flare and wheal respectively.

Technique

Gently stroke the skin over the body (preferably the back) with a smooth blunt object/a calibrated dermatographometer ($\leq$36 g/mm^3) **(Fig. 2)**. Observe for 5–10 minutes.

Positive Result

The appearance of a wheal along the line of stroke **(Fig. 3)**.

Delayed Dermographism

It is characterized by the appearance of wheals 3–6 hours later over the area of skin stroking and may persist up to 48 hours.[1]

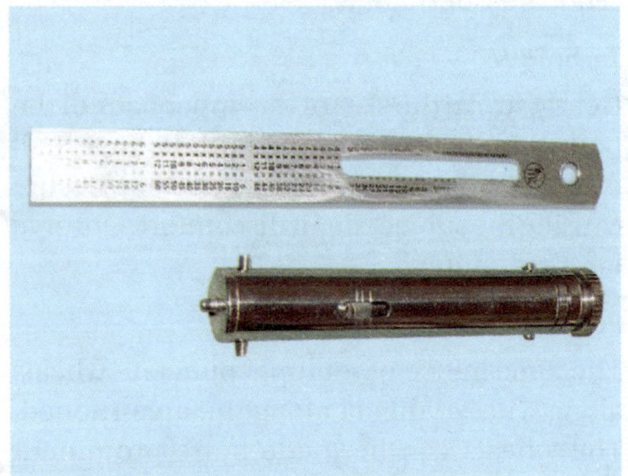

FIG. 2: Dermatographometer.

Technique

Gently stroke the skin over the body (preferably the back) with a smooth blunt object/a calibrated dermatographometer ($\leq$36 g/mm^3). Observe for the next 3–6 hours.[2]

Positive Result

The appearance of a wheal along the line of stroke.

Cholinergic Dermographism

It elicits a clinical response in the form of an erythematous line comprising of punctate wheals. This subtype develops shortly after

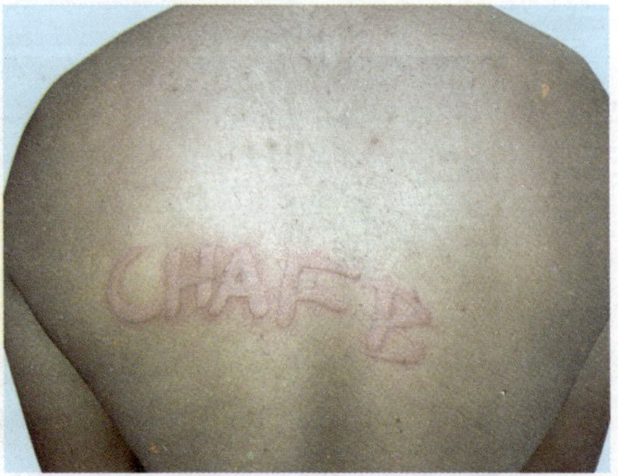

FIG. 3: Dermographism.
Courtesy: Department of Dermatology, Command Hospital Airforce, Bengaluru, Karnataka, India.

stimuli and disappears mostly within 30 minutes.[3]

Technique

Gently stroke the skin over the body of a patient with cholinergic urticaria with a smooth blunt object/a calibrated dermatographometer ($\leq$36 g/mm^3). Observe for 5–10 minutes.

Positive Result

The appearance of a wheal along the line of a stroke.

Red Dermographism

It is a form of dermographism seen with repeated rubbing, predominantly over the trunk. This condition is seen in cases of seborrheic dermatitis.[4]

Technique

Gently stroke the skin of the upper back of the body with the back of the middle fingernail over 2–3 cm length with a degree of pressure causing the subject slight discomfort. Observe for 3–5 minutes.[5]

Positive Result

The appearance of multiple punctate wheals along with erythema along the area rubbed. The wheals can be made more prominent by stretching the involved skin. The wheals appear usually in 1–2 minutes and disappear in 15 minutes and erythema persists for 1 hour.[5]

Cold Precipitated Dermographism

It develops wheals only over the chilled skin.[6] The wheals disappear on rewarming the involved skin.

Technique

Gently stroke the skin over the body with a smooth blunt object/a calibrated dermatographometer ($\leq$36 g/mm^3). Expose the skin to cold water. Observe it for 5–10 minutes.[7,8]

Positive Result

The appearance of a wheal along the line of stroke on cooling.

False Dermographism

It conditions mimic dermographism but is caused due to a different mechanism. Various types are as follows:

- *White dermographism* is a condition seen in cases of atopic dermatitis[9] characterized by the development of a white line/pallor surrounded by an area of blanching due to capillary vasoconstriction triggered by the stroking of the skin.
- *Yellow dermographism,* as implied by the name is characterized by yellowish discoloration of skin due to bile deposition. Usually, seen in cases of obstructive jaundice **(Fig. 4)**.
- *Black/green dermographism,* this entity is characterized by black/greenish discoloration of the skin due to abrasive

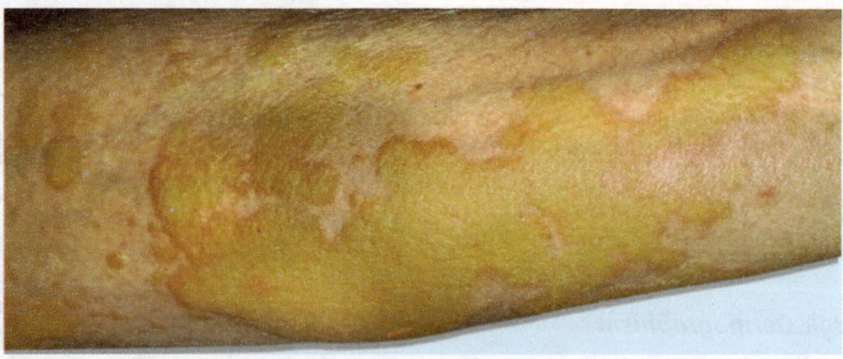

FIG. 4: Yellow dermographism.
Source: Koumaki D, Demetriou G, Krasagakis K. Yellow urticaria in a patient with alcohol-related liver cirrhosis and jaundice. Indian J Dermatol Venereol Leprol. 2021;87(5):676-7.

contact with metallic objects (rings/bracelets/wristbands, etc.) containing zinc or titanium oxide.

Delayed Pressure Urticarial

This type of urticaria is characterized by deep dermal wheals that appear in a continuously compressed region with a latent period of 30 minutes or a few hours after the release of compression. The condition may be associated with a burning sensation or pain in contrast to itching which is seen in cases of chronic spontaneous urticaria[1] **(Fig. 5)**.

Technique

- Gently stroke the skin over the anterior thigh with a weighed rod (1.5 cm in diameter weighing 2.5 kg for a duration of 15 minutes).[10]
  Or
- Gently stroke the skin over the body with a calibrated dermographometer (100 g/mm^3 for 70 seconds).[10]
  Or
- Tie the cuff of a sphygmomanometer around the arm and raise the pressure to 100 mm Hg, and maintain for 1 minute or till the patient feels discomfort, whichever is earlier.[11]

Positive Result

The appearance of a wheal along the line of stroke after 2–6 hours and also the following day.

Cold Urticaria

It is characterized by the appearance of wheals and flare in response to cold. These skin lesions usually occur during rewarming and not during chilling.

Technique

- Gently apply a cold stimulus over the body (usually volar forearm) in the form of a melting ice cube placed in a thin polythene bag for 5–20 minutes. If no wheal develops, fan the area for another 10 minutes.[6]
  Or
- Use *TempTest*® **(Fig. 6)**

Positive Result

The appearance of a wheal over the area after 10 minutes.

Heat Urticaria

This is a type of physical urticaria involving the appearance of wheals and flares within

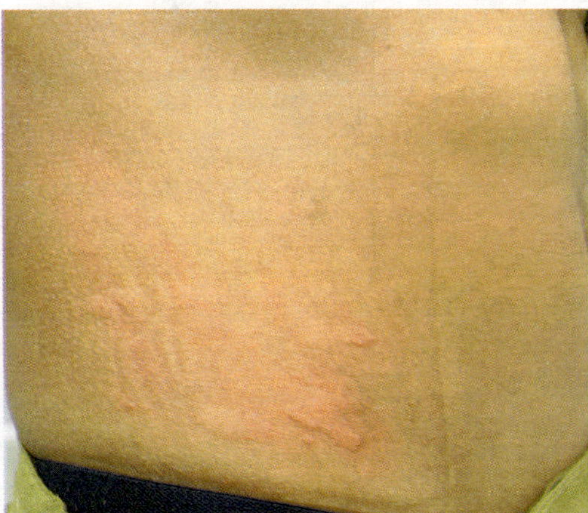

FIG. 5: Delayed pressure urticaria due to pressure of uniform belt in an army recruit.

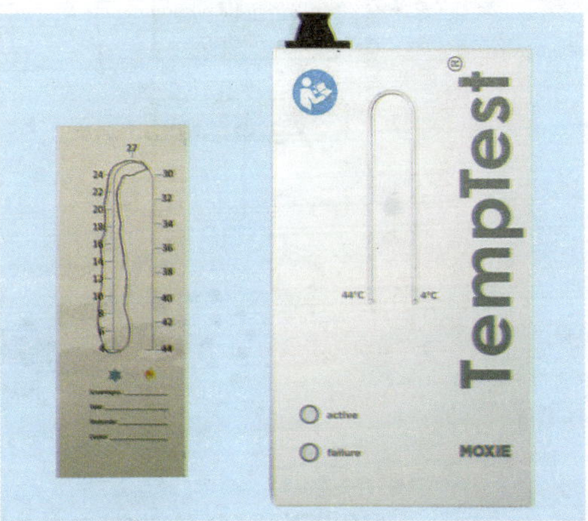

FIG. 6: TempTest®.

minutes of local heat exposure to the skin. In contrast to cholinergic urticaria that involves small punctate eruptions in response to sweating, heat urticaria develops eruptions in response to skin exposure to heat regardless of sweating/core body temperature.

Technique

- Gently apply a hot stimulus over the body (usually volar forearm) in the form of warm water in a copper/glass beaker at 38–44°C for 5 minutes.[10]
  Or
- Use TempTest

Positive Result

The appearance of a wheal over the area after 10 minutes.

> **What is TempTest®?**
> It is a device used to provide temperatures of 4–44°C to the patient's skin by placing the inner forearm on a U-shape aluminum stencil on the device for 5 minutes. The U-stencil indicates the temperature range. This method helps to assess the threshold temperature for cold urticaria.
>
> **Threshold Temperature in TempTest®**
> Cold urticaria is indicated by the highest temperature and heat urticaria by the lowest temperature.

Cholinergic Urticaria

Cholinergic urticaria is induced by stimuli that cause sweating and is characterized by small urticarial eruptions.

Mechanism

The mechanism of cholinergic urticaria is enumerated in **Flowchart 1**.

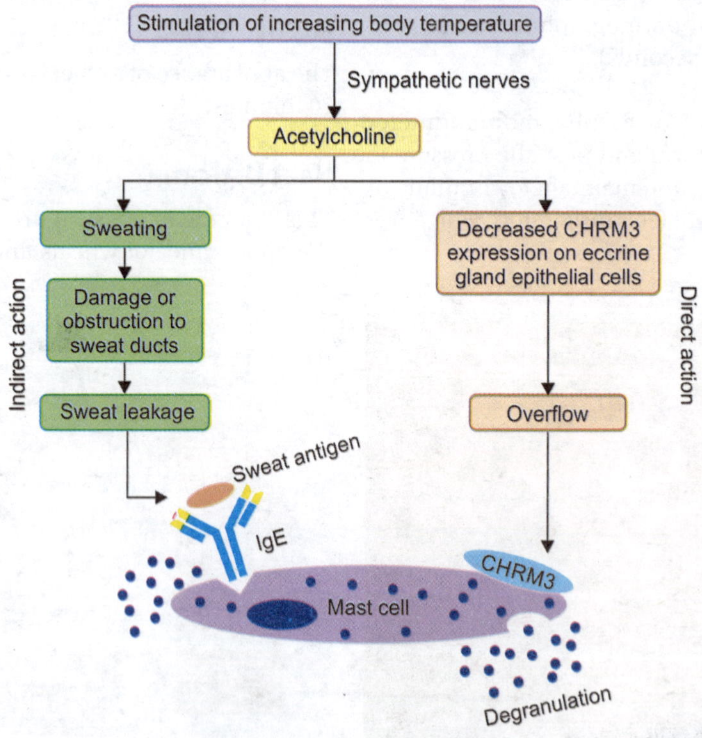

FLOWCHART 1: Mechanism of cholinergic urticaria.
(CHRM3: cholinergic receptor M3; IgE: immunoglobulin E)

Technique

- Passive heating of the body in a bath/hot shower (maximum temperature 42°C).
  Or
- Exercise to the point of sweating in a warm environment (jogging/cycling).

Positive Result

The appearance of a wheal over the area after 10 minutes.[7]

Solar Urticaria

This type of urticaria is characterized by wheals and flare that develop within minutes after local exposure of skin to a certain wavelength of light **(Fig. 7)**.

Mechanism

The mechanism of solar urticaria is enumerated in **Flowchart 2**.

Technique

Expose the part of the body to sunlight/solar stimulator.

Source of Stimulation

- Ultraviolet A (UVA) (2.4–4.2 J/cm^2)
- Broadband ultraviolet B (BBUVB) (0.024–0.042 J/cm^2)

- Monochromator light testing (specific wavelength of UVB and UVA)

Positive Result

The appearance of a wheal over the area after 10 minutes.

Aquagenic Urticaria

Aquagenic urticaria is a type of urticaria induced by exposure to water at any temperature. The skin lesion is characterized by small wheals **(Fig. 8)**.

Technique

- Apply a wet towel/cloth to the part of the body for 5 minutes.
  Or
- Immerse the part of the body in water collected in a tub for 5 minutes.

Positive Result

The appearance of a wheal over the area after 5–10 minutes.[10]

Vibratory Angioedema

Vibratory angioedema, which is a form of physical urticaria, may be inherited by

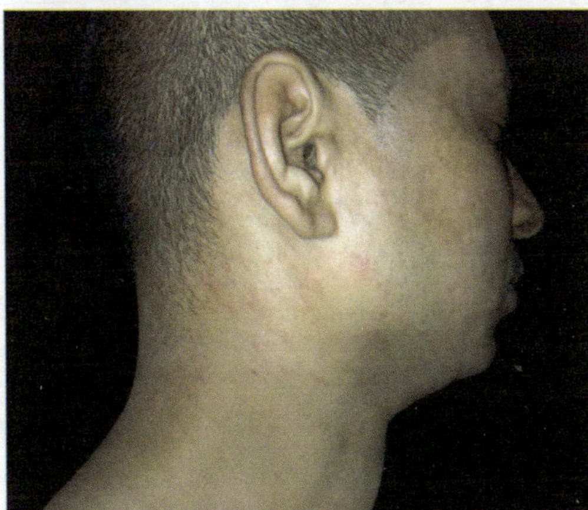

FIG. 7: Solar urticaria postexposure to sunlight.
Courtesy: Department of Dermatology, Command Hospital Airforce Bangalore, Bengaluru, Karnataka, India.

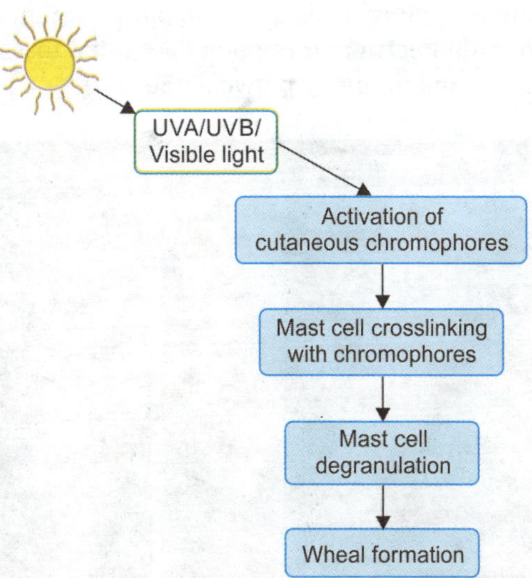

FLOWCHART 2: Mechanism of solar urticaria.
(UVA: ultraviolet A; UVB: ultraviolet B)

adhesion g protein-coupled receptor E2 (*ADGRE2)* gene mutation, an autosomal dominant trait or may be acquired after prolonged occupational vibration exposure. The condition is characterized by dermographism, cholinergic urticarial, and pressure urticaria.[10]

Technique

- Apply a vibratory stimulus to the body part in the form of some vigorous physical activity
  Or
- Use the *laboratory vortex mixer* **(Fig. 8)**. The volar surface of the forearm should be exposed to the vibration for 5 minutes by placing it over the flat plate of the laboratory vortex mixer with readings taken at 10 minutes once the stimulus has stopped.

Positive Result

The appearance of a wheal over the area after 5–10 minutes. According to the [European Academy of Allergology and Clinical Immunology (EAACI)/Global Allergy and Asthma European Network (GA²LEN)] consensus guidelines, inflammation is quantified by measuring the circumference of the forearm at three points (cubital fossa, wrist, and midpoint between the two).

The measurement is taken with a measuring tape before the application of the vibratory stimulus and 5 minutes afterward.

The various urticarial subtypes as determined by the morphological feature of wheals are as given in **Table 1**.

> Vortex mixer is a device used in laboratories to mix small vials of liquid. It consists of an electric motor with the drive shaft oriented vertically and attached to a cupped rubber piece mounted slightly off-center. As the motor runs the rubber piece oscillates rapidly in a circular motion resulting in vibrations. The patient's arm was placed on a flat plate laid on the vortex mixer, which runs between 780 and 1,380 revolutions per minute (RPM) for 10 minutes.

TABLE 1: Urticarial subtypes determined by the morphological feature of wheals.

Type of urticaria	Morphology
Spontaneous urticaria	Polymorphic (common)/annular/purpuric/small-sized wheals (<5 mm)
Cold, solar, heat, and pressure urticaria	Localized
Mechanical urticaria/symptomatic dermographism	Linear
Cholinergic/aquagenic/adrenergic urticaria	Small-sized wheals (<5 mm)

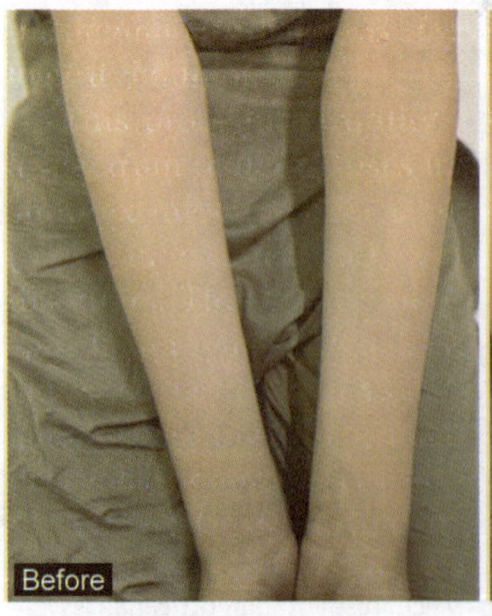

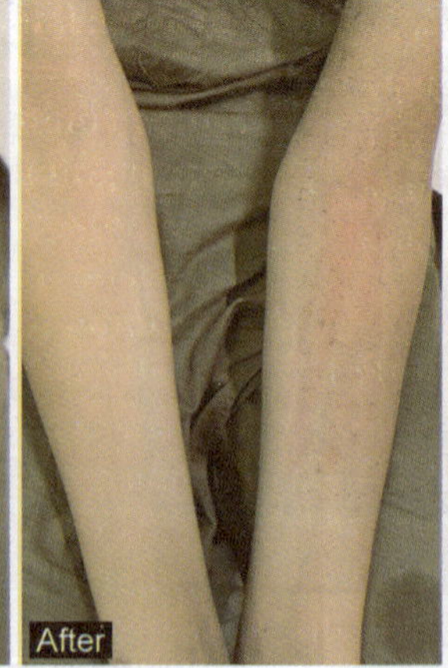

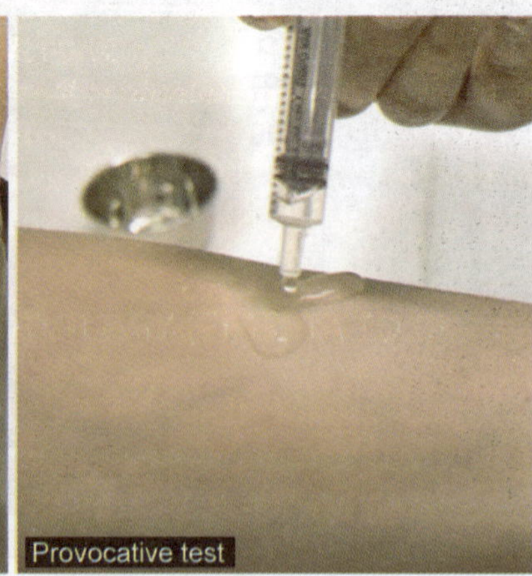

FIG. 8: Aquagenic urticaria.
Courtesy: Dr Sahana Srihari, Department of Dermatology, Adesh Institute of Medical Sciences and Research, Bathinda, Punjab, India.

BEDSIDE TESTS FOR AUTOIMMUNE URTICARIA

Autologous Serum Skin Test

Autologous serum skin test (ASST) is a simple *in vivo* clinical test for the detection of basophil histamine-releasing activity. The test is essential to screen the presence of autoantibodies against immunoglobulin E (IgE) or high-affinity IgE receptors.[11]

Indication

To diagnose autoimmune urticaria and differentiate it from chronic idiopathic urticaria.

Prerequisites

- Antihistamines (e.g., cetirizine and fexofenadine) to be withdrawn at least 2–3 days prior to the test.
- Doxepin and astemizole should be withdrawn 2–6 weeks before the procedure.[12]
- Patient should not take immunosuppressants 6 weeks to 3 months prior to the test.[13]
- Test area should be free of wheals at least 24 hours prior.

Technique

- Take 2 mL of venous blood from the antecubital vein of the patient.
- Allow the blood to clot at room temperature.
- The serum is to be separated by centrifugation [2,000 revolutions per minute (RPM) for 10–15 minutes].
- Take 0.05 mL of obtained serum and inject intradermally into the volar aspect of the forearm, avoiding the areas of wheals.
- Equal amounts of normal saline (negative control) and histamine (10 µg/mL) (positive control) are injected intradermally 3–5 cm apart in the volar aspect of the same forearm.
- The wheal and flare responses are measured after 30 minutes.

Result

The diameter of wheal (D) is measured as the average of the maximum vertical (d_1) and horizontal (d_2) diameters of the wheal **(Fig. 9)**.

$$Average\ diameter\ (D) = (d_1 + d_2)/2$$

Serum-induced wheal response with a diameter of ≥1.5 mm than that of the saline-induced response at 30 minutes is considered a positive ASST **(Fig. 10)**.

Interpretation

Positive ASST Denotes

- Increased potential to develop urticaria due to endogenous causes.

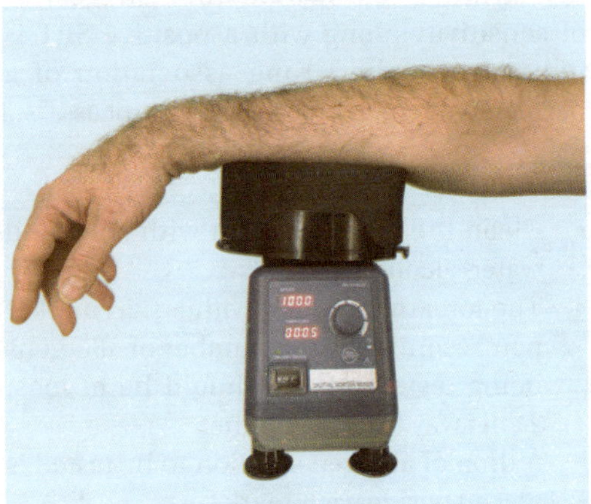

FIG. 9: Laboratory vortex mixer.

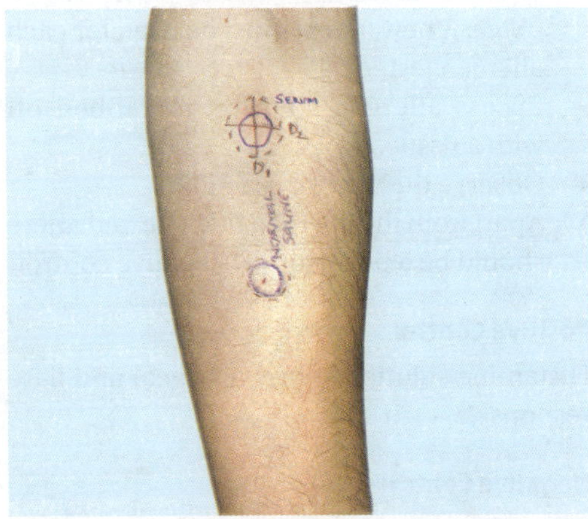

FIG. 10: Measurement of the wheal diameter in vertical (D_1) and horizontal (D_2) directions.

- Correlation with disease severity and duration.

False Positive ASST

- Demographic variation
- Varied injection techniques

BEDSIDE TEST FOR SPONTANEOUS URTICARIA

Skin Prick Tests

Skin prick tests (SPTs) refer to the most effective and cheapest method to diagnose IgE-mediated type 1 allergic reactions (e.g., urticaria). A clinical history suggestive of sensitivity along with a positive SPT is indicative of the strong association of a particular allergen to the disease process.

Technique

- Clean the inner forearm with soap and water/alcohol.
- The forearm is coded with a skin marker pen according to the number of allergens being tested. Marks should be at least 2 cm away from each other.
- A drop of allergen solution to be tested is placed beside each mark.
- A small prick through the drop is made to the skin using a sterile prick lancet. (*Note*: A new lancet must be used for each allergen tested)
- Excess allergen solution is dabbed off with a tissue.
- Observe the skin for reaction.
- Apart from the allergen being tested, there should be a positive and negative control.

Positive Control

Histamine solution shows a "wheal and flare response."

Negative Control

Saline solution shows no response.

Results

The sensitivity to the test is assessed by the degree of redness and swelling and the size of the wheal produced. It usually takes about 15–20 minutes to reach a maximum size and thereafter fades over the next few hours **(Fig. 11)**.

Interpretation of the SPT results are depicted in **Table 2**.

- *False-positive results* may be due to a positive reaction from one test site that may affect the result of a neighboring test site (place test sites at least 2 cm apart) or by an irritant reaction.
- A *false-negative result* can be caused by the medications taken before the procedure such as antihistamines and decreased skin reactivity in infants and elderly patients or due to a diluted allergen extract.

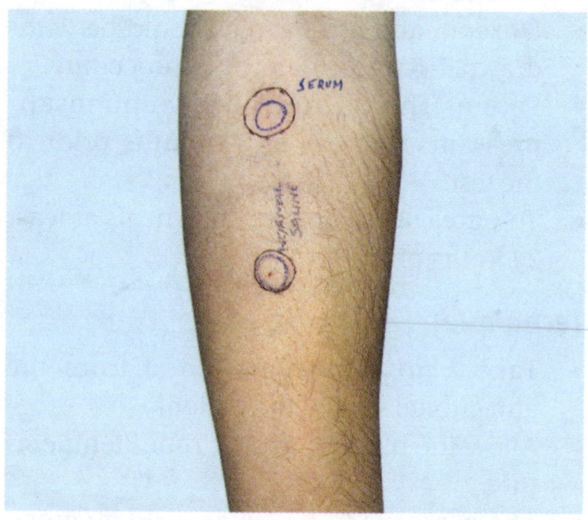

FIG. 11: Positive autologous serum skin test (ASST) result.

TABLE 2: Interpretation of the skin prick test results.

Wheal size (mm)	Old (+ scale)	Interpretation
<4	0+	Negative
5–10	2+	Mildly sensitive
10–15	3+	Moderately sensitive
>15	4+	Very sensitive

BEDSIDE TESTS FOR MAST CELL DISORDERS

Darier's Sign

Darier's sign is considered a pathognomonic sign for cutaneous mastocytosis. Its elicitation being easy and noninvasive gives a clinical clue for the diagnosis of mastocytosis. This bedside test refers to whealing, erythema, and pruritus which is elicited after mechanical stimulus to a lesion owing to an increase in the number of mast cells in the dermis. It was first described by *Ferdinand–Jean Darier* in 1905.

Mechanism

The mechanism of a positive skin prick test to progesterone is depicted in **Figure 12**.

Technique

Gentle rubbing/stroking of the skin lesions for 2–5 minutes with a blunt object (e.g., wooden tongue depressor, dull edge of a pen, fingernail, or a metallic key) approximately five times with moderate pressure.[14]

Positive Result

Local itching, erythema, and wheal formation may develop within 2–5 minutes on the involved area which may persist from 30 minutes to several hours. Occasionally vesicles may be seen[15] **(Flowchart 3)**.

Points to note:

- Positive Darier sign response is reduced if the patient is already on antihistamines.
- Positive Darier's is better elicited in pediatric patients than in adults.
- Exercise caution while performing this bedside test with adequate backup for anaphylaxis. Management since sudden degranulation of mast cells may incite a systemic response in these patients, such as nausea, diarrhea, abdominal pain, flushing, hypotension, and bronchospasm.
- Positive Darier's sign seen in 88–92% of cutaneous mastocytosis.

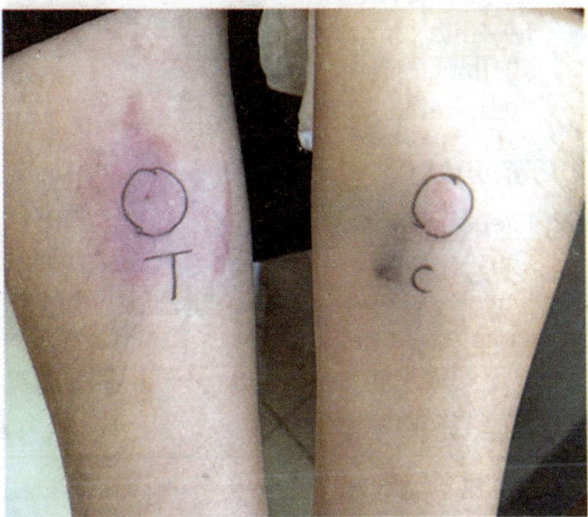

FIG. 12: Positive skin prick test to progesterone in a case of progesterone-induced urticaria.

Courtesy: Dr Siddharth Bhatt, Department of Dermatology, INHS Asvini, Mumbai, Maharashtra, India.

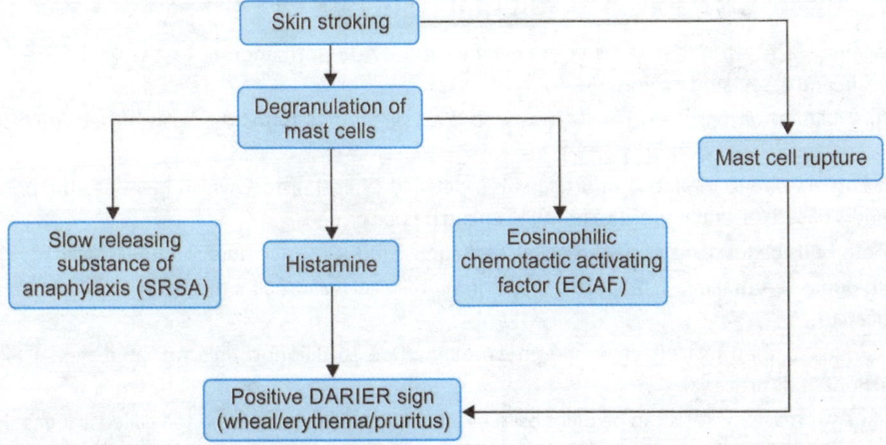

FLOWCHART 3: Mechanism of Darier's sign.

Variants of Darier's Sign[16]

- *Nonlesional Darier's sign*: Classical Darier's sign is seen in lesional skin as whealing, erythema, and pruritus, but this sign may even be demonstrated on clinically normal skin in patients of mastocytosis.
- Erythema only without urtication on rubbing the skin lesions is seen in *pseudoxanthomatous mastocytosis*, a variant of diffuse cutaneous mastocytosis.

Conditions Associated with Darier's Sign

- Cutaneous mastocytosis
- Leukemia cutis
- Juvenile xanthogranuloma
- Histiocytosis X
- Lymphoma

Differentials

- Pseudo-Darier's sign
- Dermographism[17,18]

  Darier's sign in a case of solitary mastocytoma is depicted in **Figures 13A and B**.

CONCLUSION

Urticaria is a skin disorder characterized by local transient skin or mucosal edema (wheal) and an area of redness (erythema) that typically accompanies itchy sensations

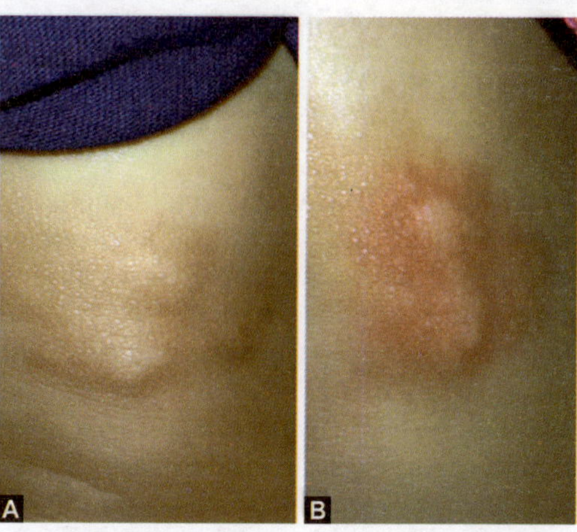

FIGS. 13A AND B: Darier's sign in a case of solitary mastocytoma. (A) Lesion of solitary mastocytoma and (B) Erythema and wheal formation over the lesion after gentle skin stroking.

Courtesy: Dr Brijesh Nair, Department of Dermatology, Command Hospital (EC), Kolkata, West Bengal, India.

and lesions usually diminish within a day. Bedside tests play a significant role in aiding clinicians through the intricate landscape of urticaria. They not only assist in confirming the diagnosis but also contribute to unraveling the underlying causes, thereby facilitating tailored treatment strategies. Most of these tests are easy to perform, noninvasive and quick eliminating the requirement of expensive and elaborate investigations.

Key Messages

- Urticaria is a heterogeneous disorder characterized by the formation of erythema, edema, raised wheals, and associated itching.
- Degranulation of mast cells results in wheals over skin which forms the basis of bedside tests for urticaria and related disorders.
- The cornerstone to diagnosis of urticaria is a detailed clinical history which identifies the potential triggers based on which specific clinical tests can be performed.
- Various bedside tests are discussed below to diagnose inducible and autoimmune urticaria.
- Autologous serum skin test (ASST) is a simple in vivo clinical test used for the diagnosis of autoimmune urticaria.
- SPTs refer to the most effective and cheapest method to diagnose IgE-mediated type 1 allergic reactions (e.g., urticaria).
- Cutaneous mastocystosis can be diagnosed by a bedside clinical phenomenon called Darier's sign.

REFERENCES

1. Hide M, Takahagi S, Hiragun T. Urticaria and angioedema. In: Kang S, Amagai M, Bruckner AL, Enk AH, Margolis DJ, McMichael AJ, et al (Eds). Fitzpatrick's Dermatology, 9th edition. New York: McGraw Hill; 2019. pp. 684-90.

2. Paller AS, Mancini AJ. 3 - Eczematous Eruptions in Childhood. In: Hurwitz Clinical Pediatric Dermatology, 4th edition. London: WB Saunders; 2011. pp. 37-70.

3. Warin RP. Clinical observations on delayed pressure urticaria. Br J Dermatol.1989;121(2):225-8.

4. Baughman RD, Jilson OF. Seven specific types of dermographism. With special reference to delayed persistent dermographism. Ann Allergy. 1963;21:248-55.

5. Bhute D, Doshi B, Pande S, Mahajan S, Kharkar V. Dermatographism. Indian J Dermatol Venereol Leprol. 2008;74(2):177-9.

6. Warin RP. Factitious urticaria: Red Dermographism. Br J Dermatol. 1981;104(3):285-8.

7. Kaplan AP. Unusual cold-induced disorders: cold-dependent dermatographism and systemic cold urticaria. J Allergy Clin Immunol. 1984;73(4):453-6.

8. Evans CD. South West of England of the and Wales Society of Dermatology. Br J Dermatol. 1970;82(1):91-3.

9. James WD, Berger T, Elston DM. Andrews' diseases of the skin Clinical Dermatology, Dermatographism, 10th edition. WB Saunders Co Ltd; 2006. pp. 153.

10. Grattan C, Marsland A. Urticaria. In: Griffiths CEM, Barker J, Bleiker TO, Chalmers R, Creamer D (Eds). Rooks Textbook of Dermatology, 9th edition. New Jersey: Wiley-Blackwell; 2016; p. 9.

11. Godse KV. Diagnosis of delayed pressure urticaria. Indian J Dermatol Venereol Leprol. 2006;72(2): 155-6.

12. George M, Balachandran C, Prabhu S. Chronic idiopathic urticaria: Comparison of clinical features with positive autologous serum skin test. Indian J Dermatol Venereol Leprol. 2008;74(2): 105-8.

13. Ghosh SK, Ghosh S. Autologous serum skin test. Indian J Dermatol. 2009;54(1):86-7.

14. Sabroe RA, Grattan CEH, Francis DM, Barr RM, Black AK, Greaves MW. The autologous serum skin test: A screening test for autoantibodies in chronic idiopathic urticaria. Br J Dermatol. 1999;140(3):446-52.

15. Hartmann K, Escribano L, Grattan C, Brockow K, Carter MC, Alvarez-Twose I, et al Cutaneous manifestations in patients with mastocytosis: Consensus report of the European Competence Network on Mastocytosis; the American Academy of Allergy, Asthma, & Immunology; and the European Academy of Allergology and Clinical Immunology. J Allergy Clin Immunol. 2016;137(1): 35-45.

16. Surjushe A, Jindal S, Gote P, Saple DG. Darier's sign. Indian J Dermatol Venereol Leprol. 2007;73(5): 363-4.

17. Nobles T, Muse ME, Schmieder GJ. Dermato-graphism. In: StatPearls [Internet]. Treasure Island (FL): StatPearls Publishing; 2024.

18. Komarow HD, Arceo S, Young M, Nelson C, Metcalfe DD. Dissociation between history and challenge in patients with physical urticaria. J Allergy Clin Immunol Pract. 2014;2(6):786-90.e2.

Bedside Tests for Peripheral Vascular Disease

Bhabani Singh, Siddhartha Dash, Abhinav Kumar Verma

INTRODUCTION

Peripheral vascular disease (PVD) occurs due to damage, occlusion, or inflammation of arteries or veins or both and causes significant morbidity and mortality globally. The most common causes of PVDs include peripheral arterial disease (PAD), chronic venous insufficiency (CVI), and deep vein thrombosis.

Peripheral arterial disease affects more than 20% of the population over 60 years.[1] It occurs due to narrowing or blockage of arteries, leading to pain, numbness, gangrene, and ultimately amputation. The symptoms of CVI include swelling of the legs, pigmentation over the skin in the lower extremities, eczematous changes, and ulcers **(Fig. 1)**, mostly around medial malleolus. The loss of productive work hours due to CVI is estimated to be 2 million workdays/year.[1] The annual incidence of DVT is estimated to be around 0.5–1 per 1,000. DVT may present as pain, tenderness, swelling, and redness or asymptomatic. The most serious complication of DVT is pulmonary embolism, which occurs in approximately one-third of cases of DVT and results in the death of around 20% of patients.[1]

Therefore, early diagnosis and management are of utmost importance to prevent morbidity and mortality in PVDs. Detailed history taking and examination can help in the early diagnosis of PVDs **(Box 1)**.

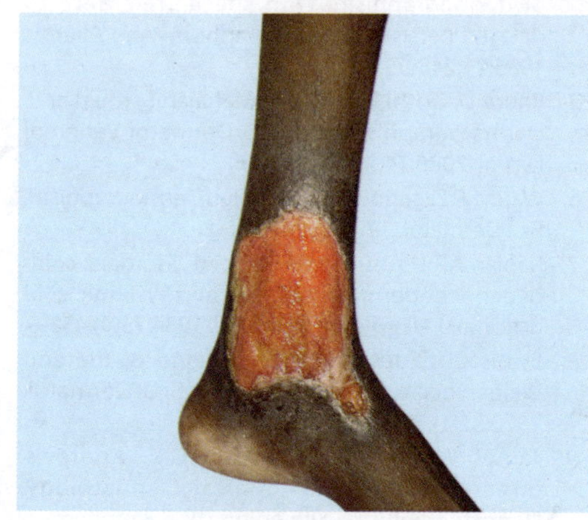

FIG. 1: Venous ulcer over the medial side of ankle with background hyperpigmentation

BEDSIDE TESTS IN ARTERIAL DISEASES

- *Buerger's postural test*: While supine, the patient is asked to raise the legs one after the other, keeping the knees straight. The legs of a normal individual remain pink even after raising the leg to 90°. But in cases of ischemic limb, elevation to a certain degree will cause marked pallor. This angle is called "Buerger's angle" or "vascular angle." A vascular angle of <30° indicates severe limb ischemia. In case of no pallor and strong suspicion of occlusive arterial disease, the elevated limb is supported, and the patient is asked to do alternate flexion and extension of

BOX 1	**Examination of the peripheral vascular system.**

- *Pre-requisites*:
  - Hands should be thoroughly washed
  - The patient should be given a brief explanation about the examination
  - Patient should be in a supine position
  - Patient should be assessed from the end of bed for signs of apparent vascular compromise
  - Examination should start from the upper limbs, followed by the neck, abdomen, and upper limbs
- *Examination of arms*:
  - Inspection should be done for signs of peripheral cyanosis, nicotine stains, and anemia
  - Capillary refill time should be assessed
  - Palpation of pulse should be done in the order of radial, ulnar, brachial, and subclavian
  - Radial-radial delay should be assessed
- *Examination of neck*:
  - Carotid pulse should be assessed for character and volume
  - Auscultation over carotids to be done for any carotid bruits
- *Examination of the abdomen*:
  - Inspection should be done to look for any scars and pulsations
  - Palpate the abdomen to feel for any pulsations
- *Examination of lower limbs*:
  - Legs should be exposed from the waist below and observed from the end of the bed
  - Inspection should be done for scars, xerosis, loss of hairs, skin pigmentation, eczematous changes, atrophie blanche, and ulcers
  - Assess the temperature along the legs and capillary refill time
  - Palpation for distal pulses in the order of femoral, popliteal, dorsalis pedis, and posterior tibial
  - A sensory examination of the lower limbs should be done
- Peripheral vascular system examination is incomplete without cardiovascular examination, capillary glucose, fundoscopy, and ankle-brachial pressure index (ABPI)

the ankle and toes to the point of fatigue. Cadaveric pallor appears over the sole if there is an occlusive arterial disease. The patient is now asked to lower the feet and assume a sitting posture, causing a cyanotic hue over the affected limb due to cyanotic congestion.[2]

- *Capillary refill time (CRT)*:
  - After elevating the limbs, the patient is asked to assume a sitting posture and hang his legs to the side of the table. In the ischemic limb, pallor will develop, and the leg will become pink in a horizontal position. This gradual process of color change from pale to pink is called "capillary filling time." A capillary filling time of 20–30 seconds indicates severe ischemia.[2]
  - Pressure is applied for 10 seconds over the distal phalanx of fingers or toes until the nail bed blanches and then released. The time taken from pressure release to the nail bed returning to normal color is called CRT. Normal CRT is <3 seconds.[3]
- *Crossed leg test or Fuchsig's test*: This test is done to demonstrate popliteal pulsation. The patient is asked to sit with crossed legs one above the other. The crossed leg will show oscillatory movement synchronous with popliteal pulsation. If the popliteal artery is blocked, the oscillatory movement will be absent.[2]
- *Cold and warm water test and cold stimulation test*: This test is done to demonstrate Raynaud's phenomenon. The patient is asked to dip his hand in ice-cold water. This will cause the hand to become white due to arteriospasm in primary and secondary Raynaud's disease cases. The normal recovery time of fingers is <15 minutes. Longer recovery time indicates a positive cold stimulation test and vascular pathology.[4] If the patient is asked to dip his hand in warm water after cold exposure, the hand will become blue due to cyanotic congestion.[2]
- *Elevated arms test*: This test is performed in thoracic outlet syndrome. The patient is asked to abduct his shoulders to 90° and externally rotate the upper limbs. In thoracic outlet syndrome, the patient will complain of fatigue and pain in forearm muscles, paresthesia of the forearm, tingling, and numbness of fingers.[2]

- *Modified Allen's test*: This test assesses the patency of the radial and ulnar arteries of the hand. The patient is asked to flex the elbow and clench his fist tightly to exsanguinate the blood. The examiner simultaneously compresses the ulnar and radial artery, and the patient is asked to unclench the fist. The palm should appear white. The pressure over the ulnar artery is released, keeping the radial artery compressed and vice-versa. If the arteries are patent, the normal color should return within 10 seconds after the release of the artery. If the pallor persists, it indicates occlusion of the artery that is released.[5]
- *Branham's or Nicoladoni's sign*: This test is done in suspected arteriovenous fistula (AVF). In this test, the examiner compresses the artery proximal to AVF, which causes a decrease in the size of swelling, the disappearance of bruit, a decrease in pulse rate, and normalization of pulse pressure.[2]
- *Costoclavicular compressive maneuver or military brace test*: The examiner palpates the radial pulse and pulls the patient's shoulder down and backward. Disappearance of radial pulse indicates costoclavicular syndrome.[2]
- *Adson's test*: It is done to detect thoracic outlet syndrome. The patient is asked to hold their breath in deep inspiration and extend and rotate the neck to either side. The examiner palpates the radial pulse. The radial pulse is lost when the patient rotates the neck to the symptomatic side.[6]
- *Halstead's maneuver or Reverse Adson's test*: While palpating the radial pulse, the examiner gives downward traction to the shoulder, and the patient is asked to keep the neck hyperextended and rotated to the opposite side. Absence or disappearance of pulse indicates thoracic outlet syndrome.
- *Roos' test or elevated arm stress test (EAST)*: The patient is asked to abduct the arm to 90° with external rotation of the shoulder and flexion of the elbow to 90°. The patient is then asked to open and close the hand slowly for 3 minutes. Inability to keep the arm in this position for 3 minutes, weakness or heaviness of the arm, tingling or numbness of the hand, and ischemic pain suggest thoracic outlet syndrome.[6]
- *Palpation of peripheral pulses*:[7] **Table 1** describes the procedure for palpation of peripheral pulses.

TABLE 1: Procedure for palpation of peripheral pulses.

Artery to be tested	Procedure
Radial artery	The examiner supports the patient's forearm on his left hand. With the other hand, the examiner palpates the pulse at the subject's wrist by curling his fingers around the distal radius from dorsal to volar aspect, and the ring, middle, and index finger are aligned longitudinally along the course of the radial artery **(Fig. 2A)**
Brachial artery (right side)	The examiner supports the patient's forearm. The subject's upper arm is abducted, the elbow slightly flexed, and the forearm externally rotated. The examiner's right hand is curled over the patient's elbow and palpates the artery along its course just medial to the biceps tendon and lateral to the medial condyle of the humerus. The position of the hands should be switched while examining the opposite side **(Fig. 2B)**
Common femoral artery	The examiner stands on the ipsilateral side and fingertips of the examining hand are pressed firmly at the groin one-third of the distance from the pubis and anterior superior iliac spine **(Fig. 2C)**
Popliteal artery	The patient is asked to lie supine, and the examiner's hand encircles the knee from both sides. The fingertips are pressed deeply into the popliteal space to palpate the pulse **(Fig. 2D)**

Continued

Continued

Artery to be tested	Procedure
Posterior tibial artery	The examiner curls the hand around the ankle by placing the thumb on the opposite side, and fingertips are indented between the medial malleolus and Achilles tendon **(Fig. 2E)**
Dorsalis pedis artery	The patient lies in a recumbent position. This artery is palpated near the center of long axis of the foot, just lateral to the extensor hallucis tendon **(Fig. 2F)**

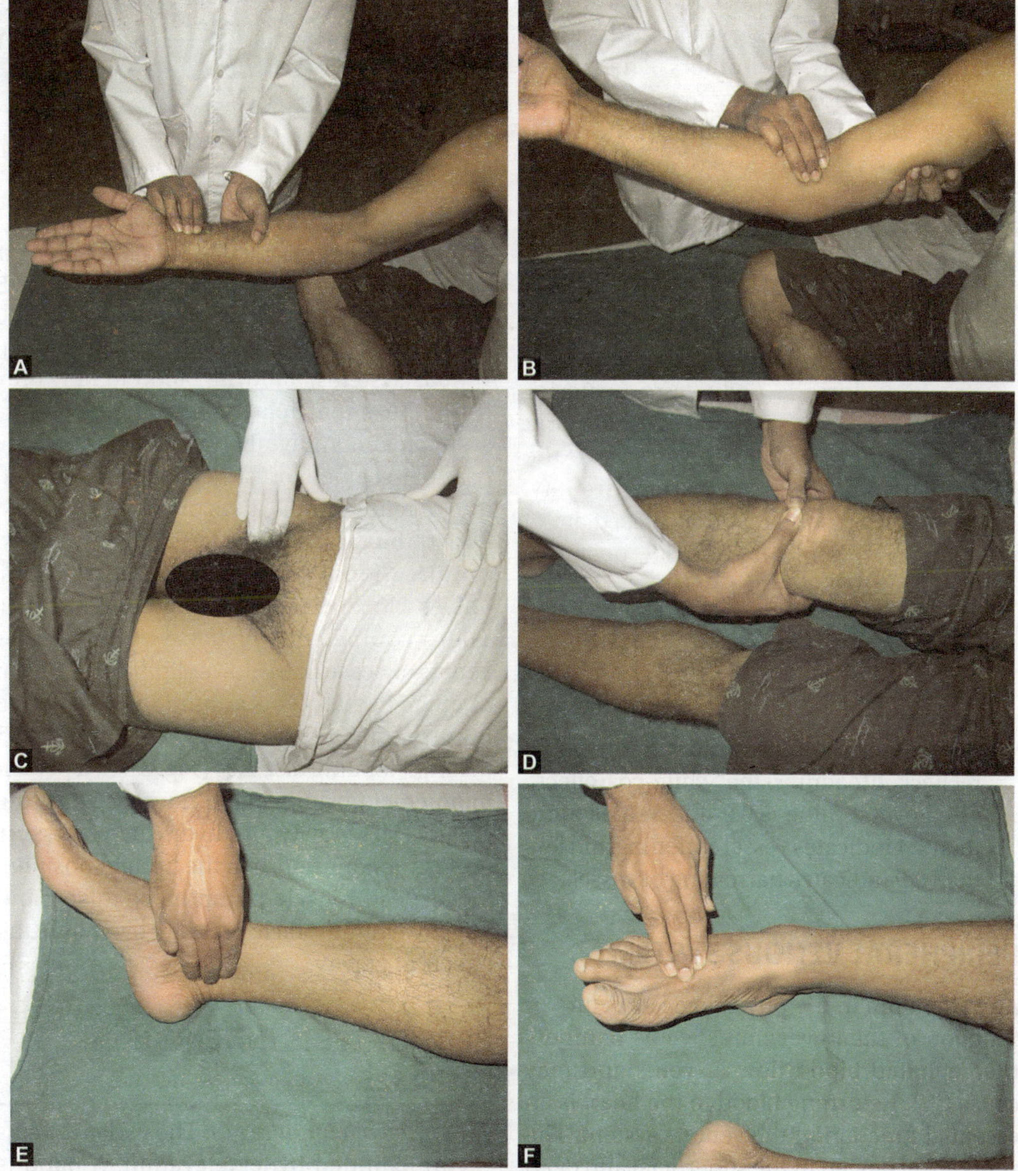

FIGS. 2A TO F: (A) Palpation of the radial artery; (B) Palpation of brachial artery; (C) Palpation of femoral artery; (D) Palpation of popliteal artery; (E) Palpation of the posterior tibial artery; and (F) Palpation of dorsalis pedis artery.

- *Radial-radial and radio-femoral delay*: The delay between two radial pulses is called radio-radial delay, and the delay between radial and femoral pulses is called radio-femoral delay. To detect these, the examiner should palpate both the radial pulse and radial and femoral pulse simultaneously. The causes of radio-radial delay are thoracic inlet syndrome, aortic aneurysm, Takayasu arteritis, aortic atherosclerosis, and others. The causes of radio-femoral delay are coarctation of the aorta, atherosclerosis of the aorta, thrombosis or embolism of the aorta, and aortoarteritis.

- *Ankle-brachial pressure index (ABPI)*: It is the ratio of the systolic blood pressure of the ankle and the upper extremity. It is used to assess the vascular status. The pressure of three arteries is measured: Brachial, dorsalis pedis, and posterior tibial artery. The cuff is placed at mid-arm for the upper extremity and above the medial malleoli for the lower extremity. A stethoscope or Doppler is placed at the anatomic site of the brachial, posterior tibial, and dorsalis pedis artery. The systolic blood pressure is measured. The order of performing the measurement is first arm, same side ankle, opposite leg, and opposite arm. If there is a 10 mm Hg difference in the arm, the initial arm is rechecked to address the "white-coat effect." The normal value is 0.9–1.4. Values more than 1.4 indicates vessel stiffening and less than 0.9 indicates narrowing of vessels.[8]

PERIPHERAL VENOUS SYSTEM

Any alteration in the physiologic structure or function of the lower limbs' veins hampers the cephalad blood flow in veins and may cause CVI. Returning blood to the heart is an essential function of the venous system. The veins are arranged in the superficial and deep compartments in three patterns—superficial veins, deep veins, and perforating veins. The

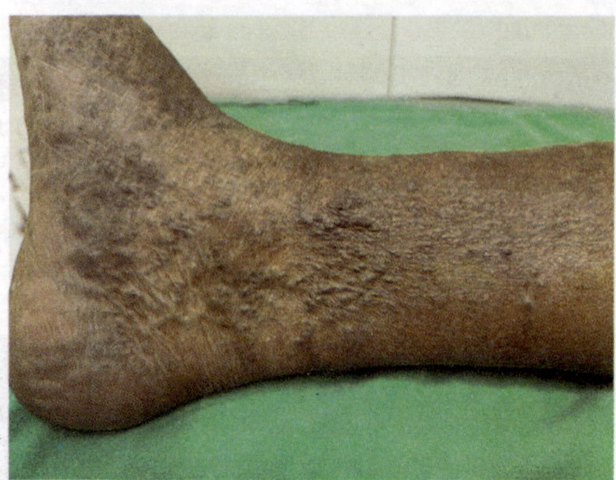

FIG. 3: Perimalleolar dilated venules.

superficial veins are the great saphenous vein (GSV) and the short saphenous vein (SSV). The perforators pierce the fascia and communicate the superficial with the deep venous systems, allowing blood to flow only from the superficial to the deep venous system. Veins have bicuspid valves at the base of a segment of the vein that is expanded into a venous sinus, thus allowing cephalad flow of blood in the superficial system and unidirectional flow through perforators. Valves close when flow begins to reverse. The incompetence of these valves causes venous disease in the lower limbs in the form of dilated small veins around the malleoli to more prominent varicosities or features of CVI in long-standing diseases **(Fig. 3)**. In a person in an erect posture, blood travels against the gravity. The gravity and hydrostatic pressure oppose venous return in the upright position. Valves, calf muscle pump mechanism, and negative intrathoracic pressure overcome the effects of gravity.

BEDSIDE TESTS IN VENOUS DISEASES

- *The cough impulse test*: The varicose veins are emptied by leg elevation. A hand is placed over the saphenofemoral junction (SFJ), which is 2–3 cm below and lateral to the pubic tubercle, and the patient is asked to cough. An impulse or a palpable thrill felt over the SFJ indicates incompetence or reflux at the SFJ. This thrill is due to a regurgitant turbulent flow. The test is cumbersome to perform in obese and vigorously coughing patients.

- *Percussion (PAP) test*: Pressure is applied onto the SFJ located 2–3 cm, and the varicose vein to be assessed is tapped. A thrill felt at the SFJ would imply incompetent valves along the continuity of the tested vein. A usual vein would prevent the transmission of the thrill due to competent valves.
- *Brodie–Trendelenburg test*: The Brodie–Trendelenburg test, described by Brodi in 1846 and made famous by Trendelenburg in 1891, primarily detects SFJ incompetence and perforator incompetence. The superficial lower extremity veins are drained by elevating the lower limbs to 45° and gently milking the more prominent visible veins along their course **(Figs. 4A and B)**.

A tourniquet is placed at the saphenous opening and applied tightly enough to prevent superficial venous reflux. The patient is asked to stand with the tourniquet in place, and the limb veins are observed. If fingers do the occlusion of the saphenous opening, it is called the Trendelenburg test, and if a tourniquet is used instead, it is called the tourniquet test.

If the distal veins fill rapidly within 30 seconds with the tourniquet in place, it implies the incompetence is at the level of perforators, and the SFJ is normal. This is considered a negative test.

If the veins remain collapsed for about 30 seconds after the patient stands with the tourniquet in place. Once the tourniquet is released, the internal saphenous vein rapidly fills with blood from above. The positive test denotes SFJ incompetence with no reflux at the perforators.

If the veins rapidly fill on standing with the tourniquet in position and again as the tourniquet is removed, the veins further distend; both SFJ and perforator incompetence are suspected.[9]

Suppose there is no venous filling with the tourniquet on and only slow filling of the veins from below even after the tourniquet is removed. In that case, this indicates a competent saphenous vein and the communicating veins.

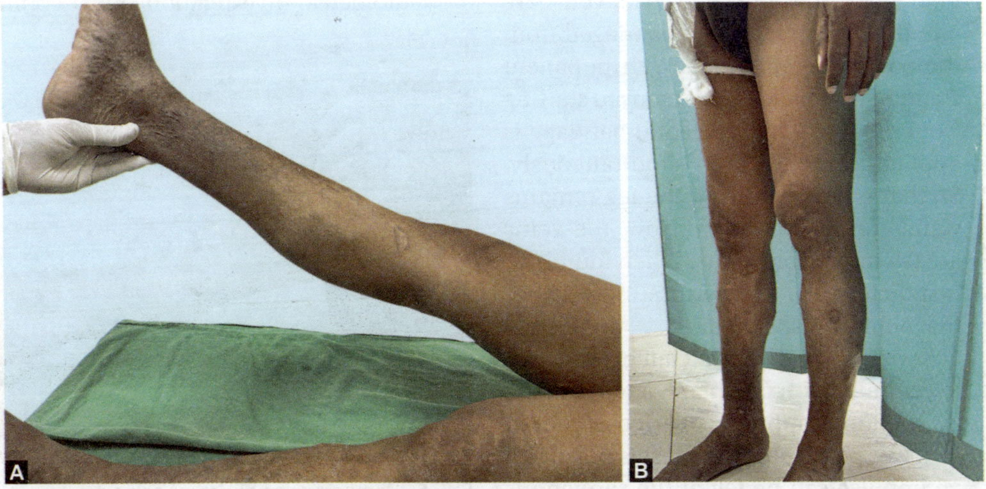

FIGS. 4A AND B: (A) Brodie–Trendelenburg test; (B) Rapidly engorged distal veins due to perforator incompetence.

The tourniquet is placed 3 cm below the SFJ level, and the test is repeated at multiple levels. The perforator above, in which there is a rapid filling of the distal veins, is considered incompetent.

The sensitivity of the Brodie–Trendelenburg test is as high as 91%, whereas this test has a poor specificity of 5%.[10]

- *Modified Perthes test*: A tourniquet is applied at the proximal mid-thigh level while the patient stands. They are asked to walk for 5 minutes or heel raise 10–20 times. If the varicose veins become less prominent, it suggests that there is no deep venous valvular insufficiency because of the calf muscle pump, which drains all the blood from the superficial venous system into a patent and competent deep venous system. This result would suggest that there is a primary problem with the superficial veins.

  If the varicose veins remain distended (or become more distended), incompetency in the deep venous system is suspected. If the patient also experiences pain in the leg, deep vein thrombosis should be ruled out.

- *Pratt test*: It is used to locate the level of perforator incompetence. First, the leg is held at 45°, and the superficial veins are emptied. Then, the leg is bandaged from the foot to the groin region. With the patient standing, the bandage is removed starting from the top, while a second bandage is applied from the groin simultaneously. So that a hand width of the leg remains visible for examination. Now, the veins are felt for any blowouts. When found, an insufficiency of the perforating veins at that point is suspected.

- *Schwartz's test*: The clinician exposes the lower limb. With one hand, a tap is made on the long saphenous varicose vein at its lower part. Schwartz's test is positive if an impulse can be felt at the saphenous opening with the other hand. This implies incompetence of the valves in the superficial venous system.

- *Fegan's test*: This test detects the site of incompetent perforators. With the patient standing, the varicosities are marked with a skin marker. The patient is then made to lie down, and the affected limb is elevated to empty the veins. Gaps or pits in the deep fascia are felt as the skin is palpated along the mark. The crescentic defects respond to the location of incompetent perforators. The principle of this test is that an incompetent perforator, being large, stretches the opening in deep fascia while it exits it.

- *Homan's sign*: This test is used to test for DVT. The patient's lower extremity is elevated to around 10° while they are in a supine position with full extension at the knee joint. The doctor then passively and abruptly dorsiflexes the foot with one hand and squeezes the calf with the other. Deep calf pain and tenderness elicited may indicate the presence of DVT and is a positive Homan's sign. The principle behind this test is that sudden dorsiflexion at the ankle causes traction on the posterior tibial vein and causes pain **(Fig. 5)**. Laboratory and radiological investigations must confirm

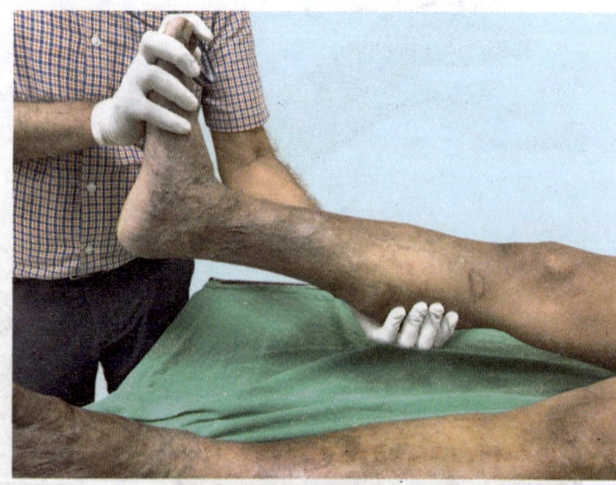

FIG. 5: Demonstration of Homan's sign.

this. False-positive Homan's sign is seen in intervertebral disc herniation, ruptured Baker's cyst, gastrocnemius spasm, and cellulitis.[11] This test has a very low sensitivity and specificity. The risk of performing this test is to dislodge any clots in the deep venous system to the pulmonary circulation.[12] This sign is estimated to have a sensitivity of 10–54% and a specificity of 39–89%.[13]

- *Moses sign*: It is elicited by compressing the calf muscle against the tibia and noticing pain. This pain is absent when squeezing the calf muscle from side to side. A positive sign indicates deep vein thrombosis in the posterior tibial veins of the lower leg.
- *Lowenberg's sign*: When a blood pressure cuff is placed around the calf and inflated to 80 mm Hg, and the patient feels pain,

Lowenberg's sign is considered positive and indicates DVT of the lower leg veins. The test was first described in 1954 by Robert I Lowenberg.

All these signs elicited in case of DVT are neither specific nor sensitive and always do need confirmation by Doppler ultrasonography or D-dimer test.

CONCLUSION

This chapter has explored the diverse array of bedside tests available for PVD. These tests' practical utility, cost-effectiveness, and noninvasiveness are paramount in modern practice. Though we continue to witness technological advancements, incorporating bedside tests is a cornerstone in providing comprehensive, patient-centered care in this new era of precision and efficiency.

Key Messages

- Peripheral vascular diseases (arterial or venous) do possess cutaneous manifestations. Dermatologists should be well versed in examining the peripheral vascular system.
- Though imaging modalities have surpassed clinical examination in PVD, bedside tests help in prompt and on-the-spot diagnosis, resulting in timely intervention and preventing potential complications.
- These tests can be done in diverse healthcare settings, ensuring its broader implementation across patients.
- These tests offer cost-effective means of screening.
- The bedside tests contribute to a patient's comprehensive vascular health assessment.

REFERENCES

1. Shabani Varaki E, Gargiulo GD, Penkala S, Breen PP. Peripheral vascular disease assessment in the lower limb: a review of current and emerging non-invasive diagnostic methods. Biomed Eng Online. 2018;17:61.
2. Das S. Examination of peripheral vascular disease and gangrene. In: Das S (Ed). A Manual on Clinical Surgery, 9th edition. Kolkata; 2011. pp. 80-99.
3. McGuire D, Gotlib A, King J. Capillary Refill Time. In: StatPearls [Internet]. Treasure Island (FL): StatPearls Publishing; 2023.
4. Aleksiev T, Ivanova Z, Dobrev H. Cold stimulation test in patients with plaque psoriasis. Skin Res Technol. 2023;29:e13421.
5. Zisquit J, Velasquez J, Nedeff N. Allen test. In: StatPearls [Internet]. Treasure Island (FL): StatPearls Publishing; 2023.
6. Povlsen S, Povlsen B. Diagnosing Thoracic Outlet Syndrome: Current Approaches and Future Directions. Diagnostics (Basel). 2018;8:21.
7. Hill RD, Smith RB III. Examination of the extremities: Pulses, bruits, and phlebitis. In: Walker HK, Hall WD, Hurst JW (Eds). Clinical Methods: The

History, Physical, and Laboratory Examinations, 3rd edition. Boston: Butterworths; 1990.

8. Clary KN, Massey P. Ankle Brachial Index. In: StatPearls [Internet]. Treasure Island (FL): StatPearls Publishing; 2023.

9. Browse NL, Burnand KG, Irvine AT, Wilson N (Eds). Diseases of the Veins, 2nd edition. London: Arnold Publishers; 1999. pp. 169-89.

10. Kim J, Richards S, Kent PJ. Clinical examination of varicose veins: a validation study. Ann R Coll Surg Engl. 2000;82:171-5.

11. Hirsh J, Hull RD, Raskob GE. Clinical features and diagnosis of venous thrombosis. J Am Coll Cardiol. 1986;8:114B-127B.

12. Homans J. Thrombosis of the deep veins of the lower leg, causing pulmonary embolism. N Engl J Med. 1934;211:993-7.

13. McGee S (Ed). Evidence-Based Physical Diagnosis. Philadelphia, USA: Saunders; 2012. pp. 472-3.

Demonstration of Ectoparasites

Senkadhir Vendhan, Karthi Kishore, Prince Malla

INTRODUCTION

Within the field of dermatology, the demonstration of ectoparasites serves as a crucial diagnostic and educational tool, offering a revealing glimpse into the world of organisms that thrive on the exterior of their hosts. Ectoparasites, encompassing a diverse range of arthropods, mites, ticks, and insects, play a significant role in dermatological conditions, making their identification and understanding pivotal in-patient care and management.

These demonstrations involve various methodologies, from direct visual identification to intricate microscopic examination, aimed at unraveling the morphological intricacies and life cycles of these organisms. By showcasing ectoparasites through live specimens, preserved samples, or microscopic slides, dermatologists and healthcare practitioners gain invaluable insights into their biology, behavior, and the implications they bear on dermatological health.

The demonstration of ectoparasites not only aids in accurate identification and diagnosis of conditions such as scabies, pediculosis, and tick-borne diseases but also broadens our understanding of their epidemiology, transmission patterns, and potential therapeutic interventions. Furthermore, these demonstrations serve as invaluable educational tools, enlightening dermatology students, researchers, and healthcare professionals about the intricate world of ectoparasitism.[1]

DEMONSTRATIONS OF SCABIES

- *Equipment required*:
  - Microscope: Use a compound light microscope with various magnification levels (typically 10×, 40×, and 100×).
  - Slides and cover slips: Clean glass slides and coverslips for preparing specimens.
  - Potassium hydroxide (KOH) or mineral oil: To facilitate the examination by enhancing transparency and clearing debris.
- *Clinical examination*:
  - Burrows identification:
    - Look for characteristic burrows, which are thin, wavy, and may have a grayish or reddish appearance **(Figs. 1 and 2)**.
    - Common locations include the webs of fingers, wrists, elbows, armpits, waistline, buttocks, genitalia, and feet.
  - Papules and excoriations: Note the presence of red papules (small, raised bumps) and excoriations (scratch marks) around burrows due to intense itching **(Fig. 3)**.

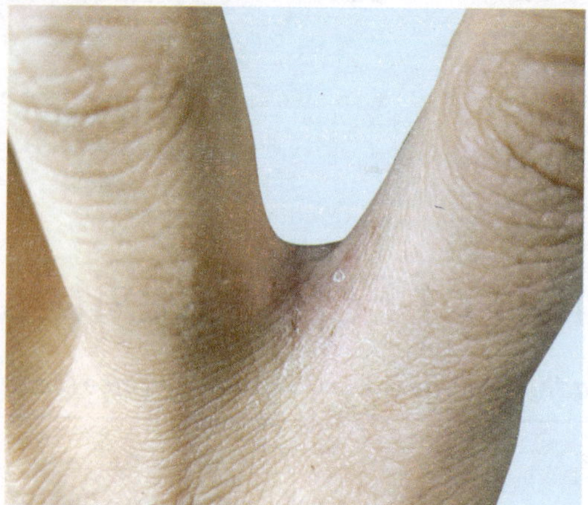

FIG. 1: Burrows on the webspace of hand.

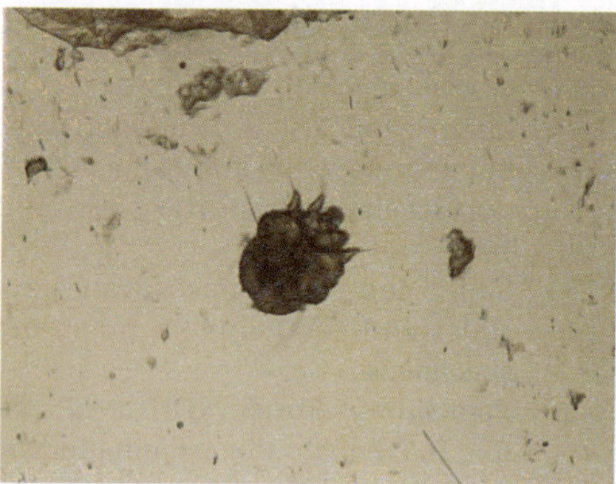

FIG. 2: Dermoscopy of scabies mite.

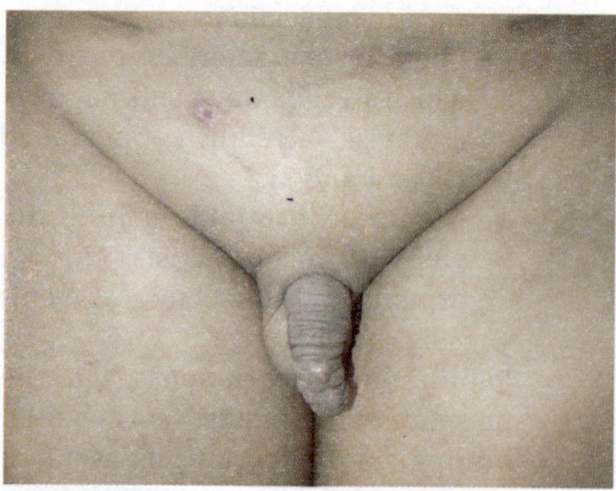

FIG. 3: Young adult with papule and excoriation marks.

- *Skin scraping*:
  - Equipment preparation: Ensure a clean glass slide, a blunt scalpel, or a skin scraping tool.
  - Procedure:
    - Gently scrape the suspected burrows or lesions using a scraping tool or the edge of a slide.[2]
    - Collect the scraped material onto the glass slide. Avoid causing discomfort or bleeding to the patient.
- *Microscopic examination*:
  - Slide preparation:
    - Apply a small amount of mineral oil or KOH to the collected material on the slide.
    - Cover the sample with a coverslip to prevent drying.
  - Microscopy:
    - Begin examination under a microscope at lower magnification (10× or 20×) to locate areas of interest **(Fig. 4)**.
    - Gradually increase the magnification (40× or higher) for detailed observation.
- *Additional considerations*:
  - Staining techniques: Giemsa stain or acetic acid can improve visibility and make the mites and eggs more discernible under the microscope.

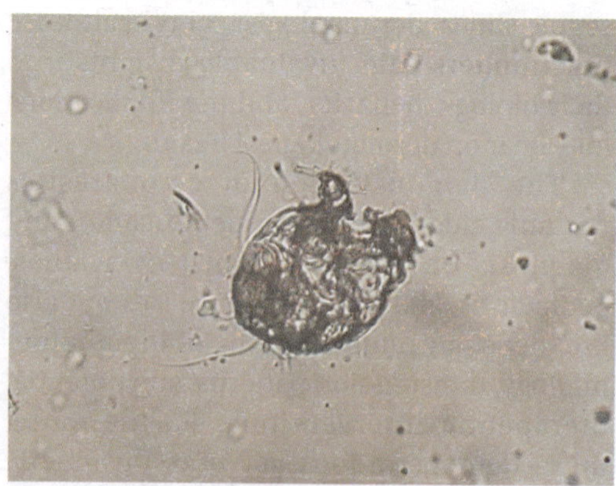

FIG. 4: Low power view of the scabies mite.

- ○ Higher magnification: Use higher magnification settings to ensure accurate identification due to the mites' small size.
- The microscopic examination of scabies involves careful observation of skin scrapings under a microscope to identify the presence of scabies mites, their eggs, or fecal matter. Here is a detailed breakdown of the microscopic examination process.

  Characteristics of sarcoptic scabies under a microscope:
  - ○ Size and shape:
    - – Tiny size: Sarcoptic scabies mites are extremely small, measuring around 0.2–0.4 mm in length.[3]
    - – Oval or rounded body: They typically have an oval or rounded body shape when viewed from above **(Fig. 5)**.
  - ○ Legs and appendages:
    - – Eight legs: These mites have eight legs, visible when viewed from below.
    - – Pincer-like structures: Their legs might exhibit pincer-like structures or hooks, particularly noticeable in males.
  - ○ Cuticle and surface texture:
    - – Translucent cuticle: The mites often appear translucent or semitransparent under the microscope due to their thin cuticle.
    - – Fine striations: Their body surface might display fine, linear striations when observed closely.
  - ○ Mouthparts and sensory organs:
    - – Chelicerae and pedipalps: Sarcoptic scabies have distinct mouthparts, including chelicerae and pedipalps, visible under higher magnification.
    - – Sensory organs: Sensory setae or bristles might be observable around the mite's body.
  - ○ Identification of gender (male vs. female):
    - – Sexual dimorphism: Males are generally smaller than females and might display more prominent structures like the pincer-like appendages.
    - – Presence of sperm sacs: In females, visible under the microscope and filled with spermatozoa.
  - ○ Movement and behavior:
    - – Slow movement: When observed under the microscope, *Sarcoptes scabiei* typically exhibit slow, deliberate movements.
    - – Burrowing activity: They might display characteristic burrowing behavior if observed within skin scrapings.
  - ○ Location and observation technique:
    - – Skin scrapings: *S. scabiei* mites are usually observed within skin scrapings collected from affected areas like burrows or lesions.
    - – Higher magnification: Detailed observation often requires higher magnification levels (40× or higher) due to their tiny size.
- Recording and documentation:
  - ○ Documentation: Take notes and document findings, including the number of mites observed and their

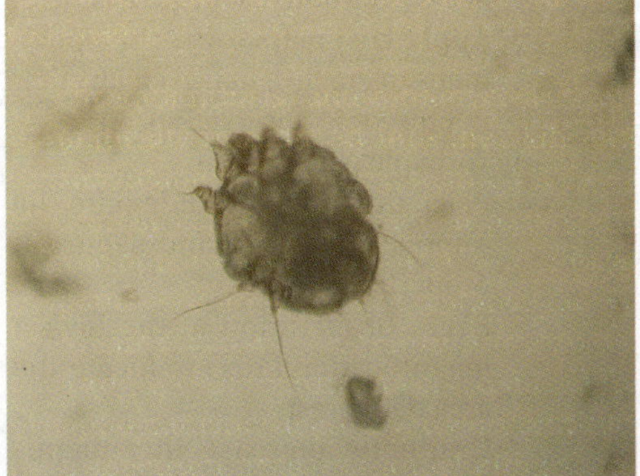

FIG. 5: High power view of the microscope showing *Sarcoptes scabiei* mite.

location in relation to the scraped material.

- o Photography: Consider taking photomicrographs for record-keeping or consultation purposes.
- o Safety measures:
  - – Handling precautions: Use gloves and follow proper laboratory safety protocols to avoid contact with potentially infectious materials.
  - – Disposal: Dispose of used slides and contaminated materials following biohazard disposal guidelines.

DEMONSTRATION OF PEDICULOSIS

Sample Collection

- *Equipment required*:
  - o Fine-toothed lice comb: Specifically designed for lice detection and removal
  - o Magnifying glass or handheld microscope: Optional, for closer examination
  - o Clean glass slides and coverslips: For specimen preparation
  - o Fine-tipped forceps: For handling samples during preparation
  - o Good lighting: Adequate lighting for clear visibility
- *Procedure*:
  - o Preparation:
    - – Ensure the individual's hair is dry and detangled for efficient examination.
    - – Choose a well-lit area to conduct the examination and collection process.
  - o Sectioning and inspection:
    - – Divide the hair into smaller segments using clips or hair ties to facilitate a systematic examination.
    - – Examine each section of hair, starting from the scalp, for the

presence of adult lice, nits, or nymphs.[4]

- o Extraction of samples:
  - – Using the fine-toothed lice comb, comb through a small section of hair near the scalp.
  - – Extract any live lice or nits found during combing using fine-tipped forceps or fingers if necessary.
- o Collection for microscopic examination:
  - – Place the collected live lice or nits onto clean glass slides for further examination.
  - – Arrange the specimens on the slides in a manner that allows for clear observation under the microscope.

Microscopic Examination

- *Equipment required*:
  - o Microscope: Compound light microscope with varying magnification levels (10×, 40×, and 100×).
  - o Clean glass slides and coverslips: For specimen preparation
  - o Proper lighting: Adequate illumination for precise observation
- *Procedure*:
  - o Slide preparation:
    - – Carefully transfer the collected live lice or nits onto clean glass slides.
    - – Apply coverslips over the specimens to create a flat, even layer for microscopic observation.
  - o Microscopic observation:
    - – Place the prepared slide onto the microscope stage and secure it properly.
    - – Begin observation at the lowest magnification (10×) to locate the area of interest.
    - – Gradually increase the magnification (40×, 100×) for detailed examination of the lice or nits.

- *Identification of pediculosis mite and nits*: Characteristics of nits under a microscope—
  - Oval shape:
    - Distinctive shape: Nits appear as small, elongated, and oval-shaped structures.[5]
    - Consistent size: They typically maintain a uniform size, although variations might occur.
  - Color and transparency:
    - Whitish or yellowish hue: Nits often display a whitish or yellowish coloration **(Fig. 6)**.
    - Translucency: They might appear translucent, allowing some light to pass through, especially if the egg is viable.
  - Attachment to hair shaft:
    - Firm adherence: Nits are firmly attached to the hair shaft near the scalp.
    - Proximity to scalp: They are found very close to the scalp due to the warmth necessary for incubation.
  - Location and distribution:
    - Specific placement: Nits are typically located on one side of the hair shaft, firmly glued in place.
    - Consistent pattern: They are often arranged in rows along the hair shaft.
  - Size:
    - Variation in size: They may vary slightly in size, but generally maintain a consistent size range.
  - Texture and appearance:
    - Smooth surface: Nits generally have a smooth, glossy appearance when observed closely.
    - Imperfections: Some may display minor irregularities or imperfections on the surface.
  - Viability:
    - Viability check: Under a microscope, viable nits might show signs of an embryo or developing louse within the egg.
  - Magnification level:
    - Optimal magnification: The characteristics are best observed at higher magnification levels, typically 40× or higher, for clear identification **(Figs. 7 and 8)**.

Caution

Differentiation from debris: It is crucial to differentiate nits from other particles like

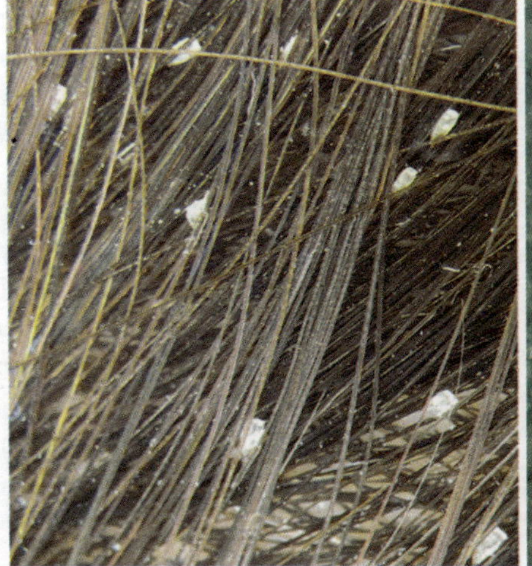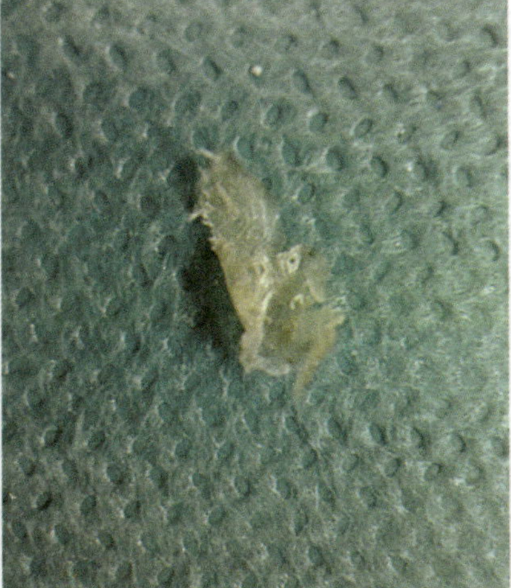

FIG. 6: Demonstration of empty and full nits under a microscope.

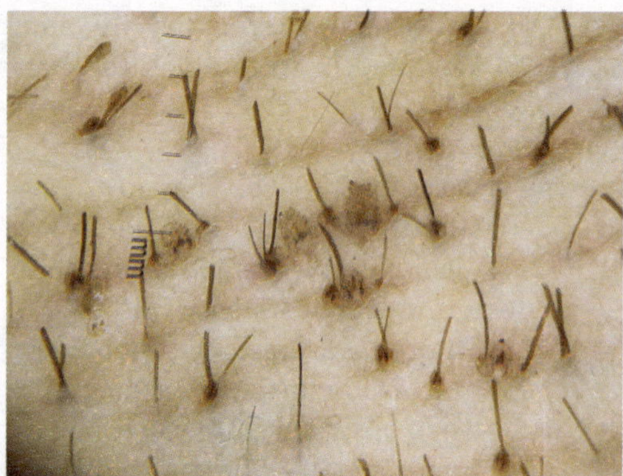

FIG. 7: Dermoscopy of pediculosis.

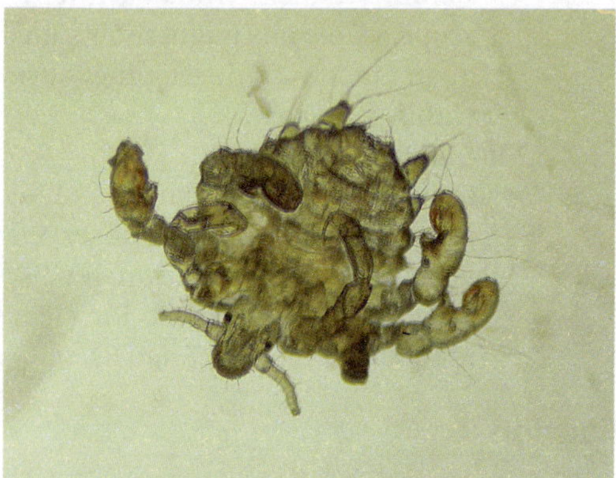

FIG. 8: Pediculosis lice in higher magnification.

dandruff or debris. Proper lighting and close examination aid in accurate identification.

Conclusion

Demonstrating pediculosis mites involves a thorough process starting from sample collection to meticulous microscopic examination. Careful extraction and observation of live lice and nits enable accurate identification and confirmation of lice infestation. This detailed demonstration aids in understanding the characteristics and features of pediculosis mites, contributing to effective diagnosis and treatment strategies.

DEMONSTRATION OF TICKS

Ticks, arachnids of the order Ixodidae, are important vectors of diseases. Identifying these parasites requires a keen eye and microscopic examination.

Identification Techniques

- *Size and morphology:*
  - Use a magnifying lens for preliminary examination. Note their size, varying from 1 mm to 1 cm, and distinct spider-like appearance with an oval- or pear-shaped body.
  - Distinguish the anterior capitulum from the posterior idiosoma, housing mouthparts and legs, respectively.
- *Mouthparts and appendages:*
  - The capitulum houses the mouthparts: The hypostome, a barbed structure aiding attachment, and paired chelicerae for cutting skin during feeding.
  - Observe four pairs of legs, each with jointed segments. Note specialized structures like sensory organs, claws, or Haller's organs, pivotal for tick sensory perception.

Microscopic Examination

- *Preparation:* Secure ticks with fine-tipped tweezers, placing them on a microscope slide. Cover delicately with a coverslip to avoid distortion or damage.
- *Magnification and observation:*
  - Start at lower magnifications (10× to 40×) to visualize overall size, shape, and anatomical orientation.
  - Increase to higher magnifications (100× to 400×) for detailed observation.
- *Detailed features:*
  - Legs: Focus on the legs to identify segments, sensory structures, and specialized adaptations aiding attachment.

- ○ Capitulum: Analyze the capitulum, highlighting the hypostome's structure, its barbed edges, and the arrangement of palps and chelicerae.
- ○ Idiosoma: Examine the idiosoma for distinctive patterns, color variations, and specialized structures like festoons, and identifying characteristics for species differentiation.
- *Species differentiation:*
  - ○ Utilize taxonomic keys or atlases specific to tick identification.
  - ○ Note species-specific variations in mouthpart morphology, festoon patterns, and specialized structures for accurate species identification.

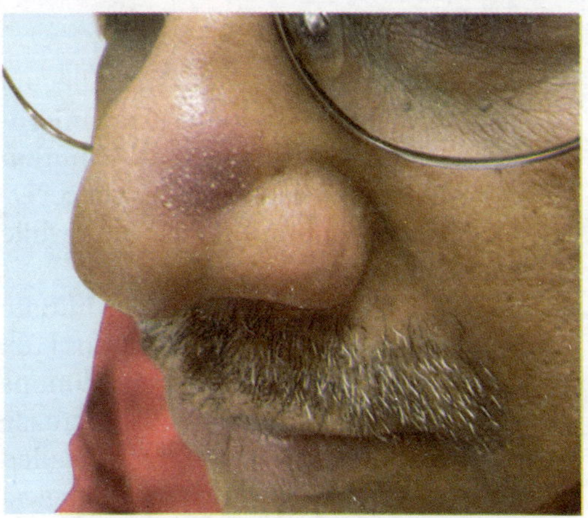

FIG. 9: Clinical image of demodicosis.

Conclusion

Microscopic identification of ticks involves meticulous examination, focusing on anatomical details crucial for precise species classification.

DEMONSTRATION OF DEMODEX

- *Skin scraping method*:
  - ○ Utilize a sterile scalpel blade or curette to gently scrape the affected skin area, focusing on regions prone to *Demodex* infestation (e.g., cheeks and eyelids) **(Fig. 9)**.
  - ○ Collect the obtained material onto a glass microscope slide or a sterile collection vial for subsequent examination.
- *Follicular extraction*:
  - ○ Employ fine forceps to delicately pluck several vellus hairs or eyelashes from the affected area.
  - ○ Transfer the extracted hairs onto a microscope slide or into a collection vial, ensuring minimal trauma.
- *Adhesive tape stripping*:
  - ○ Apply transparent adhesive tape onto the affected skin area and gently peel it off to collect superficial material containing *Demodex*.
  - ○ Attach the tape to a microscope slide for microscopic examination.
- *Eyelash sampling*:
  - ○ Use sterile forceps to remove several eyelashes from the eyelid margin, targeting areas suspected of *Demodex* involvement.
  - ○ Place the collected eyelashes onto a microscope slide or into a collection vial for subsequent analysis.

Considerations for Successful Sample Collection

- *Site selection*: Choose sampling sites based on clinical manifestations and areas where *Demodex* infestation is suspected, ensuring representative samples **(Fig. 10)**.
- *Sterility and patient comfort*: Maintain aseptic techniques during sample collection to minimize contamination and prevent potential infection. Prioritize patient comfort and minimize discomfort during the sampling procedure.

Microscopy Techniques

- *Sample preparation:* Transfer collected *Demodex* specimens onto glass microscope slides, ensuring even distribution and avoiding overlapping. Apply a coverslip delicately to prevent distortion while maintaining sample integrity.
- *Magnification and observation*: Initiate examination at lower magnifications (10× to 40×) to locate *Demodex* specimens within the sample. Gradually increase magnification (100× to 400×) for detailed observation and analysis of morphological features.

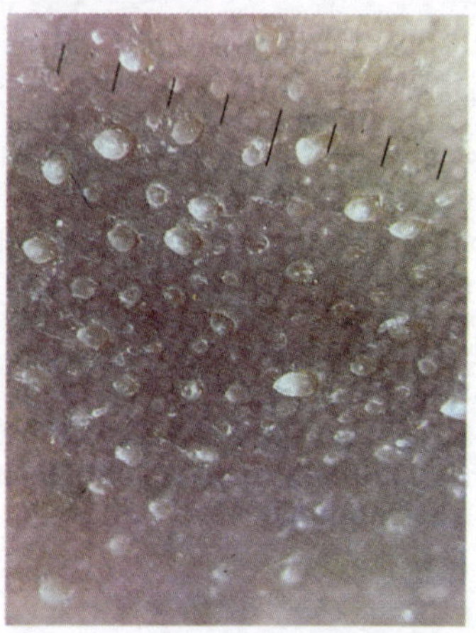

FIG. 10: Dermoscopy of *Demodex*.

Key Observations and Analysis

- *Morphological characteristics*:
  - Body structure: Identify elongated, cigar-shaped bodies, typically measuring between 0.1 and 0.4 mm, comprising segments and tapering ends **(Fig. 11A)**, which can be double checked with biopsy characteristics **(Fig. 11B)**.
  - Appendages: Focus on the eight appendages, highlighting four pairs of legs equipped with specialized structures like claws and sensory organs.
  - Habitat localization: Note specific positioning within hair follicles or sebaceous glands, distinguishing between *Demodex* folliculorum and *Demodex* brevis.
- *Differential characteristics*:
  - Species identification: Discriminate between *Demodex* species based on size, appendage structures, and habitat preference, crucial for accurate species-level diagnosis.

Advanced Microscopy Techniques

High-powered magnification: Utilize advanced microscopy systems, such as

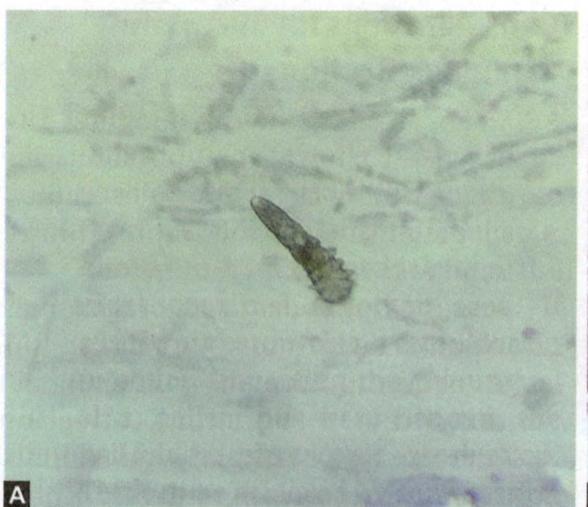

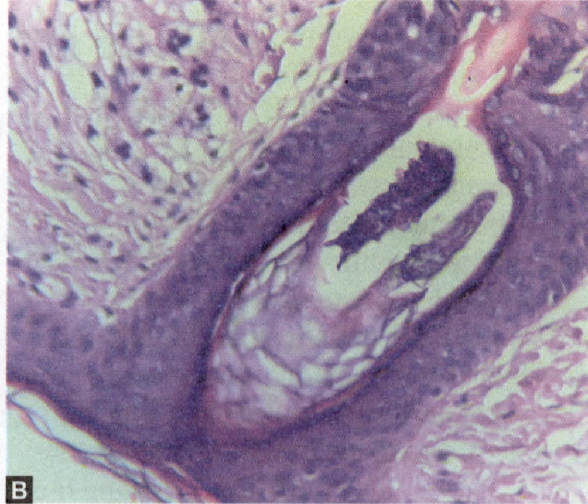

FIGS. 11A AND B: *Demodex* under light microscopy and hematoxylin and eosin (H&E) stain.
Courtesy: Dr Rashmi Jindhal.

confocal microscopy or scanning electron microscopy (SEM), for enhanced visualization of fine details and three-dimensional imaging of *Demodex* structures.

Clinical Significance and Conclusion

Microscopic examination enables precise characterization of *Demodex* morphology, aiding in accurate diagnosis and understanding of associated dermatoses.

MISCELLANEOUS

Worms

- *Filariasis*:
  - Microscopic analysis: Examine blood samples for microfilariae using microscopy, identifying characteristic sheathed larvae. Utilize thick and thin blood smears stained with Giemsa or hematoxylin and eosin (H&E) for visualization and identification of microfilariae species.
  - Key features*:* Observe microfilariae morphology (e.g., *Wuchereria bancrofti and Brugia malayi*) such as nuclei, sheath presence, and tail morphology aiding species differentiation.
- *Larva migrans (cutaneous)*:
  - Microscopic examination: Analyze skin scrapings or biopsy specimens under a microscope to detect larval structures. Utilize histopathological techniques with H&E staining to visualize and identify larvae (e.g., *Ancylostoma braziliense and Ancylostoma caninum*).
  - Characteristics*:* Observe larval structures within the epidermis or dermis, identifying hookworm larvae based on size, morphology, and distinctive hook-like structures.

Maggots

- *Myiasis*:
  - Microscopic analysis: Examine extracted larvae or wound secretions under a microscope. Utilize microscopy to identify larval features, including size, mouthparts, and segmentations.
  - Identification: Observe morphological characteristics, such as posterior spiracles or cephalopharyngeal skeleton, aiding in the identification of maggot species (e.g., *Lucilia sericata and Cochliomyia hominivorax*).

Leeches

- *Leech infestation*:
  - Microscopy techniques: Examine skin or tissue samples to detect leech attachment sites. Employ microscopy to visualize leech mouthparts and segments extracted from wounds.
  - Identifying features*:* Observe the presence of characteristic anterior and posterior suckers, identifying leech species based on morphological features and size variations.

Insect Bites, Spider Bites, and Scorpion Stings

- *Insect bites*:
  - Microscopic examination: Examine skin biopsy samples or lesion scrapings to visualize insect parts or venom deposits using microscopy.
  - Identification: Identify characteristic insect structures (e.g., mouthparts, hairs, or venom sac remnants) for insect bite diagnosis and differentiation.
- *Spider bites*:
  - Microscopy analysis: Utilize skin biopsy samples to identify spider

venom deposits or histopathological changes associated with spider bite reactions.

- ○ Key observations: Identify necrotic tissue, inflammatory changes, or characteristic spider venom components using microscopy.
- *Scorpion stings*:
  - ○ Microscopic examination: Examine skin tissue samples to detect scorpion venom deposits or histopathological changes post-sting.
  - ○ Characteristic features: Identify venom components or tissue reactions indicative of scorpion envenomation, aiding in diagnostic confirmation.

CONCLUSION

The demonstration of ectoparasites stands as a pivotal facet in dermatology, aiding in the identification, understanding, and management of numerous dermatoses. The integration of clinical presentations with microscopic findings enriches the diagnostic process. Visual demonstrations of characteristic skin lesions, bites, or infestation patterns alongside microscopic images enhance dermatologists' proficiency in recognizing ectoparasitic involvement. Continuous refinement of demonstration techniques and knowledge dissemination remain essential for the evolving landscape of ectoparasitology in dermatology.

Key Messages

- Identifying these ectoparasites is essential for effective patient care and management.
- The integration of clinical presentations with microscopic findings enhances the diagnostic process.
- Continuous refinement of demonstration techniques and knowledge dissemination is emphasized.
- Adaptation to the evolving landscape of ectoparasitology in dermatology is crucial for staying current and effective in diagnosis and management.

REFERENCES

1. Mathison BA, Pritt BS. Laboratory identification of arthropod ectoparasites. Clin Microbiol Rev. 2014;27(1):48-67.

2. Kandi V. Laboratory Diagnosis of Scabies Using a Simple Saline Mount: A Clinical Microbiologist's Report. Cureus. 2017;9(3):e1102.

3. Bandi KM, Saikumar C. Sarcoptic mange: a zoonotic ectoparasitic skin disease. J Clin Diagn Res. 2013;7(1):156-7.

4. Meister L, Ochsendorf F. Head Lice. Dtsch Arztebl Int. 2016;113(45):763-72.

5. Sweileh WM. Global output of research on epidermal parasitic skin diseases from 1967 to 2017. Infect Dis Poverty. 2018;7(1):74.

Bedside Laboratory Tests in Hair Diseases

Shrikant Kumavat, Siddharth Mani, Lalita Kumari

INTRODUCTION

Hair loss is a common problem and major cause of distress to patients. Hair consultations are nowadays becoming a major part of daily dermatology practice. To find out the cause of hair loss clinician should first take a detailed history, do a clinical examination and then perform investigations. There are many hair tests which can help to diagnose and monitor hair loss. These tests can be categorized into noninvasive, semi-invasive, and invasive tests. These tests are listed in **Box 1**. In this chapter we are going to focus on tests which can be done bedside. Hence, invasive tests like scalp biopsy are not discussed here.

NONINVASIVE TESTS

Hair Pull Test[1] (Traction Test)

It is a simple bedside test to evaluate severity and location of hair loss. A group of 20–50 scalp hairs are pulled together with index finger and thumb by a gentle force **(Fig. 1)**. The fingers are moved from the base of hairs till the distal end. Hairs which are epilated during the process are counted. If the count is >10% it constitutes a positive pull test and indicates active hair loss. Washing and brushing hair before the test may alter the results, hence, patients should avoid head wash at least 24 hours before the test. The test is positive in telogen effluvium, anagen effluvium, advancing edge of alopecia areata, and androgenetic alopecia (AGA). In cases of acute telogen effluvium, the pull test is positive over the entire scalp whereas in cases of AGA, it could usually be positive over the area of thinning.

BOX 1	Bedside tests in hair diseases.

- *Noninvasive tests:*
  - Daily hair count
  - Standardized wash test
  - 60 seconds hair test
  - Hair pull test
  - Global photography
  - Hair feathering
  - Wood's lamp
  - Trichoscopy
  - Contrasting felt examination
  - Hair weight estimation
  - Trichometry
  - Trichotillometry
  - Light microscopy
  - Polarizing microscopy
  - Confocal microscopy
  - Phototrichogram
- *Semi-invasive test:*
  - Trichogram
  - Unit area trichogram
- *Invasive test:*
  - Scalp biopsy

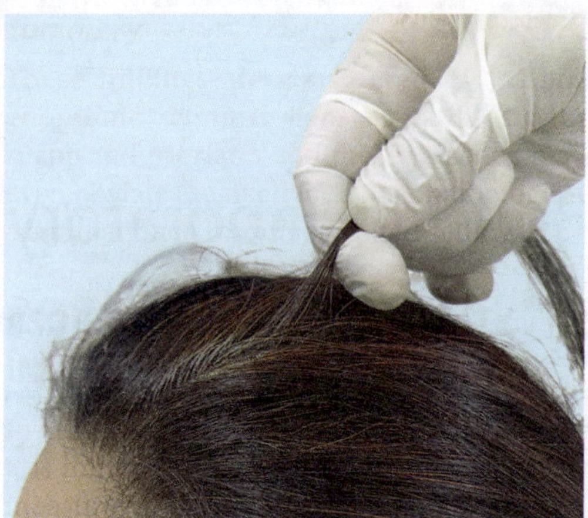

FIG. 1: Demonstration of hair pull test.

It is a very rough estimate and difficult to standardize because the force applied by the examiner is different for every hair which is pulled together.

Daily Hair Counts[2]

A healthy adult loses around 100 hairs per day. This is a result of normal hair growth cycle activity in which telogen hairs are shed and new anagen hair comes out from empty follicles. In this test, patients are instructed to collect and count the shed hairs in 1 day. The test is positive if the daily shed hair count goes beyond 100 hairs. It indicates pathological hair loss and is seen in telogen effluvium, alopecia areata, and AGA.

Sixty Seconds Hair Count[2]

Before washing the hair, it is gently combed for 60 seconds over a contrasting-colored pillow or sheet. Start at the top back of the scalp and move the comb forward to the front of the scalp. This process is repeated before three consecutive hair washes. The patient should use same comb/brush. After each session the number of hairs on the comb or brush and on the pillow are noted.

Wash Test or Rebora Test[1]

In the wash test, the individual abstains from shampooing for a period of 5 days. Subsequently, they shampoo and rinse their hair in a basin with the hole covered by gauze. The hairs retained in the water and on the gauze are gathered and submitted for examination. It is crucial to count the hairs and categorize them into two groups: Those measuring ≤3 cm and those measuring ≥5 cm in length. The hairs that were 3 cm or shorter were considered telogen vellus hairs, and patients having at least 10% of them were classified as having AGA. This technique plays a significant role in distinguishing telogen effluvium from female-pattern hair loss.

The observations are interpreted as shown in **Table 1**.

Contrasting Felt Examination[1,2]

This examination is employed to observe small, miniature hairs on the scalp. An index card, featuring black felt on one side and white felt on the other, is utilized. After creating a part in the hair, the index card is positioned along the scalp. Delicate short hairs with broken or tapered distal tips become visible along the edges of the felt. These miniature hairs are observable in the androgen-dependent regions of both men

TABLE 1: Interpretation of hair wash test.

Observation	Interpretation
≤100 hairs and with ≥10% vellus hair (≤3 cm in length)	AGA
>100 hairs and with <10% vellus hair as TE	TE
>100 hairs and with ≥10% vellus hair as AGA combined with TE	AGA with TE
≤100 hairs with <10% vellus hair	TE in remission

(AGA: androgenetic alopecia; TE: telogen effluvium)

and women experiencing AGA. In cases of regrowing telogen effluvium, a distinctive short frontal fringe is evident.

Hair Feathering[3]

This test is also known as tug test. This test is used for demonstrating hair shaft fragility. A group of hairs (around 50) are held in one hand and the other hand pulls away the distal end. If the hair shaft breaks it is considered a positive test. This test is positive in trichorrhexis nodosa, monilethrix, pili torti, trichorrhexis invaginata, trichthiodystrophy, and bubble hair.

Wood's Lamp Examination[4]

The color of the fluorescence emitted by hair with help of Wood's lamp can be used to detect infection of hair **(Figs. 2A and B)**. Woods lamp is helpful to detect tinea capitis and trichomycosis axillaris. Infection from *Microsporum* species such as *M. audouinii*, *M. canis*, *M. ferrugineum*, *M. distortum* produces blue-green fluorescence while *M. gypseum* produces dull-yellow fluorescence. Most of the *Trichophyton* species do not produce fluorescence except *Trichophyton schoenleinii* which produces dull-blue fluorescence. *Trichomycosis axillaris* which infects axillary hair produces dull-yellow fluorescence.

Hair Weight Estimation[5]

A fixed dimension area is marked on the scalp. The hairs from the marked area are cut 1 mm above the surface. All those cut hairs are collected and the weight is noted. This procedure is repeated again after a fixed interval. The change in weight indicates hair growth. This method is useful in the assessment of the efficacy of hair growth promoters like minoxidil or finasteride.

Trichometry[6]

Trichometry is the measurement of hair diameter. The dermoscope or laser beam diffraction can be used to measure hair diameter. Cross-sectional trichometry can quantify the hair mass in defined area and used to compare in subsequent visit. Commercially available device measures the cross-sectional area of the bundle of hair growing within the 2×2 cm (4 cm^2) scalp area, and displays the hair mass index. This test can be used to assess conditions such as male and female androgenic alopecia, postpartum effluvium, and effects of drugs such as minoxidil and finasteride.

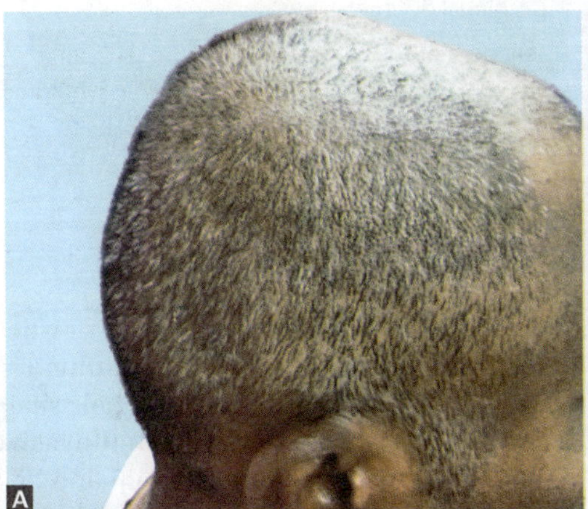
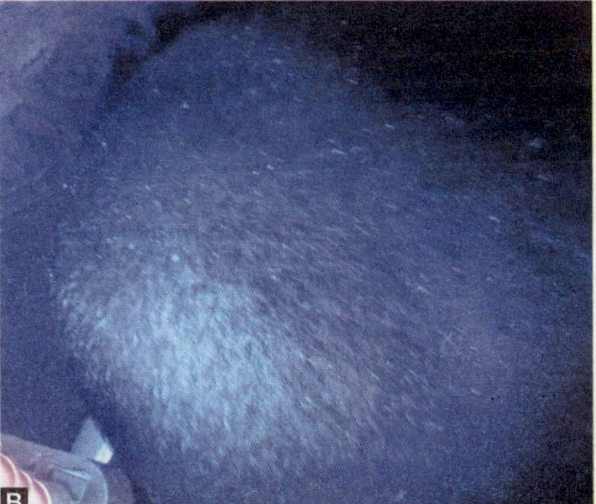

FIGS. 2A AND B: Fluorescence demonstrated by Wood's lamp in tinea capitis.

Trichotillometry[7]

Trichotillometer measures the force required for epilation. The epilation force is decreased in malnutrition and loose anagen syndrome.

Light Microscopy of Hair[2]

Hairs are plucked and are mounted on a glass side. These hairs are fixed firmly by cello tape. The proximal 2 cm part of hair is observed under a light microscope. If fungal infection is suspected, a drop of 20% KOH should be placed on the glass slide to observe fungal hyphae and spores.

It is a simple, cheap, and commonly done bedside test. Various indications are mentioned in **Table 2**. **Table 3** encompasses the characteristic features seen on light microscopy of the hair.

Polarizing Microscopy of Hair[8]

Thallium poisoning causes empty spaces in a disorganized cortex producing dark bands on the shaft of hair. Polariscopic examination of the hair in trichothiodystrophy (sulfur-deficient brittle hair) shows characteristic alternate dark and white bands of hair shaft called as "tiger tail" appearance which is not visualized on light microscopic examination.

Confocal Microscopy of Hair[9]

Confocal microscopy is also known as confocal laser scanning microscopy (CLSM) or laser scanning confocal microscopy (LSCM). Confocal microscope uses a laser to illuminate samples. It can provide a three-dimensional image of the transverse section of hair without taking the physical section. Confocal scanning microscopy (CSM) can be used to study the surface of the cuticle, identify and quantify exogenous deposits, and obtain high-quality 3D images of hair. This relatively noninvasive, nondestructive technique is routinely used to monitor the efficiency of shampoos or hair cosmetics.

TABLE 2: Various indications of light microscopy.

Indication	Example
Infections and infestations	• Tinea capitis • Piedra • Pediculosis • Trichomycosis axillaris
Hair shaft anomalies—structural defect	• Monilethrix • Pili torti • Bubble hair • Pohl–Pinkus constrictions • Pili annulati
Hair shaft anomalies—fractures	• Trichoptilosis • Trichoclasis • Trichoschisis
Hair shaft anomalies—nodes	• Trichorrhexis nodosa • Trichonodosis • Trichorrhexis invaginata • Hair casts
Bands	• Pili annulati • Kwashiorkor
Narrowings	• Monilethrix • Pohl–Pinkus constrictions • Tapered hair • Exclamation mark hair
Assessment of hair loss	• Androgenetic alopecia • Telogen effluvium
Metabolic and nutritional disorders	Kwashiorkor
Genodermatosis	• Netherton syndrome • Loose anagen syndrome • Menkes kinky hair syndrome

Trichoscopy[2,10]

Conventional handheld dermoscope or video dermoscope can be used for examination of scalp skin, follicular ostia, and hair shaft. Trichoscopy is an important noninvasive tool used to diagnose various scalp and hair disorders. It is useful not only in diagnosis

TABLE 3: Light microscopic features of common hair diseases.

Hair disease	Features on light microscopy
Tinea capitis (ectothrix variant)	Fungal spores are found on surrounding the shaft
Tinea capitis (endothrix variant) **(Fig. 3)**	Fungal spores are seen inside the hair shaft
White piedra	Fungal hyphae are arranged perpendicular to hair shaft
Black piedra	Hair shaft is studded with acrospores and fungal hyphae are arranged in parallel fashion
Trichorrhexis invaginata **(Fig. 4)**	The shaft is invaginated into itself resulting in a ball and socket type defect seen as a bamboo tree appearance
Trichorrhexis nodosa	Bulging of shaft where the cuticle is lost and the frayed cortical fibers project out giving the appearance of two paint brushes thrust into one another
Monilethrix	Beaded appearance
Pili torti	Twisted appearance
Loose anagen syndrome	Rumpled sock appearance

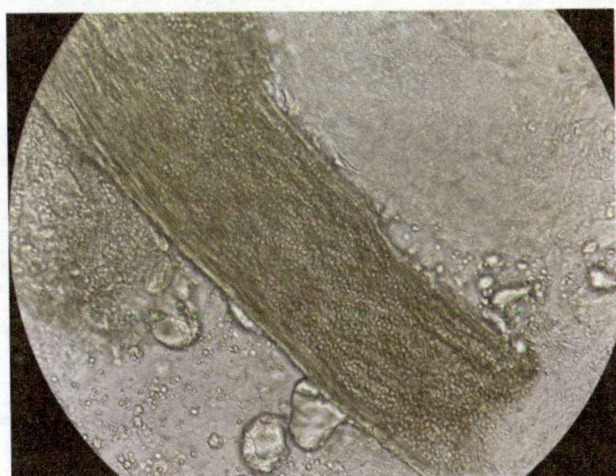

FIG. 3: Multiple spores inside hair shaft (endothrix) (KOH, 40×).
Courtesy: Dr Vikrant Saoji, Nagpur, Maharashtra, India.

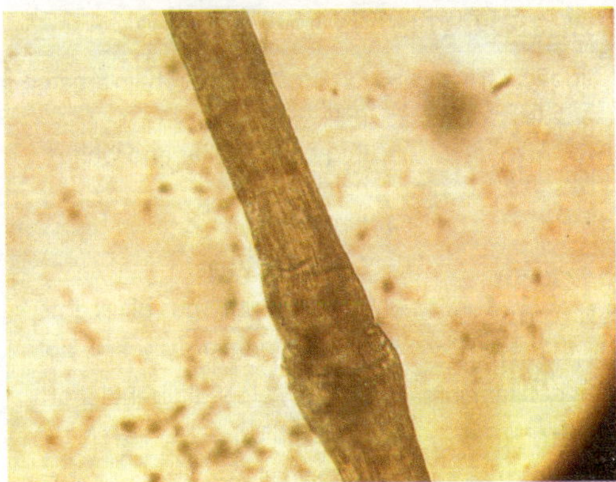

FIG. 4: Trichorrhexis invaginata.

but it also serves as an important tool in post treatment monitoring. Video dermoscope [universal serial bus (USB) attached dermoscope] has a digital camera which is connected to a computer via USB **(Fig. 5)**. It shows focused areas on a computer screen in real time with several magnifications. Images can be recorded in digital format and used for follow-up treatment. Important trichoscopic features of various disorders are mentioned in **Tables 4 and 5**.

Global Photography[11]

This technique is commonly used in androgenic alopecia. Photographs of the scalp are taken before and after the treatment to compare the results. Four standard views (vertex, midline, frontal, and temporal) are recorded. A stereotactic positioning device is used for taking photos. Patient's forehead and chin are fixed on the device and a camera with flash light is mounted on the other end. Before clicking the photograph of the vertex view the hairs are combed away from the

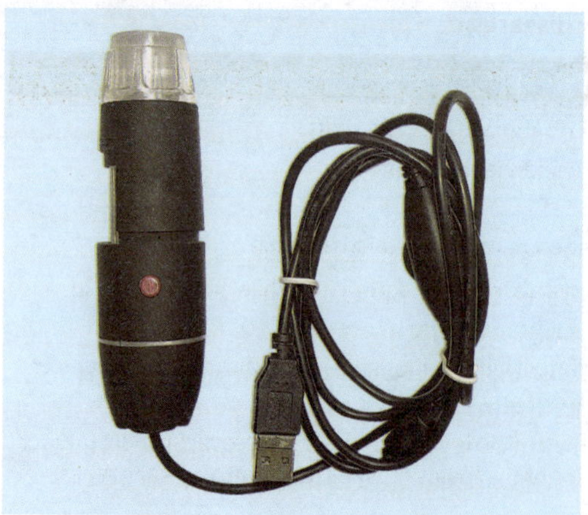

FIG. 5: Universal serial bus (USB) attached dermoscope.

TABLE 4: Trichoscopic features of nonscarring alopecia.

Nonscarring alopecia	Trichoscopic features
Alopecia areata (Fig. 6)	• Exclamation mark hair/tapered hair • Regrowing vellus and white hairs • Pigtail hair • Coudability hair • Regular, numerous black dots • Regular, numerous yellow dots
Trichotillomania (Fig. 7)	• Broken hair of different length • Trichoptilosis • Flame hairs • V-sign • Coiled hair/hook hair/question mark hair • Mace hair • Burnt matchstick sign/hair • Perifollicular hemorrhage
Androgenetic alopecia (Fig. 8)	• Short vellus hair • Hair diameter variation • Yellow dots • Honeycomb pigmentation • Peripilar sign
Telogen effluvium	• Decreased hair density • Presence of empty follicles • Upright regrowing hair

Continued

Continued

Nonscarring alopecia	Trichoscopic features
Tinea capitis (Fig. 9)	• Comma hairs • Corkscrew hairs • Zig-zag hairs • Morse code-like hairs • Bent hair • Block hairs • Black dots • Perifollicular and interfollicular scales
Temporal triangular alopecia	• Short vellus hairs (in tufts) • Length diversity in vellus hairs • White dots with slight perifollicular scaling • Honeycomb pattern pigmentation

TABLE 5: Trichoscopic features of scarring alopecia.

Nonscarring alopecia	Trichoscopic features
Lichen planopilaris	• Peripilar casts • Absence of follicular openings/scarring • Broken hairs • White dots situated amidst honeycomb pigment pattern give a "starry sky" pattern • Perifollicular blue-gray dots
Discoid lupus erythematosus	• Follicular plugs • Areas of scarring • Broken hair • Red dots • Different vascular patterns in active disease as arborizing vessels
Folliculitis decalvans (Fig. 10)	• Tuft of hairs • Broken hairs • Yellow dots and blacks dots
Pseudopelade of Brocq	• Loss of follicular ostia • Ivory-white areas • Occasionally solitary dystrophic hairs

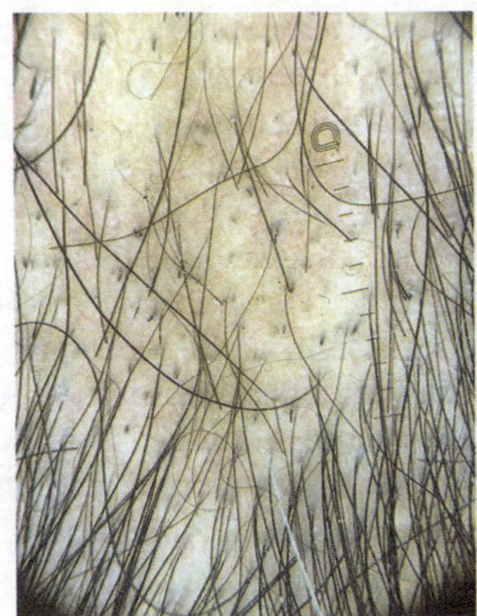

FIG. 6: Black dots, broken hair in alopecia areata seen on dermoscope.
Courtesy: Dr Hiloni Chokshi, Dr Vasantrao Pawar Medical College, Hospital, and Research Center, Nashik, Maharashtra, India.

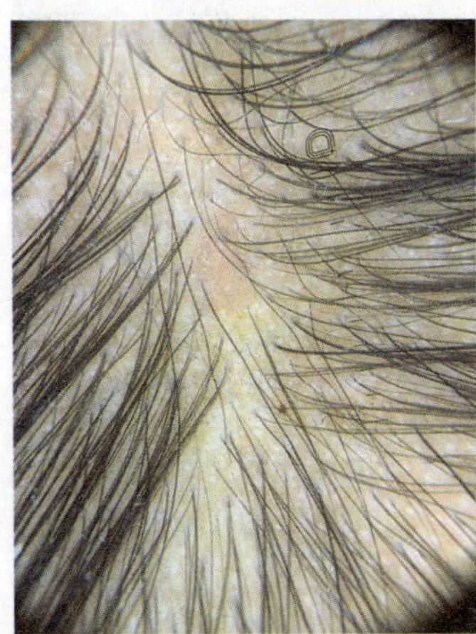

FIG. 8: Hair miniaturization in androgenic alopecia seen on dermoscope.
Courtesy: Dr Hiloni Chokshi, Dr Vasantrao Pawar Medical College, Hospital, and Research Center, Nashik, Maharashtra, India.

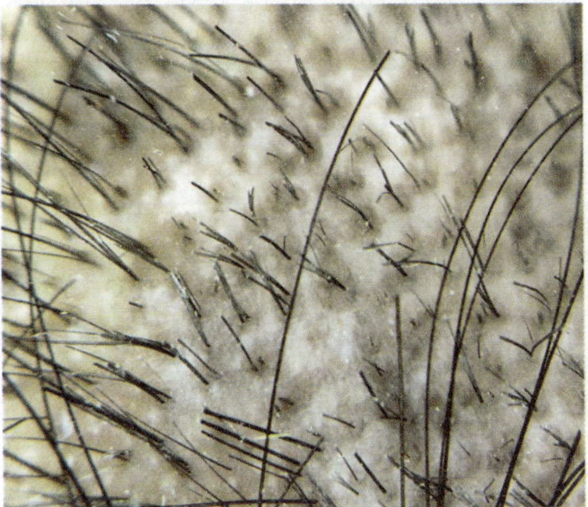

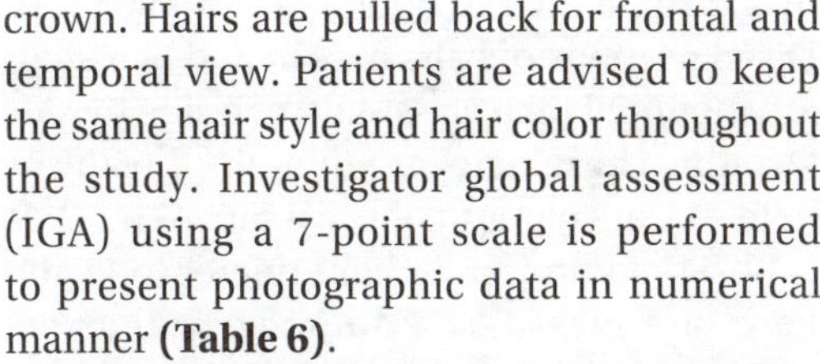

FIG. 7: Broken hair of different length seen in trichotillomania seen on dermoscope.

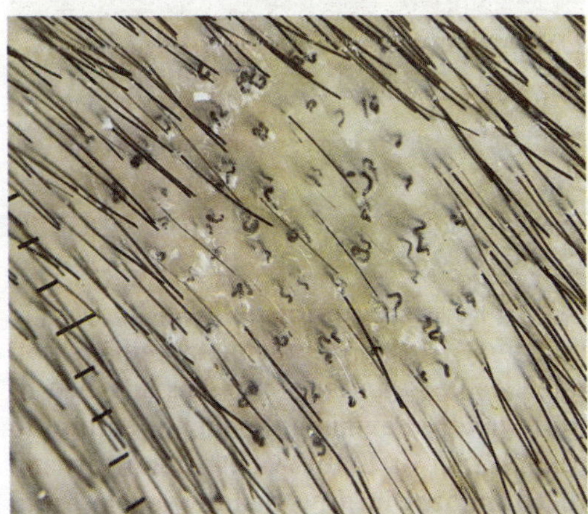

FIG. 9: Corkscrew hairs seen in tinea capitis seen on dermoscope.

crown. Hairs are pulled back for frontal and temporal view. Patients are advised to keep the same hair style and hair color throughout the study. Investigator global assessment (IGA) using a 7-point scale is performed to present photographic data in numerical manner **(Table 6)**.

This technique creates a permanent record of hair growth. Photographs of before and after treatment are compared to evaluate the effect of treatment. It also motivates the patients to continue treatment.

Photographic Trichogram[12,13]

Phototrichogram allows the in vivo study of hair growth cycle and takes measurements of hair such as hair density, hair length, and hair diameter. A fixed area of 2 cm^2 is marked by a marker over the scalp (mid vertex). All hairs

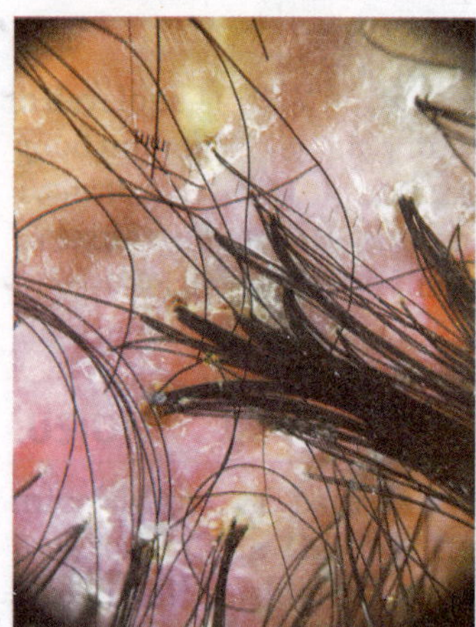

FIG. 10: Tuft of hairs seen in folliculitis decalvans seen on dermoscope.

TABLE 6: Investigator global assessment scale.

Hair density	Grade
Greatly decreased	−3
Moderately decreased	−2
Slightly decreased	−1
No change	0
Slightly increased	1
Moderately increased	2
Greatly increased	3

of marked area are trimmed about 1 mm from the surface. A close-up photograph of this area is taken by camera or video dermoscope. Hair density, diameter, and length are measured manually or with help of computer software. The same area is photographed again after 48 hours. This time hair length, hairs showing growth (anagen hairs), and hairs not showing growth (telogen hairs) are measured.

Modifications of Phototrichogram

Contrast-enhanced Phototrichogram

Gray hairs are difficult to visualize in routine photographic methods. In this modified procedure, black color hair dye is applied before taking photographs. Less pigmented and thin hairs are better visualized due to black hair dye.

Scalp Immersion Proxigraphy

Immersion oil is applied and cover slip is put on the area to be photographed. The oil improves the visualization of hairs.

Trichoscan[14]

This procedure uses an inbuilt dermoscope attached to a digital camera to take photographs. Hair dye is applied to the target area before shaving. The area is dot tattooed. Approximately 1.8 cm^2 area is photographed by the instrument with 20-fold magnification on day 1 and 3. The digital photographs are stored in a computer and are analyzed by software. The software can calculate hair density (n/cm^2), hair diameter (μm), hair growth rate (mm/day), and anagen/telogen ratio. This method is simple and gives fast results. Tricoscan can be used to compare effectiveness of different hair growth promoting substances and study androgenic or other forms of diffuse hair loss.

SEMI-INVASIVE TESTS

Trichogram/Hair Pluck Test[1,2]

It is also known as hair root analysis or hair pluck test. The test is performed after 5 days of shampooing. Hairs are selected from a specific site. The hairs are cut 0.5 cm above the surface. Around 5–10 hairs are grasped in artery forceps whose tips are covered by rubber tubing **(Fig. 11)**. A firm and sudden pull is exerted in the direction of emergence of those hairs. This procedure is repeated in the same area to obtain around 50 hairs. Distal portions of hairs are cut and hair roots are mounted on a glass slide in a side by side fashion. These hairs are then fixed with the help of transparent adhesive tape. The slide is observed under the light microscope and hairs are classified into anagen, telogen, catagen, and dystrophic hairs **(Table 7)**.

For a given patient trichogram is interpreted according to the predominant pattern observed. Telogen pattern is seen in telogen effluvium, dystrophic pattern in anagen effluvium, and mixed dystrophic-telogen pattern is seen in alopecia areata.

Unit Area Trichogram[1,2]

This is a variation of trichogram in which hairs are collected only from a defined area (60 mm²). In addition to light microscopy, other hair measurements such as hair density, hair length, and hair diameters are also noted. The results of this method are reproducible and clinically relevant. Hence, it can be used to compare results in clinical trials.

CONCLUSION

In conclusion, bedside tests stand as indispensable tools in the diagnosis of hair disorders, offering a practical and efficient means of evaluation. Their simplicity, cost-effectiveness, and accessibility make them valuable for initial assessments, aiding healthcare professionals in distinguishing between various conditions such as scarring and nonscarring alopecia or differentiating between different subtypes of earlier mentioned alopecia. By incorporating these

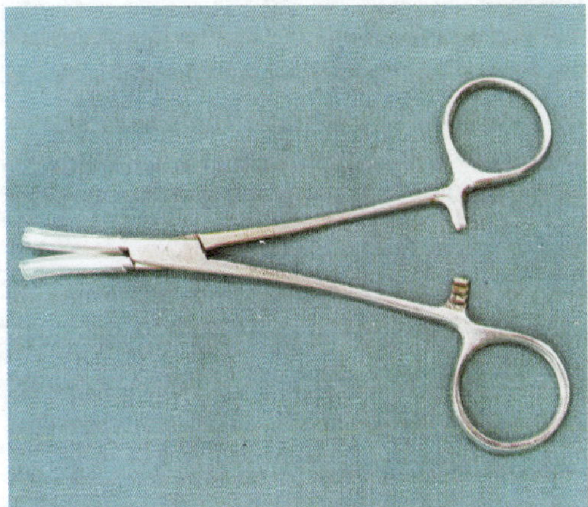

FIG. 11: Artery forceps with tips covered by polyvinyl chloride (PVC) tubing obtained from IV set.

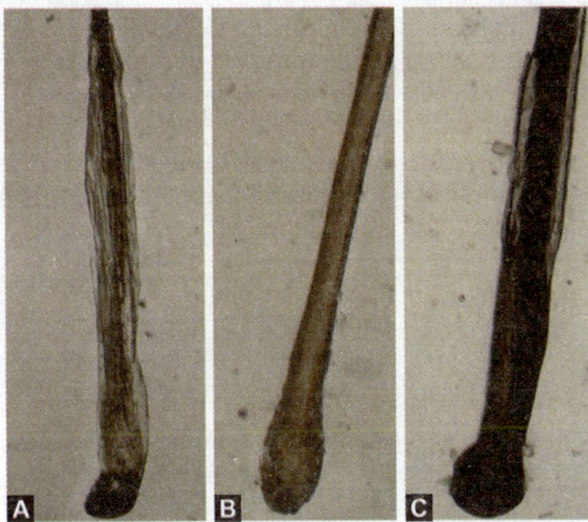

FIGS. 12A TO C: (A) Anagen hair; (B) telogen hair; (C) catagen hair.

TABLE 7: Light microscopic features of hair in a trichogram.

Type of hair (normal values)	Characteristics of hair
Anagen (80–88%) (Fig. 12A)	• Thick and dark base • Inner and outer root sheath are preserved • Angle of 20° is found between the hair bulb and hair shaft
Telogen (10–20%) (Fig. 12B)	• Hairs are thin • Club shaped and smoothly contoured straight shaft • Bulb is nonpigmented covered by loose or absent outer root sheath.
Catagen (1–2%) (Fig. 12C)	Similar to telogen hairs except their bulb is not smooth and is covered by loose and thick inner and outer root sheath.
Dystrophic	• Absent outer root sheath and sometimes inner root sheath also • Root is tapered severely to a point

bedside tests into diagnostic protocols, clinicians can streamline the diagnostic journey, facilitating timely, and accurate identification of underlying issues. This, in turn, allows for the formulation of targeted and personalized treatment plans, ultimately improving patient outcomes. The utility of bedside tests extends beyond mere convenience; they represent a crucial step toward enhancing the precision and efficacy of diagnostic practices in the realm of hair disorders.

Key Messages

- There are three types of hair tests which include noninvasive, semi-invasive, and invasive. Noninvasive and semi-invasive tests can be performed at bedside.
- In cases of acute telogen effluvium, the hair pull test is positive over the entire scalp whereas in cases of AGA, it could usually be positive over the area of thinning.
- The daily hair count test is positive if the daily shed hair count goes beyond 100 hairs. It indicates pathological hair loss and is seen in telogen effluvium, alopecia areata, and AGA.
- In hair wash test, the hairs that were 3 cm or shorter were considered telogen vellus hairs, and patients having at least 10% of them were classified as having AGA. This technique plays a significant role in distinguishing telogen effluvium from female-pattern hair loss.
- Hair feathering is important test use for demonstrating hair shaft fragility. This test is positive in trichorrhexis nodosa, monilethrix, pili torti, trichorrhexis invaginata, trichthiodystrophy, and bubble hair.

REFERENCES

1. Falcon CS, Espinoza N, Gunman D. Pull test and trichogram. In: Alves R, Grimalt R (Eds). Techniques in the Evaluation and Management of Hair Diseases. India: CRC press; 2001. pp. 30-43.
2. Dhurat R, Saraogi P. Hair evaluation methods: merits and demerits. Int J Trichology. 2009;1(2): 108-19.
3. Mubki T, Rudnicka L, Olszewska M, Shapiro J. Evaluation and diagnosis of the hair loss patient: part I. History and clinical examination. J Am Acad Dermatol. 2014;71(3):415.e1-415.e15.
4. Gupta LK, Singhi MK. Wood's lamp. Indian J Dermatol Venereol Leprol. 2004;70(2):131-5.
5. Olsen EA. Current and novel methods for assessing efficacy of hair growth promoters in pattern hair loss. J Am Acad Dermatol. 2003;48(2): 253-62.
6. Wikramanayake TC, Mauro LM, Tabas IA, Chen AL, Llanes IC, Jimenez JJ. Cross-section Trichometry: A Clinical Tool for Assessing the Progression and Treatment Response of Alopecia. Int J Trichology. 2012;4(4):259-64.
7. Chase ES, Weinsier RL, Laven GT, Krumdieck CL. Trichotillometry: the quantitation of hair pluck-ability as a method of nutritional assessment. Am J Clin Nutr. 1981;34(10):2280-6.
8. Rudnicka L, Olszewska M, Waśkiel A, Rakowska A. Trichoscopy in Hair Shaft Disorders. Dermatol Clin. 2018;36(4):421-30.
9. Hadjur C, Daty G, Madry G, Corcuff P. Cosmetic assessment of the human hair by confocal microscopy. Scanning. 2002;24(2):59-64.
10. Ross EK, Vincenzi C, Tosti A. Videodermoscopy in the evaluation of hair and scalp disorders. J Am Acad Dermatol. 2006;55(5):799-806.
11. Rakowska A. Photography in hair diseases. In: Alves R, Grimalt R (Eds). Techniques in the Evaluation and Management of Hair Diseases. India: CRC press; 2001. pp. 24-9.
12. Van Neste MD. Assessment of hair loss: clinical relevance of hair growth evaluation methods. Clin Exp Dermatol. 2002;27(5):358-65.
13. Dhurat R. Phototrichogram. Indian J Dermatol Venereol Leprol. 2006;72(3):242-4.
14. Hoffmann R. TrichoScan: combining epiluminescence microscopy with digital image analysis for the measurement of hair growth in vivo. Eur J Dermatol. 2001;11(4):362-8.

Bedside Tests to Detect Sweat Disorders

Prachi Verma, Smriti Sharma, K Lekshmipriya

INTRODUCTION

Sweat glands are epidermal appendages widely distributed over the body except over the nipples, lips, and external genital organs. Their major function is thermoregulation via perspiration and to act as an excretory organ for drugs and their metabolites. Sweat glands are eccrine glands where the secretion of sweat occurs without pinching off of outer cell parts. Sweat disorders may present in innumerable ways, such as essential hyperhidrosis, complete anhidrosis with heat intolerance, and compensatory hyperhidrosis due to anhidrosis or hypohidrosis.[1-3]

Analysis of sweat disorders includes various quantitative tests used for sweat examination. The thermoregulatory sweat test (TST) was formulated for the objective evaluation of sweat disorders. It is considered to be the gold standard for sweat-related studies of the entire anterior body surface. Later several other objective tests were developed for evaluation of sweating. These include the quantitative sudomotor axon reflex test, silicone impressions test, sympathetic skin response, gravimetry/ evaporimetry, and quantitative direct and indirect axon reflex test. However, all of these tests require specialized equipment and are expensive and time-consuming. For the patient, the TST is uncomfortable and requires disrobing and covering the whole body with the color indicator. It is advisable to initially screen the suspected patients with an appropriate and effective bedside test to validate the need for further in-depth evaluation.[4-6]

QUALITATIVE SWEAT ESTIMATION TESTS

Direct Visualization of Sweat

This is the simplest test used for subjective evaluation of sweating in a person. Unclothed patients are made to sit in a sauna room in conditions mimicking the bedside setting of 80°F (26.7°C) and 35% humidity for 10–15 minutes so as to cause sweating. The examiner now assesses the patient's skin for the presence of sweat droplets by reflection of light. A bright pen light is shone onto the patient's skin at an angle and perpendicular to the skin surface. The sweat droplets reflecting the light are visualized. The detection of light reflection was marked as a positive finding for the presence of sweat at that site. We should avoid using a low-intensity penlight or a very bright light near to the skin surface to help prevent artifacts **(Table 1)**.

Palpation of Skin

Another crude test that can be done for detection of sweating is palpation of the patients' skin. This is primarily an extension

TABLE 1: Advantages and disadvantages of direct visualization of sweat method.[7]

Advantages	Disadvantages
• Easy to perform • No specific equipment or set up required	• Subjective findings with observer variation • No objective quantification possible

TABLE 2: Advantages and disadvantages of palpation of sweat method.

Advantages	Disadvantages
• Easy to perform • No specific equipment or set up required	• Subjective in nature • May be considered unhygienic by evaluators

TABLE 3: Advantages and disadvantages of gravimetry method.

Advantages	Disadvantages
• Easy to perform and fast • Objective and absolute evaluation possible	• Difficult to do in generalized hyperhidrosis • Wide and erratic variations

to the direct visualization test. The subjects are made to undress and sit in a room in a temperature setting of 80°F (26.7°C) and 35% humidity for 10–15 minutes. The skin is then palpated with bare hands using the tips of index and middle fingers sliding over the patient's body. The palpating fingers feel a yank at the site of moisture caused by excessive sweating. Dry dorsum of the fingers can be used to brush the patient's skin to detect moisture in case the fingers of the examiner are moist **(Table 2)**.[7]

Gravimetry (Blotting Paper Test)

The blotting paper technique is a quantitative measure of the amount of sweat over a certain period of time. It is easy to perform and helps in a somewhat objective quantification of sweating in localized areas. The blotting paper is weighed in dry state prior to applications over areas to be tested. The paper is then applied to the areas that need to be evaluated, for 1 minute and then weighed again after sweating. The weight change is taken to represent the amount of sweat absorbed and expressed as milligrams/ minutes. The blotting paper test is primarily used for gustatory sweating in cases such as Frey's syndrome. It also finds it application in assessing localized hyperhidrosis especially palmoplantar hyperhidrosis **(Table 3)**.[1,8]

Starch–iodine Test

The Minor's starch–iodine test is an unpretentious and inexpensive method for recognizing the presence of perspiration, identifying the affected surface area and assessing the severity of sweat overproduction. It is the most widely used test performed in dermatology outpatient department (OPD) for sweat-related disorders. It is principally useful in locating areas of focal perspiration for planning injectable treatments like botulinum toxin. It also finds its use in assessing the treatment efficacy (i.e., botulinum toxin injection or surgery). The Minor's test is not used to quantify hyperhidrosis severity, but it can identify different perspiration intensities.

The methodology includes thorough cleaning and drying of the skin area that needs to be evaluated. 1–5% iodine in alcohol solution is applied over the area. The starch–iodine test was modified with use of Betadine™ solution as the marker solution. The solution applied over the skin is then thoroughly dried. A starch powder (e.g., cooking corn starch) is lightly sprinkled on the skin area using a cotton ball, brush, or loose gauze. The moisture from the sweat dissolves the iodine and starch, consequential in forming a polyiodide chain via a chemical reaction. This reaction turns the light brown iodine color into a dark purple color. The purple area indicates the sweat gland orifices, which appear as small dots.

There are multiple modifications to Minor's test which have been formulated over the years. Paper saturated with starch–iodine placed over the sweat area also produces similar results. Alizarin or ponceau red dye has also been used in place of iodine solution for iodine-sensitive patients. The sweat area here turns pink. The limitation to Minor's test includes appearance of false-positives such as dark pigments, if the skin has not been thoroughly dried of sweat or if the iodine solution is not thoroughly dried prior to starch application. There are also false-negatives if excess amount of starch is applied.

The Minor's test is not helpful in determining the severity of hyperhidrosis. However, it can help in determining the different perspiration intensities by using the intensity visual scale. It is a six-grade visual scale, the concluding color from the Minor's test is categorized as follows: 0, no sweating; 1, initial; 2, mild; 3, moderate; 4, intense; and 5, excess sweating. The appearance of areas with great sweating would be homogenous and highly pigmented (scores 3–5), whereas areas with less sweating would be heterogeneous and speckled (scores 0–2) **(Table 4; Figs. 1 and 2)**.[1,5,9,10]

TABLE 4: Advantages and disadvantages of starch–iodine test.

Advantages	Disadvantages
• Topographic test which helps in accurate charting of sweat points • Easy record maintenance with the help of photography	• Cumbersome process of application of multiple layers of reagents and the hassle of removing the iodine paint • Chances of allergic reaction to iodine • Lack of dynamic testing

Spoon Test

The spoon test has been in use since ancient times for sweat disorders. An alcohol swab is used to sterilize a simple kitchen soup spoon and then dried. The clean and dry spoon is to be held with the thumb and forefinger and its convex surface is gently glided across the skin surface, with the weight of the spoon providing the only source of pressure. The spoon glides smoothly across the skin at all sites unless it comes in contact with the moist skin. Here the friction causes the spoon to stop. During the test wherever the spoon sticks to the moist skin, it is quickly dried and reapplied at the next site. There is a chance of false-positive test when the spoon glides perpendicularly to the loose skinfold. To overcome this, it is to be noted that the spoon is glided along the skinfold and not against them. The examiner should try and avoid any excess external pressure to not increase the contact area and create a false sense of friction. The neck is kept hyperextended during the procedure to maximize smoothness of the skin. Patients are advised to avoid frowning, which causes skinfolds and pseudofriction at the forehead **(Table 5)**.[7,9,11,12]

QUANTITATIVE SWEAT ESTIMATION TESTS

Ninhydrin Test

It is a quantification method that counts on the chemical reaction that occurs between ninhydrin reagents and amino acids present in the sweat. Methodology begins with cleaning the hand thoroughly to remove all dirt and sweat and then drying it. The ninhydrin reagent is sprayed onto a paper, which is then placed over the area to be tested firmly for 15–30 seconds. The paper is then analyzed digitally. The image produced on the paper helps in detection of amount of sweat **(Table 6)**.[5,13]

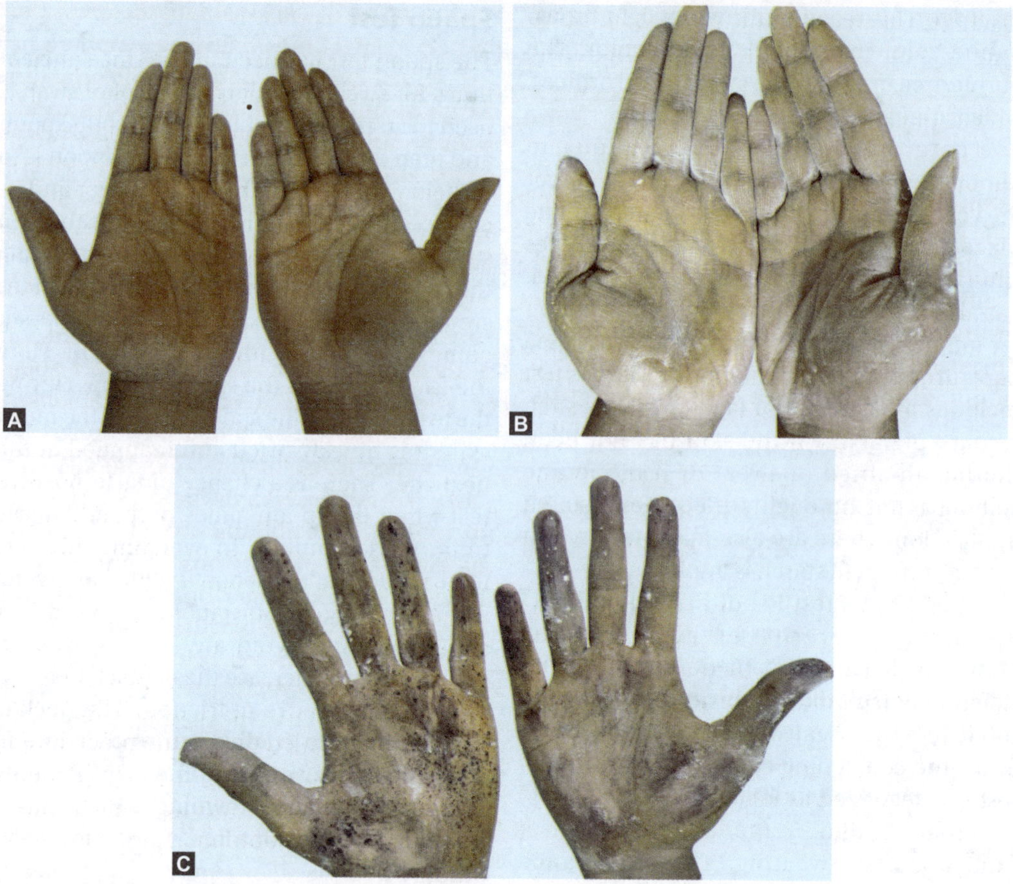

FIGS. 1A TO C: Demonstration of Minor's starch test: (A) Application of Betadine on both palms; (B) Sprinkled corn starch on dried hands after Betadine application; and (C) Positive starch–iodine test with blue-brown discoloration.

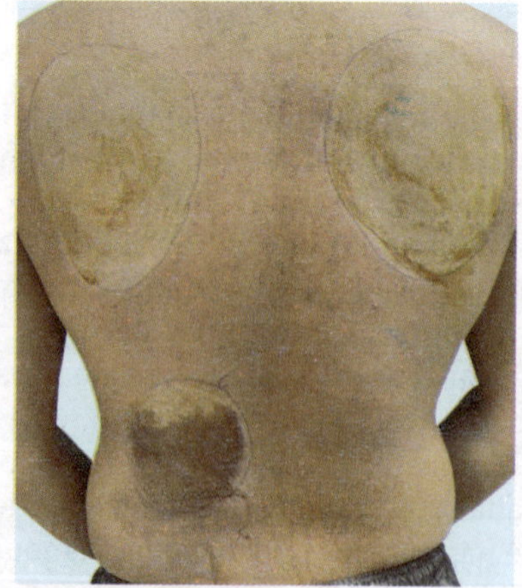

FIG. 2: Starch–iodine test in a patient with Ross syndrome with hypohidrosis.

TABLE 5: Advantages and disadvantages of the spoon test.

Advantages	Disadvantages
• Easy to perform • No specific equipment or set up required	• Subjective findings with observer variation • No objective quantification possible

TABLE 6: Advantages and disadvantages of ninhydrin test.

Advantages	Disadvantages
• Objective detection of sweat • Record maintenance in the form of digital image	Requirement of a digital analyzer

Evaporimetry

It is a quantitative test that measures transepidermal water loss (TEWL) through the skin using a vapor pressure gradient. TEWL for normal skin under ambient conditions ranges between 4 and 10 $g/h/m^2$. This amounts to a total of about 500 mL of water loss per day, however, this may rise up to 30 times higher when the epidermis is damaged or in case of excessive sweating disorders. There are various methods for measuring TEWL such as the open-chamber, closed chamber methods like ventilated-chamber and unventilated-chamber. In closed-chamber devices, TEWL is measured by calculating the evaporation rate (evaporimetry) based on the increased relative humidity in the closed chamber. The final value is stated in weighed amount of water (g)/area of evaporation (m^2)/time (hours). Various evaporimetry measurement devices have been reported **(Figs. 3A and B; Table 7)**.[5,6,14]

Silicone Impressions

The silicone impression method is used to detect sweat release. It has been primarily used in ascertaining postganglionic sympathetic cholinergic sudomotor function by measuring the direct and axon-reflex facilitated sweat response. The method includes stimulating the sweat glands by iontophoresis with acetylcholine, pilocarpine, or methacholine. The skin is then dried thoroughly and a thin moldable layer of silicone is applied over the skin. Sweat droplets formed by the triggered sweat glands displace the silicone material resulting in permanent impressions. These impressions are assessed for number, distribution, and droplet size either directly under a light microscope or through computer-assisted analysis. Dental impression material is typically used, which has a working time of approximately 2 minutes and fully polymerizes within 5 minutes. Data are reported as droplet number, size, and distribution. Volume of sweat production can be estimated by assuming the droplets form a hemisphere **(Table 8)**.[9]

CONCLUSION

Sweat disorders are a major cause of concern among the patients attending dermatology clinics across the globe. The need for correctly assessing and diagnosing the condition is imperative to improve the quality of life of these patients. The diagnostic gold standard tests for sweat disorders, such as TST, the quantitative sudomotor axon reflex test, silicone impressions test, sympathetic skin response, and quantitative direct and indirect axon reflex test are equipment heavy requiring a specific setup and trained

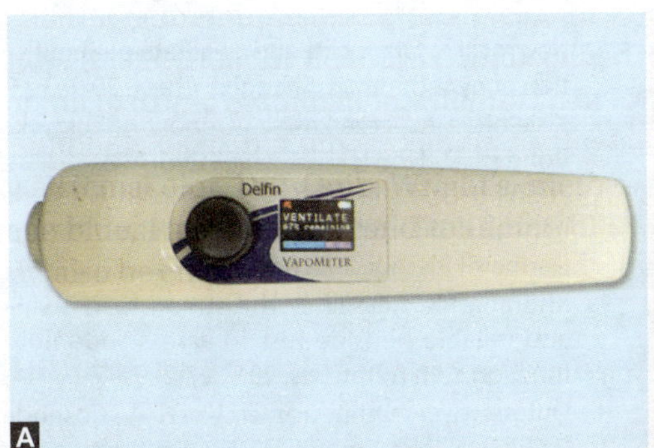

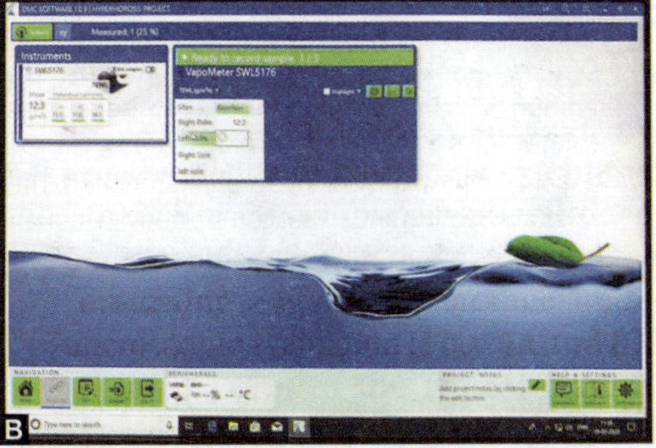

FIGS. 3A AND B: (A) Vapometer for measuring transepidermal water loss (TEWL) and (B) Delphin modular core software used to collect and assess data from Vapometer.

TABLE 7: Advantages and disadvantages of evaporimetry.

Advantages	Disadvantages
• Objective calculation of sweat response • Comparison with normal sweat response possible	• Heavy costly equipment required. • Cannot be done bedside

TABLE 8: Advantages and disadvantages of the silicon impression test.

Advantages	Disadvantages
• Objective sweat analysis done. • Record keeping in the form of silicone impressions	Prone to artifacts left by hairs, dirt, skin surface texture, and air bubbles

personnel. Bedside tests, such as Minor's starch–iodine test and blotting paper test have evolved as quick and useful simple to do tests that help in making early diagnosis of various skin conditions. They are primary helpful in eliminating the need for complex and costly laboratory tests and reducing the waiting period for the laboratory test results. However, they are subjective with low accuracy.

Key Messages

- Sweat glands are epidermal appendages distributed all over the body except over the lips, areolae, and external genital organs.
- Sweat disorders can be classified into essential hyperhidrosis, complete anhidrosis with heat intolerance, and compensatory hyperhidrosis.
- Objective tests for sweat estimation include the TST (gold standard test), quantitative sudomotor axon reflex test, silicone impressions test, sympathetic skin response, gravimetry/evaporimetry, and quantitative direct and indirect axon reflex test. But, these tests require specialized equipment, expertise, time, and can be cumbersome to perform, and therefore hold more of an academic value.
- Simpler to do effective bedside tests that can be employed to screen patients with suspected sweat-related disorders include the direct visualization test, palpation method, gravimetry, Minor's starch–iodine test, spoon test, ninhydrin test, evaporimetry, and silicone impressions.

REFERENCES

1. Griffiths C, Barker J, Bleiker T, Chalmers R, Creamer D, (Eds). Rook's Textbook of Dermatology, 9th edition. Chichester, West Sussex ; Hoboken, NJ: John Wiley & Sons Inc; 2016. p. 1.

2. Baker LB. Physiology of sweat gland function: The roles of sweating and sweat composition in human health. Temperature (Austin). 2019;6(3):211-59.

3. Bovell D. The human eccrine sweat gland: Structure, function and disorders. J Local Global Health Sci. 2015;2015(1):5.

4. Jadoon S, Karim S, Akram MR, Kalsoom Khan A, Zia MA, Siddiqi AR, et al. Recent Developments in Sweat Analysis and Its Applications. Int J Analytic Chem. 2015;2015:e164974.

5. Nawrocki S. Diagnosis and qualitative identification of hyperhidrosis. Shanghai Chest. 2019;3:35.

6. Kisielnicka A, Szczerkowska-Dobosz A, Purzycka-Bohdan D, Nowicki RJ. Hyperhidrosis: disease aetiology, classification and management in the light of modern treatment modalities. Postepy Dermatol Alergol. 2022;39(2):251-7.

7. Khurana RK, Russell C. The spoon test: a valid and reliable bedside test to assess sudomotor function. Clin Auton Res. 2017;27(2):91-5.

8. Dulguerov P, Quinodoz D, Vaezi A, Cosendai G, Piletta P, Lehmann W. New objective and quantitative tests for gustatory sweating. Acta Otolaryngol. 1999;119(5):599-603.

9. Illigens BMW, Gibbons CH. Sweat testing to evaluate autonomic function. Clin Auton Res. 2009;19(2):79-87.

10. Hansen C, Wayment B, Klein S, Godfrey B. Iodine-Starch test for assessment of hyperhidrosis in amputees, evaluation of different methods of application. Disabil Rehabil. 2018;40(25):3076-80.

11. Tsementzis SA, Hitchcock ER. The spoon test: a simple bedside test for assessing sudomotor autonomic failure. J Neurol Neurosurg Psychiatry. 1985;48(4):378-80.

12. Bors E. Simple methods of examination in paraplegia: I. the spoon test. Spinal Cord. 1964;2(1): 17-9.

13. Friedman M. Applications of the ninhydrin reaction for analysis of amino acids, peptides, and proteins to agricultural and biomedical sciences. J Agric Food Chem. 2004;52(3):385-406.

14. Klotz T, Ibrahim A, Maddern G, Caplash Y, Wagstaff M. Devices measuring transepidermal water loss: A systematic review of measurement properties. Skin Res Technol. 2022;28(4):497-539.

Index

Page numbers followed by *b* refer to box, *f* refer to figure, *fc* refer to flowchart, and *t* refer to table.